EMERGING

INFECTIONS

3

EMERGING

INFECTIONS

3

Edited by

W. Michael Scheld
Division of Infectious Diseases
University of Virginia Health Sciences Center
Charlottesville, Virginia

William A. Craig
William S. Middleton Memorial Veterans Hospital
Madison, Wisconsin

James M. Hughes
National Center for Infectious Diseases
Centers for Disease Control and Prevention
Atlanta, Georgia

ASM PRESS *Washington, D.C.*

Cover photo: Nipah virus encephalitis. Viral antigens in neurons and neuronal processes are seen by immunostaining of central nervous system tissue from a patient who died of encephalitis. Naphthol-fast red with hematoxylin counterstain was used. Original magnification, ×158. Courtesy of Sherif R. Zaki, Division of Viral and Rickettsial Diseases, National Center for Infectious Diseases, Centers for Disease Control and Prevention.

To our parents:

William H. and Lucille L. Scheld,
John A. and Dorothy B. Craig,
and
James P. and Adelaide M. Hughes

CONTENTS

CONTRIBUTORS

Corrie Brown • Department of Pathology, College of Veterinary Medicine, University of Georgia, Athens, Georgia 30602-7388

Ralph T. Bryan • National Center for Infectious Diseases, Centers for Disease Control and Prevention, Albuquerque, New Mexico 87110

Salvatore T. Butera • HIV/AIDS and Retrovirology Branch, Division of AIDS, STD, and TB Laboratory Research, National Center for Infectious Diseases, Centers for Disease Control and Prevention, Mail Stop G-19, 1600 Clifton Road NE, Atlanta, Georgia 30333

Louisa E. Chapman • HIV/AIDS and Retrovirology Branch, Division of AIDS, STD, and TB Laboratory Research, National Center for Infectious Diseases, Centers for Disease Control and Prevention, Mail Stop G-19, 1600 Clifton Road NE, Atlanta, Georgia 30333

Michael O. Favorov • Hepatitis Branch (World Health Organization Collaborating Center for Research and Reference in Viral Hepatitis), Division of Viral and Rickettsial Diseases, National Center for Infectious Diseases, Centers for Disease Control and Prevention, Atlanta, Georgia 30333

Thomas M. Folks • HIV/AIDS and Retrovirology Branch, Division of AIDS, STD, and TB Laboratory Research, National Center for Infectious Diseases, Centers for Disease Control and Prevention, Mail Stop G-19, 1600 Clifton Road NE, Atlanta, Georgia 30333

J. Fuller • Department of Microbiology, Mount Sinai Hospital, 600 University Avenue, Toronto, Ontario M5G 1X5, Canada

Lynn M. Grattan • Department of Neurology, University of Maryland School of Medicine, Baltimore, Maryland 21201

Walid Heneine • HIV/AIDS and Retrovirology Branch, Division of AIDS, STD, and TB Laboratory Research, National Center for Infectious Diseases, Centers for Disease Control and Prevention, Mail Stop G-19, 1600 Clifton Road NE, Atlanta, Georgia 30333

James M. Hughes • National Center for Infectious Diseases, Centers for Disease Control and Prevention, Mail Stop C-12, 1600 Clifton Road NE, Atlanta, Georgia 30333

Louis V. Kirchhoff • Department of Internal Medicine, University of Iowa, and Department of Veterans Affairs Medical Center, Iowa City, Iowa 52242

James W. LeDuc • National Center for Infectious Diseases, Centers for Disease Control and Prevention, Mail Stop C-12, 1600 Clifton Road NE, Atlanta, Georgia 30333

Scott Lillibridge • National Center for Infectious Diseases, Centers for Disease Control and Prevention, Mail Stop C-12, 1600 Clifton Road NE, Atlanta, Georgia 30333

E. Liu • Department of Microbiology, Mount Sinai Hospital, 600 University Avenue, Toronto, Ontario M5G 1X5, Canada

D. E. Low • Department of Microbiology, Mount Sinai Hospital, 600 University Avenue, Toronto, Ontario M5G 1X5, Canada

James H. Maguire • Division of Infectious Disease, Brigham and Women's Hospital, and Department of Immunology and Infectious Diseases, Harvard School of Public Health, Boston, Massachusetts 02115

Harold S. Margolis • Hepatitis Branch (World Health Organization Collaborating Center for Research and Reference in Viral Hepatitis), Division of Viral and Rickettsial Diseases, National Center for Infectious Diseases, Centers for Disease Control and Prevention, Atlanta, Georgia 30333

Joseph E. McDade • National Center for Infectious Diseases, Centers for Disease Control and Prevention, Mail Stop C-12, 1600 Clifton Road NE, Atlanta, Georgia 30333

A. McGeer • Department of Microbiology, Mount Sinai Hospital, 600 University Avenue, Toronto, Ontario M5G 1X5, Canada

J. Glenn Morris • Department of Medicine, University of Maryland School of Medicine, Baltimore, Maryland 21201

Kurt B. Nolte • Office of the Medical Investigator, University of New Mexico School of Medicine, Albuquerque, New Mexico 87131-5091; Medical Examiner/Coroner Information Sharing Program, Division of Environmental Hazards and Health Effects, National Center for Environmental Health, Centers for Disease Control and Prevention, Atlanta, Georgia 30341; and Infectious Disease Pathology Activity, Division of Viral and Rickettsial Diseases, National Center for Infectious Diseases, Centers for Disease Control and Prevention, Atlanta, Georgia 30333

David W. Oldach • Department of Medicine and Institute of Human Virology, University of Maryland School of Medicine, Baltimore, Maryland 21201

James G. Olson • Division of Viral and Rickettsial Diseases, National Center for Infectious Diseases, Centers for Disease Control and Prevention, Mail Stop A-26, 1600 Clifton Road NE, Atlanta, Georgia 30333

Stephen M. Ostroff • National Center for Infectious Diseases, Centers for Disease Control and Prevention, Mail Stop C-12, 1600 Clifton Road NE, Atlanta, Georgia 30333

Christopher D. Paddock • Division of Viral and Rickettsial Diseases, National Center for Infectious Diseases, Centers for Disease Control and Prevention, Mail Stop G-32, 1600 Clifton Road NE, Atlanta, Georgia 30333

Didier Raoult • Unité des Rickettsies, Faculté de Médecine, Université de la Méditerranée, CNRS UPRES A 6020, 27, Boulevard Jean Moulin, 13385 Marseille Cedex 05, France

Paul A. Sandstrom • HIV/AIDS and Retrovirology Branch, Division of AIDS, STD, and TB Laboratory Research, National Center for Infectious Diseases, Centers for Disease Control and Prevention, Mail Stop G-19, 1600 Clifton Road NE, Atlanta, Georgia 30333

David A. Schwartz • Department of Pathology, Emory University School of Medicine, Atlanta, Georgia 30335

William M. Switzer • HIV/AIDS and Retrovirology Branch, Division of AIDS, STD, and TB Laboratory Research, National Center for Infectious Diseases, Centers for Disease Control and Prevention, Mail Stop G-19, 1600 Clifton Road NE, Atlanta, Georgia 30333

Robert V. Tauxe • Foodborne and Diarrheal Diseases Branch, Division of Bacterial and Mycotic Diseases, National Center for Infectious Diseases, Centers for Disease Control and Prevention, Mail Stop A-38, 1600 Clifton Road NE, Atlanta, Georgia 30333

Mitchell I. Wolfe • Surveillance and Programs Branch, Division of Environmental Hazards and Health Effects, National Center for Environmental Health, Centers for Disease Control and Prevention, Atlanta, Georgia 30341

Sherif R. Zaki • Division of Viral and Rickettsial Diseases, National Center for Infectious Diseases, Centers for Disease Control and Prevention, Mail Stop G-32, 1600 Clifton Road NE, Atlanta, Georgia 30333

FOREWORD

When we reflect on the impressive gains in health status over the 20th century, it is clear to most of us that they can largely be tied to improvements in public health. We estimate that at least 25 of the 35 years of life expectancy gained during the 20th century can be tied to public health actions. The results have been dramatic. For example, smallpox has been eradicated in nature; polio has been eliminated from the Western Hemisphere, and progress is being made toward the goal of global eradication; childhood vaccine-preventable diseases are at record lows in the United States; and, in the last decade alone, *Haemophilus influenzae* type b disease has gone from among the most common causes of childhood meningitis to such a rarity that it is used as a teaching case in our medical schools.

Even as we take great pride in what we have achieved, our job is far from done, and we face significant challenges as we enter the next century and the next millennium. Although infectious diseases do not have the same impact on mortality in the United States as they did in 1899, they remain far and away the leading cause of death in the developing world. Even in the United States, infections account for about one in every six health care dollars spent and are the leading cause of outpatient visits in this country. Despite our successes, many challenges remain if we are to ultimately control infectious diseases.

We are constantly reminded of our vulnerability to emerging infectious diseases. AIDS, now only 18 years into the epidemic, will almost certainly go down in history as one of the worst plagues that humankind has ever faced. More than 25 pathogens of public health importance have been recognized in the past 25 years. They range from *Legionella pneumophila* to Ebola virus to *Escherichia coli* O157: H7 to hepatitis C virus. Just this year, we have recognized a new cause of encephalitis in Malaysia (Nipah virus) and seen a different strain of avian influenza virus in Hong Kong produce human illness for the first time (influenza A virus H9N2). Even in areas where we have had the greatest success in controlling infectious diseases, there are warning signs on the horizon. Antimicrobial resistance threatens to reverse many of the gains of the past 50 years in infectious disease control. Food-borne diseases represent another emerging threat.

As we know, not all infectious disease threats come from nature. There is also the growing threat of intentional use of biological agents, either state sponsored or by terrorist groups. The specter of bioterrorism is real. There is a need for better surveillance, improved laboratory diagnostic capability, training, development of rapid communications systems, and development of a national, deployable stockpile of essential drugs and biologics to ensure their prompt availability should an event of bioterrorism occur.

Successfully meeting the challenges of the next century requires building upon the successes of the present one while being mindful of new challenges. In order to continue our progress, I have developed four priorities for action during my tenure at the Centers for Disease Control and Prevention. They are as follows: (i) strengthen science for public health action, (ii) collaborate with health care partners for prevention, (iii) promote healthy living at every stage of life, and (iv) work with partners to improve global health. All of these are highly applicable to infectious disease control and prevention.

Today the disparities in health between the developed world and developing world are startling. In no area is this more apparent than in infectious diseases. Respiratory infections, diarrheal disease, human immunodeficiency virus infection, measles, and malaria all continue to be major killers and causes of disability in developing-world populations. We must extend our prevention successes to the populations of these countries, or else the prevention gap will continue to grow. To do so, we must work more closely with both traditional and new global partners to help shape the science, design the policy, and provide the support to promote global public health.

Jeffrey P. Koplan
Director
Centers for Disease Control and Prevention

PREFACE

As a result of improvements in sanitation and overall living conditions during the early part of the 20th century and the subsequent introduction of many vaccines and antibiotics, tremendous progress has been made in the prevention and control of infectious diseases. Globally, smallpox has been eradicated and target dates have been established for the eradication of poliomyelitis and dracunculiasis. In the United States, the annual incidence of several vaccine-preventable diseases is at an all time low.

In spite of these successes, infectious diseases remain the leading cause of death worldwide. The World Health Organization (WHO) estimated that approximately 16 million (30%) of the 54 million deaths that occurred worldwide in 1998 were caused by microbial agents. In the United States, infectious diseases are the third leading cause of death.

The Institute of Medicine (IOM) published a report entitled "Emerging Infections: Microbial Threats to Health in the United States" in the fall of 1992. This report, developed under the leadership of Joshua Lederberg and Robert Shope, identified the important factors that contribute to disease emergence and reemergence. These factors include changes in human demographics and behaviors, advances in technology and industry, economic development and changes in land use, increases in travel and commerce, microbial adaptation and change, and deterioration in the public health system at the local, state, national, and global levels.

Recognizing the intense interest and scientific and public health importance of new and emerging infectious diseases, the program committee of the Interscience Conference on Antimicrobial Agents and Chemotherapy (ICAAC) and the officers of the Infectious Diseases Society of America (IDSA) organized joint sessions during ICAAC and the IDSA annual meeting beginning in 1995. These joint sessions on new and emerging pathogens were immensely popular, attracting audiences in excess of 4,000, and were planned carefully to span the gamut among new and emerging bacteria, viruses, fungi, and parasites with appropriate discussions on national and international strategies for control.

The chapters in *Emerging Infections 3* were derived primarily from presentations given at the sessions on new and emerging infections at the 1998 ICAAC and are updated and fully referenced for this volume. These chapters focus on a variety of diseases that pose major clinical and public health challenges today; some have been recognized for a century or more, while others have been identified during the past 25 years. Some affect healthy persons, while others primarily affect immunosuppressed persons. Some are important problems in the United States, while others cause disease primarily in other parts of the world. The epidemiology of each has been influenced by one or more of the factors identified in the IOM report.

Because of the nature of the "global village" in which we live, we cannot afford to be ignorant or complacent about any of them.

Experiences with these diseases dramatically remind physicians, microbiologists, researchers, public health officials, policy makers, and the public of the critical importance of ensuring the availability of the capacity to detect, respond to, and control these infections. The ability to address these emerging and reemerging microbial threats requires adequate surveillance and response capacity, ongoing research and training programs, strengthened prevention and control programs, and rebuilding of the public health system at the local, state, national, and international levels. The challenges that these diseases will continue to pose demand a multidisciplinary approach and a supply of trained clinicians, microbiologists, pathologists, biomedical researchers, rodent and vector biologists, ecologists, behavioral scientists, and public health officials. The challenges also require funds to support the people and facilities needed to meet them. This is especially true in the developing world because poverty and malnutrition make populations especially susceptible to emerging and reemerging infections.

Future challenges are difficult to predict but certainly include more problems with antimicrobial-resistant infections, the threat of another influenza pandemic, and the increasingly complex challenges of food-borne disease resulting from the globalization of the food supply. The global human immunodeficiency virus epidemic will put large numbers of people at risk for currently recognized and new opportunistic infections. The roles of hepatitis B and C viruses in chronic liver disease and hepatocellular carcinoma, human papillomavirus in cervical cancer, and *Helicobacter pylori* infection in peptic ulcer disease and gastric cancer are now well established. Additional chronic diseases will certainly be found to have an infectious etiology, providing important new opportunities for disease prevention in the future. Food safety and blood safety will continue to be priorities and to pose challenges. Recent events provide a grim reminder of the threat of bioterrorism, further emphasizing the need to strengthen infectious disease surveillance and response capacity. The final chapter in this volume provides a public health perspective on this issue.

Based on the continued importance of new and emerging infectious diseases as defined by the 1992 IOM report, symposia on these topics are planned for future ICAACs. We plan production of an annual volume on new and emerging infections based on the presentations at each year's ICAAC. This volume, the third in the series, should serve as a valuable source of current information for persons responsible for coping with infectious diseases in the new millennium.

W. Michael Scheld
William A. Craig
James M. Hughes

ACKNOWLEDGMENTS

We thank everyone who has helped us in the preparation of this volume. Most importantly, we thank all of the authors for their outstanding contributions. As editors, we are particularly grateful to those members of the Interscience Conference on Antimicrobial Agents and Chemotherapy (ICAAC) Program Committee and others who assisted us in coordinating topic and speaker selection for and/or moderating the joint symposia on emerging infections during the 1998 ICAAC: Eduardo Gotuzzo, André Lomar, and Barbara Murray. Numerous other colleagues provided helpful discussion, advice, and criticism. We are also grateful to our secretaries, Natalie Regensburg, Susan Waisner, and Darlene Shannon. We thank Ken April of ASM Press for coordinating production of the book. And, finally, we thank our families for their understanding and support during this undertaking.

Emerging Infections 3
Edited by W. M. Scheld, W. A. Craig, and J. M. Hughes
© 1999 ASM Press, Washington, D.C.

Chapter 1

Hepatitis E Virus Infection: an Enterically Transmitted Cause of Hepatitis

Michael O. Favorov and Harold S. Margolis

Hepatitis E virus (HEV) is the most recently characterized of five viruses known to produce the majority of cases of hepatitis worldwide. Each hepatitis virus belongs to a different taxonomic family, and each type of viral hepatitis has unique epidemiologic characteristics and can be considered to have recently emerged or reemerged (Table 1) (56). Worldwide, viral hepatitis is a common problem, and its acute and/or chronic consequences produce substantial morbidity and mortality in both developed and developing countries. The availability of vaccines offers the realistic potential to prevent and control the morbidity and mortality associated with hepatitis A virus (HAV) and hepatitis B virus (HBV) infections. However, those forms of viral hepatitis for which an effective vaccine is not available (i.e., viral hepatitis caused by hepatitis C virus [HCV] and HEV) pose a greater challenge for prevention and control.

EPIDEMIOLOGY

Geographic Distribution of Infection

Limited studies suggest that a substantial proportion of cases of acute viral hepatitis in Asia, the Indian subcontinent, and Africa is due to HEV infection (21, 31, 43, 47, 48, 65, 105). Within these regions, acute hepatitis E occurs in epidemics, sporadic cases occur between epidemics, and most cases are primarily associated with ingestion of contaminated drinking water.

Hepatitis E does not appear to be a new disease; however, its presence became evident only with the development of diagnostic tests that differentiate acute HAV and acute HBV infections. In 1955, 29,000 cases of hepatitis occurred in New Delhi, India, following fecal contamination of the city's drinking water (61, 104).

Michael O. Favorov and Harold S. Margolis • Hepatitis Branch (World Health Organization Collaborating Center for Research and Reference in Viral Hepatitis), Division of Viral and Rickettsial Diseases, National Center for Infectious Diseases, Centers for Disease Control and Prevention, Atlanta, GA 30333.

Table 1. Emerging and reemerging nature of diseases associated with hepatitis viruses, United States

Disease	Yr in which characterized (reference)		Incidence (estimated no. of infections/yr [reference])	Criteria for emergence
	Disease	Virus		
Hepatitis A	1940s–1952	1973 (36)	150,000–200,000 (17)	Periodic nationwide epidemics, 1950s to present; most recent epidemic, 1991; communitywide epidemics are common
Hepatitis B	1940s–1952	1965 (10)	200,000–300,000 (22)	National increase in disease incidence from 1983 to 1985
Hepatitis C	1975–1989	1989 (19)	150,000–220,000 (5)	Newly discovered virus; age-specific prevalence of infection indicative of highest disease incidence 10 to 20 yr ago
Hepatitis D	1977	1977 (76)	No estimates	Newly discovered virus; epidemiology similar to that of HBV
Hepatitis E	1953–1980	1990 (75)	Rare in United States	Newly discovered virus; large epidemics in developing countries

At the time of the epidemic, virus-specific diagnostic tests were not available and the disease was thought to be due to a variant of HAV that overwhelmed host immunity (61). Subsequent testing of stored specimens demonstrated that these patients did not have acute HAV or acute HBV infection. This newly identified disease was called enterically transmitted non-A, non-B hepatitis and suggested the presence of at least one other hepatitis virus (105).

Epidemics of hepatitis E have been reported from all parts of the Asian continent, from Africa, and from the Americas (Table 2). Cases have been imported into the United States from areas where HEV infection is known to occur, but with no evidence of subsequent spread (29). More recently, several acute cases of hepatitis E have been identified in the United States, but their sources have not been identified (69).

The precise worldwide endemicity of HEV infection has not been determined due to a lack of standardized, readily available serodiagnostic tests (see "Detection of HEV Infection" below). For instance, prevalence studies suggest that 1 to 5% of persons in the United States and Western Europe may have been infected with HEV (59, 89). However, these findings are inconsistent with the almost complete absence of reported cases of hepatitis E, unless the vast majority of infections were asymptomatic. Until a better correlation between cases of hepatitis E and prevalence of antibody to HEV (anti-HEV) can be established, endemicity of infection is probably best determined by the presence or absence of epidemics. Countries that have experienced disease outbreaks and where sporadic cases of hepatitis E occur between outbreaks can be considered to have high endemicities of infection, while countries with no data, no outbreaks, or reporting only of imported cases of hepatitis E can be considered to have low endemicities of infection.

Table 2. Epidemics of enterically transmitted non-A, non-B hepatitis (hepatitis E) worldwide

Region	Country (location)	Date	No. of cases	Reference(s)
Asia	India (New Delhi)	1955–1956	29,000	61
	India (Kashmir)	1979–1989	36,000	48, 74, 87
	Burma (Mandalay)	1982	399	65
	Nepal (Katmandu)	1973–1974	10,000	40, 83
	Nepal (Katmandu)	1980–1982	6,000	45
	Borneo	1987	2,300	23
	Pakistan (Islamabad)	1993–1994	3,827	29, 92
	China (Xinjian)	1988–1989	200,000+	106, 110
Central Asia	Kyrgyzstan	1956–1957	5,000	78
	Kyrgyzstan	1987–1988	31,000	101
	Turkmenistan (Tashauz)	1975–1976	25,000	79
	Turkmenistan (Tashauz)	1985–1986	16,700	34
	Tajikistan (Dushanbe)	1983–1984	9,800	43
	Uzbekistan	1986–1987	12,000	35
Africa	Algeria	1980–1981	788	25
	Ivory Coast	1983–1984	623	15, 77
	Sudan	1985	2,012	15
	Somalia (refugee camp)	1991	2,000	15
North America	Mexico (Huitzililla)	1986	94	16, 103
	Mexico (Telixtac)	1986	129	16, 103

Disease Incidence

In areas with high endemicities of HEV infection (e.g., Central Asia, Nepal, and India), 7- to 10-year epidemic cycles with pronounced seasonal variations have been documented from viral hepatitis surveillance data (Fig. 1) (24, 85, 104). While these epidemics occur in the face of a relatively high background rate of viral hepatitis, they often have a rapid onset, which suggests a common source of infection such as contaminated water (34, 73, 79).

Age at Infection

During epidemics and among reported cases in areas of high endemicity, disease incidence has been highest in young adults. This is inconsistent with the incidence of other enterically transmitted infections, for which attack rates are highest in young children. The mean age for persons with symptomatic infection has been 29 years, with the highest attack rates in the 20- to 30-year-old age group (16, 45, 48, 61, 65). Clinical attack rates among adults have ranged from 3 to 10%, whereas among children less than 15 years of age, attack rates have ranged from 0.2 to 3% (15, 16, 45, 47, 103). Population-based serologic studies have demonstrated that while infection occurs in children, young adults have the highest prevalence of infection. In populations with a high endemicity of HEV infection, the prevalence of anti-HEV in children less than 10 years of age is ≤5%, and this increases to 10 to 40% among adults >25 years of age (4, 54, 90). By comparison, the prevalence of antibody to HAV among children <10 years of age in most countries where

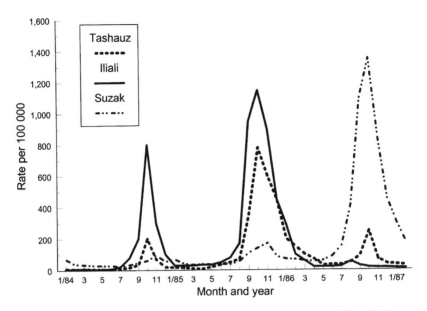

Figure 1. Seasonal variation in acute hepatitis, Central Asian republics, 1984 to 1986. Tashauz, Turkmenistan; Iliali, Turkmenistan; and Suzak, Kyrgyzstan. The figure is adapted from reference 34.

HEV is endemic is >90% (80). A higher rate of asymptomatic infection is present in children, although the precise age at which the ratio of symptomatic to asymptomatic infection changes is not known (14, 37, 54).

Most incidence and prevalence data indicate that in areas with a high endemicity of HEV infection, a large proportion of children remain susceptible to infection and that during outbreaks the highest incidence of infection occurs among young adults. Possible explanations for these findings include the possibility (i) that HEV is not easily transmitted by routes other than contaminated water, that the quality of the water used by young children in these areas is different from the quality of the water used by adults, and that person-to-person transmission is inefficient; (ii) that transmission does not generally occur between epidemics; or (iii) that susceptibility or immune response to infection is age or dose related.

Among persons with hepatitis E, the male-to-female ratio has ranged from 1:1 to 3:1 (45, 47, 61). However, epidemiologic studies have shown that sociological factors contributed to a predominance of men in some outbreaks, with temporary residence of men seeking work in a region with a high rate of hepatitis E being the most common explanation (45). In outbreaks that affected less transient populations (e.g., central Asia, Africa, and Mexico), the male-to-female ratio has reflected that of the general population (8, 35, 88).

Sources and Possible Reservoirs of Infection

Fecal contamination of water has been identified epidemiologically as the source of HEV transmission in most epidemics, and HEV RNA has been detected in water

(15, 24, 44, 70, 73). Further support for water as the primary source of infection during outbreaks has been the interruption of disease transmission by simple means of water purification such as chlorination or boiling (15, 61). However, the source or reservoir of infection during intraepidemic periods has not been defined. In contrast to other enterically transmitted infections, such as HAV, person-to-person contact does not appear to be a major source of transmission of HEV in either the epidemic or the interepidemic setting. Low (0.7 to 8.0%) secondary attack rates have been found for hepatitis E in households with patients with primary cases of infection (2, 65), whereas higher (4 to 20%) secondary attack rates have been found for hepatitis A (39, 53, 81). Also, the degree to which food-borne transmission occurs remains unclear since most investigations have lacked adequate control groups and serologic testing (82).

In areas of low endemicity, the major source of infection in anti-HEV-positive persons is unknown, but it may be due to international travel. When examined in a case-control study, anti-HEV-positive blood donors in Sacramento, Calif., were found to be more likely to have traveled to countries in which HEV is endemic and accounted for about 60% of infections (59). However, another study found that 21% of blood donors, 16% of homosexual men, and 23% of injection drug users in Baltimore, Md., were positive for anti-HEV (89).

While some human hepatitis viruses have closely related viruses that infect animals other than humans (i.e., HBV is related to a hepadnavirus that infects woodchucks, squirrels, and ducks [57], and HAV is related to a heparnavirus that infects Old World monkeys [66, 94]), these non-human-host viruses do not appear to infect humans. Experimental infection with human-derived HEV has been reported in pigs, sheep, and rodents (see "Animal Models of Infection" below) (7, 84, 100). However, the unusual epidemiology of HEV infection (e.g., the low incidence of infection in children and the low rate of person-to-person transmission) suggests that a nonhuman reservoir may exist, and HEV infection has been detected in domestic animals. Higher anti-HEV prevalence and HEV RNA were detected in pigs living in areas of Nepal that reported cases of hepatitis E than in pigs from areas where no cases were reported (20). In addition, anti-HEV was detected in 29 to 62% of domestic cattle in Turkmenistan, whereas it was detected in 12% of age-matched domestic cattle from Ukraine, an area with a low endemicity of HEV infection (30).

Recently, HEV was identified in pigs from the midwestern United States (63, 64). The open reading frame (ORF) ORF2 shared about 79 to 80% nucleotide sequence identity and 90 to 92% amino acid sequence identity with human HEV strains, and ORF3 had 83 to 85% nucleotide sequence identity and 77 to 82% amino acid sequence identity with human HEV strains. Phylogenetic analyses showed that swine HEV is closely related to, but is distinct from, human HEV, and swine HEV cross-reacted with antibody to the human HEV capsid antigen.

CLINICAL SPECTRUM OF DISEASE

The incubation period for hepatitis E has been defined from experimental infections in nonhuman primates, an experimental infection in a man, and well-studied

point source outbreaks and has ranged from 22 to 60 days, with a mode of 40 days
(6, 61). Besides jaundice, signs and symptoms have included dark urine (92 to
100%), nausea (46 to 85%), abdominal pain (41 to 85%), vomiting (50%), pruritus
(13 to 55%), joint pain (3 to 81%), rash (3%), and diarrhea (3%). Fever is present
in approximately 20% of patients, and almost all have hepatomegaly (34, 47, 48).

A high case fatality rate has been a consistent feature of hepatitis E among
pregnant women. The mortality rate among pregnant women has ranged from 17
to 33%, while the case fatality rate among nonpregnant women has been the same
as that among men (45, 50, 61). The highest rate of fulminant hepatitis has occurred
during the 20th to 32nd week of gestation and during labor. Among patients with
acute liver failure, renal failure secondary to hemoglobinuria or a hemorrhagic
diathesis has been the most common cause of death.

Pathomorphologic changes observed in patients with hepatitis E include chole-
stasis with gland-like transformation of bile ducts, portal inflammation, ballooning
degeneration, Kupffer cell hyperplasia, and liver cell necrosis that has varied from
single-cell degeneration to bridging necrosis with preservation of the lobular structure (29, 47, 48). Follow-up studies of persons with hepatitis E indicate that chronic
liver disease has not been a consequence of this infection.

ANIMAL MODELS OF INFECTION

Experimental transmission of HEV infection was performed with a human vol-
unteer (6), and experimental models of infection have been established in several
species of nonhuman primates. The most widely used nonhuman primate model of
infection has been the cynomolgus macaque (13, 97). In addition, experimental
infections have been produced in tamarins (13, 45), African green, squirrel, and
rhesus monkeys (11), and chimpanzees (3). Experimental infections have provided
a picture of the virologic, immunologic, clinical, and histopathologic events that
occur during the course of infection. Elevations in liver enzyme levels occur 24 to
38 days following inoculation (52, 91). HEV antigen is detected in the cytoplasm
of hepatocytes as early as 10 days after inoculation, precedes liver enzyme level
elevations, and may persist for as long as 21 days after peak liver enzyme level
elevation (51, 52). Viremia, as defined by the presence of HEV RNA in serum, can
be detected in infected animals prior to elevation of liver enzyme levels and is
usually present until the appearance of anti-HEV (52, 93). HEV RNA is detected
in feces and bile as early as 6 to 7 days after inoculation and has been shown to
persist in feces for as long as 35 days after inoculation. The duration and pattern
of virus excretion in humans are thought to be similar to those found in nonhuman
primate models, although there have been reports of prolonged viremia or virus
excretion (67). In contrast to the other hepatitis viruses, the severity of symptoms
appears to be directly related to the size of the inoculum. Infectivity studies with
nonhuman primates have demonstrated a direct relationship between HEV dose and
incubation period, biochemical evidence of hepatitis, and duration of hepatitis. In
addition, there is an inverse relation between dose and time to seroconversion (97).

An immunoglobulin M (IgM) antibody response to HEV (IgM anti-HEV) is
detected during the early phase of infection, coincident with liver enzyme level

elevations, and persists for 5 to 6 months after acute infection (31, 52, 54). IgG anti-HEV is generally detected almost simultaneously with IgM antibody (31, 52, 54). The duration of IgG anti-HEV was initially characterized as being relatively short (37). However, chimpanzees have been shown to have detectable antibody 4 years after infection (30), individual patients have been shown to have anti-HEV activity for at least 1 year after infection (72), and approximately 85% of persons involved in hepatitis E outbreaks have been shown to be anti-HEV positive 10 years later (30).

Experimental HEV infection has been reported in a number of nonprimate species, including pigs, sheep, and rodents. Experimental infection was first reported in pigs, as confirmed by immune electron microscopic detection of HEV in stool, seroconversion to anti-HEV, and histologic evidence of acute hepatitis in liver biopsy specimens (7). Recently, swine HEV has been shown to infect both pigs and nonhuman primates (rhesus monkeys and chimpanzees), and a swine-like HEV strain isolated from humans has been shown to infect pigs (63). In addition, infection has been produced in laboratory rats, as evidenced by histopathologic changes and shedding of HEV RNA in stools (55).

VIRUS CHARACTERIZATION

HEV is a 32- to 34-nm virus whose electron microscopic appearance resembles that of caliciviruses (27). Early characterization showed that geographically distinct virus isolates cross-reacted with convalescent-phase serum by immune electron microscopy, the computed sedimentation coefficient was 165S to 183S for virus from stool suspensions, and the buoyant density in potassium tartrate-glycerol was 1.29 g/ml (12). The molecular cloning of HEV was accomplished in 1990 with virus obtained during experimental infection of cynomolgus macaques (75). The virus has a single-stranded positive-sense 3′-polyadenylated [poly(A)$^+$] RNA genome containing three ORFs, with nonstructural genes located at the 5′ end and structural genes located at the 3′ end of the genome. ORF1 is approximately 5 kb in length and contains sequence motifs associated with nucleoside triphosphate binding, helicase function, and RNA-dependent RNA polymerase (12, 75, 86, 109). ORF2 is approximately 2 kb and contains major structural proteins. ORF3 contains 328 bp and overlaps ORF1 by 1 nucleotide and ORF2 by 327 nucleotides; its function is unclear (12, 75, 86). The genomic organization of HEV is substantially different from those of other hepatitis viruses, and recent studies of feline calicivirus suggest that HEV may belong to a larger family of single-stranded, poly(A)$^+$ RNA viruses that possess three ORFs and at least two subgenomic transcripts ranging in size from 2 to 4 kb (27).

Except for an isolate from Mexico, geographically distinct isolates of HEV have shown little genomic variability in the structural region, whereas a high degree of variability has been found in nonstructural regions (18, 38, 102, 107, 108). Several cell culture systems have been used to propagate HEV, as indicated by detection of negative-sense HEV RNA. Cell culture has not sustained expression of HEV antigen or of virus particles, although antibody neutralization of infection has been demonstrated (62).

An HEV strain that is distinct from most human HEV isolates has been isolated from swine (64). However, a swine-like HEV strain has also been isolated from humans with acute hepatitis (63). These findings suggest the existence of a larger group of viruses whose relationships in humans and animals are unknown.

DETECTION OF HEV INFECTION

Immunoassays for Anti-HEV

Prior to production of HEV antigens by recombinant DNA technology, anti-HEV was detected by immune electron microscopy with stool-derived virus (11, 13) or by blocking fluorescent microscopy with antigen from the liver of infected macaques (51). Subsequently, recombinant expressed proteins and synthetic peptides, primarily from ORF2, have been used to develop immunoblotting assays and enzyme immunoassays for the detection of anti-HEV activity (14, 31, 33, 37, 46, 54, 95).

A number of antigens have been used to configure the various assays used to detect anti-HEV activity and have included (i) recombinant proteins from the C-terminal region of ORF3 of the Mexico and Burma strains (37), (ii) recombinant proteins from ORF2 antigenic domains of two geographically distinct HEV strains (28, 41), (iii) a mosaic protein containing several linear antigenic epitopes from ORF2 (46), (iv) a complete ORF2 recombinant conformational antigen (95), and (v) mixtures of synthetic peptides (26, 32, 68). In addition, synthetic peptides have been used to block antibody binding in a confirmatory assay for specimens reactive by some of the immunoassays described above (42).

Assessment of the performance of immunoassays for detection of anti-HEV has been somewhat problematic. Almost all assays detect antibody in persons or animals with acute HEV infection or hepatitis E (58). However, the ability of these tests to accurately identify persons previously infected with HEV has been difficult to determine because of a lack of a large number of specimens from persons in the convalescent phase at known periods of time following HEV infection (58). Studies that have examined the age-specific prevalence of anti-HEV in countries with a high endemicity of infection have generally produced prevalence estimates that correlate with reported disease incidence (hepatitis E) during both epidemic and nonepidemic periods. However, studies of blood donors in countries with a low endemicity of HEV have demonstrated antibody prevalences of 1 to 10%, prevalence estimates that are difficult to rectify with essentially no reported cases of hepatitis E (58, 59, 89). Until there is better validation of serologic tests for anti-HEV, the results of studies, especially those conducted in areas with low endemicities of infection, should be interpreted with caution.

There has been a low level of concordance between most assays when they are used to identify persons with past infection in areas with a low endemicity of infection. Prevalence data for blood donors in the United States whose blood was tested by two enzyme immunoassays indicate that 1.2 to 1.4% were anti-HEV positive, with only a 27% concordance by either test among reactive specimens (59).

Immunoassays that detect IgG and IgM anti-HEV have been developed. Most (>96%) patients with acute hepatitis E have detectable IgM anti-HEV, and IgG anti-HEV is usually present soon after the onset of symptoms. IgM anti-HEV appears to be present in most patients for up to 30 days after the onset of jaundice, 50% are positive 4 to 12 months later (33), and IgM anti-HEV is not detected 20 months after acute infection (14).

Data from immunization and cross-protection studies with cynomolgus macaques suggest that anti-HEV detected by some of these assays affords some level of protection against infection (96, 98). In addition, anti-HEV has been shown to block infectivity in cell culture (62). However, it is not known whether both IgG and IgM antibodies afford protection, and HEV epitopes associated with neutralization have not been defined.

Antibody Persistence

Early studies suggested that IgG anti-HEV persisted for a year or less following acute infection (37, 54, 68, 107). However, subsequent studies found antibody among persons involved in an epidemic in Kashmir, India, 14 years after the epidemic (49). Similarly, antibody has been detected in 65 to 75% of persons residing in Mexican villages and in a Central Asian community involved in an outbreak of hepatitis E 10 years previously (30). In addition, anti-HEV has been shown to persist for over 10 years in chimpanzees experimentally infected with HEV, with significant differences in antibody detection, depending on the configuration of the immunoasay (Fig. 2).

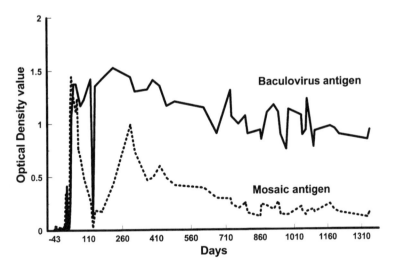

Figure 2. Detection of IgG anti-HEV following experimental intravenous inoculation of a chimpanzee with HEV (30). Baculovirus antigen, enzyme immunoassay configured with a complete ORF2 antigen expressed in insect cells (96); mosaic protein antigen, immunoassay configured with ORF2 and ORF3 immunogenic epitopes combined in a recombinant expressed mosaic protein (46).

Detection of HEV RNA

Amplification of RNA by reverse transcription-PCR (RT-PCR) has been used to detect HEV RNA in the stools of experimentally infected animals, as well as in humans with hepatitis E (1, 93, 99). A number of methods have been used to detect HEV RNA, including RT-PCR amplification following extraction of RNA, immunoprecipitation, or immunocapture of virus (9, 60, 93, 99).

PREVENTION AND CONTROL

In areas of high endemicity, outbreaks of hepatitis E are clearly related to fecal contamination of drinking water, and disease attack rates correlate with the proportion of contaminated water used by a household (16, 45, 73, 103). However, human and animal contamination often occurs, and the relation of the source of contamination to disease attack rates is unknown. Nonetheless, improvements in the quality of the water supply through chlorination or boiling have rapidly interrupted disease transmission (45, 61, 73, 103).

Passive immunization through the use of immune globulin has been used to attempt to prevent infection in various outbreaks. However, because these were generally not controlled clinical trials and were performed prior to the availability of immunoassays for the detection of anti-HEV, no conclusions as to the efficacy of passive pre- or postexposure immunoprophylaxis can be drawn (16, 87).

Early studies indicated that active immunization with recombinant ORF2 proteins provided some protection from infection in the cynomolgus macaque model (71). Subsequent studies with the cynomolgus or rhesus monkey model of HEV infection with various ORF2 recombinant proteins of HEV, including those expressed with a baculovirus vector, have demonstrated a dose-dependent antibody response to immunization. Upon intravenous challenge with homologous or heterologous virus, animals with higher levels of antibody were protected against disease (they had normal liver enzyme levels and normal liver histology), but they excreted virus in their stools, indicating that complete protection from infection did not occur (96, 98).

CONCLUSIONS

Infection with HEV, a recently characterized hepatitis virus, produces epidemics of disease associated with fecal contamination of drinking water. Although clearly an enterically transmitted virus, there appears to be a low rate of person-to-person transmission and low rates of infection among children. Serologic evidence of HEV infection in domestic animals, the recent discovery of an HEV strain in swine, and the isolation of a swine-like HEV strain from a person with hepatitis E indicate the need to determine the role that animals play in the epidemiology of HEV infection.

REFERENCES

1. **Aggarwal, R., and K. A. McCaustland.** 1998. Hepatitis E virus RNA detection in serum and feces specimens with the use of microspin columns. *J. Virol. Methods* **74:**209.

2. **Aggarwal, R., and S. R. Naik.** 1994. Hepatitis E: intrafamilial transmission versus waterborne spread. *J. Hepatol.* **21:**718–723.

3. **Arankalle, V. A., J. Ticehurst, M. A. Sreenivasan, A. Z. Kapikian, H. Popper, K. M. Pavri, and R. H. Purcell.** 1988. Aetiological association of a virus-like particle with enterically transmitted non-A, non-B hepatitis. *Lancet* **i:**550–554.

4. **Arankalle, V. A., S. A. Tsarev, M. S. Chadha, D. W. Alling, S. U. Emerson, K. Banerjee, and R. H. Purcell.** 1995. Age-specific prevalence of antibodies to hepatitis A and E viruses in Pune, India 1982 and 1992. *J. Infect. Dis.* **171:**447–450.

5. **Armstrong, G. L., M. J. Alter, G. M. McQuillan, and H. S. Margolis.** The past incidence of hepatitis C virus infection: implications for the future burden of chronic liver disease in the United States. Submitted for publication.

6. **Balayan, M. S., A. G. Andjaparidze, S. S. Savinskaya, E. S. Ketiladze, D. M. Braginsky, A. P. Savinov, and V. F. Poleschuk.** 1983. Evidence for a virus in non-A, non-B hepatitis transmitted via the fecal-oral route. *Intervirology* **20:**23–31.

7. **Balayan, M. S., R. K. Usmanov, N. A. Zamyatina, D. I. Djumalieva, and F. R. Karas.** 1990. Brief report: experimental hepatitis E infection in domestic pigs. *J. Med. Virol.* **32:**58–59.

8. **Bellabes, H., A. Benatallah, and A. Bourguermouh.** 1984. Non-A, non-B epidemic viral hepatitis in Algeria: strong evidence for its water spread, p. 637. *In* G. N. Vyas, J. L. Dienstag, and J. H. Hoffnagle (ed.), *Viral Hepatitis and Liver Disease.* Grune and Stratton, Orlando, Fla.

9. **Bi, S.-L., M. A. Purdy, K. A. McCaustland, H. S. Margolis, and D. W. Bradley.** 1993. The sequence of hepatitis E virus isolated directly from a single source during an outbreak in China. *Virus Res.* **28:**223–247.

10. **Blumberg, B. S., H. J. Alter, and S. Visnich.** 1965. A "new" antigen in leukemia sera. *JAMA* **191:** 541–546.

11. **Bradley, D. W., A. Andjaparidze, E. H. Cook, Jr., K. McCaustland, M. Balayan, H. Stetler, O. Velazquez, B. Robertson, C. Humphrey, M. Kane, and I. Weisfuse.** 1988. Aetiological agent of enterically transmitted non-A, non-B hepatitis. *J. Gen. Virol.* **69:**731–738.

12. **Bradley, D. W., M. J. Beach, and M. A. Purdy.** 1992. Recent developments in the molecular cloning and characterization of hepatitis C and E viruses. *Microb. Pathog.* **12:**391–398.

13. **Bradley, D. W., K. Krawczynski, E. H. Cook, Jr., K. A. McCaustland, C. D. Humphrey, J. E. Spelbring, H. Myint, and J. E. Maynard.** 1987. Enterically transmitted non-A, non-B hepatitis: serial passage of disease in cynomolgus macaques and tamarins, and recovery of disease-associated 27 to 34 nm virus-like particles. *Proc. Natl. Acad. Sci. USA* **84:**6277–6281.

14. **Bryan, J. P., S. A. Tsarev, M. Igbal, J. Ticehurst, S. Emerson, A. Ahmed, J. Duncan, A. R. Rafiqui, I. Malik, R. H. Purcell, and L. J. Legters.** 1994. Epidemic hepatitis E in Pakistan: patterns of serologic response and evidence that antibody to hepatitis E virus protects against disease. *J. Infect. Dis.* **170:**517–521.

15. **Centers for Disease Control.** 1987. Enterically transmitted non-A, non-B hepatitis—East Africa. *Morbid. Mortal. Weekly Rep.* **36:**241–244.

16. **Centers for Disease Control.** 1987. Enterically transmitted non-A, non-B hepatitis—Mexico. *Morbid. Mortal. Weekly Rep.* **36:**597–602.

17. **Centers for Disease Control and Prevention.** 1997. Unpublished data.

18. **Chatterjee, R., S. A. Tsarev, J. Pillot, P. Coursaget, S. U. Emerson, and R. H. Purcell.** 1997. African strains of hepatitis E virus that are distinct from Asian strains. *J. Med. Virol.* **53:**139–144.

19. **Choo, Q. L., G. Kuo, A. J. Weiner, L. R. Overby, D. W. Bradley, and M. Houghton.** 1989. Isolation of a cDNA clone derived from a bloodborne non-A, non-B viral hepatitis genome. *Science* **244:**359–362.

20. **Clayson, E. T., B. Innis, K. S. A. Myint, S. Narupiti, D. W. Vaughn, S. Biri, P. Ranabhat, and M. P. Shrestha.** 1995. Detection of hepatitis E virus infections among domestic swine in the Kathmandu valley of Nepal. *Am. J. Trop. Med. Hyg.* **53:**228–232.

21. **Clayson, E. T., M. P. Shrestha, D. W. Vaughn, R. Snitbhan, K. B. Shrestha, C. F. Longer, and B. L. Innis.** 1997. Rates of hepatitis E virus infection and disease among adolescents and adults in Kathmandu, Nepal. *J. Infect. Dis.* **176:**763–766.

22. **Coleman, P. J., G. M. McQuillan, L. A. Moyer, S. B. Lambert, and H. S. Margolis.** 1998. Incidence of hepatitis B virus infection in the United States, 1976–1994: estimates from the National Health and Nutrition Examination Surveys. *J. Infect. Dis.* **178**:954–959.

23. **Corwin, A., M. P. Putri, J. Winarno, I. Lubis, S. Suparmanto, A. Sumardiati, K. Laras, R. Tan, J. Master, G. Warner, F. S. Wignall, R. Graham, and K. C. Hyams.** 1997. Epidemic and hepatitis E virus transmission in West Kalimantan (Borneo), Indonesia. *Am. J. Trop. Med. Hyg.* **57**:62–65.

24. **Corwin, A. L., H. B. Khiem, E. T. Clayson, P. K. Sac, V. T. T. Nhung, V. T. Yen, C. T. T. Cuc, D. Vaughn, J. Mervin, T. L. Richie, M. P. Putri, J. He, R. Graham, F. S. Wignall, and K. C. Hyams.** 1996. A waterborne outbreak of hepatitis E virus transmission in southwestern Vietnam. *Am. J. Trop. Med. Hyg.* **54**:559–562.

25. **Coursaget, P., Y. Buisson, N. Enogat, M. Nahor N'Gawara, R. Roue, C. Molinie, J. Desrame, R. Bercion, A. Touze, Y. Gharbi, and R. Kastally.** 1996. Hepatitis E virus infections in France and Africa, p. 201–212. *In* Y. Buisson, P. Coursaget, and M. Kane (ed.), *Enterically-Transmitted Hepatitis Viruses.* La Simarre, Paris, France.

26. **Coursaget, P., N. Depril, Y. Buisson, C. Molinie, and R. Roue.** 1994. Hepatitis type E in a French population: detection of anti-HEV by a synthetic peptide-based enzyme-linked immunoadsorbent assay. *Res Virol.* **145**:51–57.

27. **Cubitt, D., D. W. Bradley, et al.** 1995. Virus taxonomy: classification and nomenclature of viruses. *Arch. Virol.* **10**(suppl.):359.

28. **Dawson, G. J., K. H. Chau, C. M. Cabal, P. O. Yarbough, G. R. Reyes, and I. K. Mushahwar.** 1992. Solid-phase enzyme-linked immunosorbent assay for hepatitis E virus IgG and IgM antibodies utilizing recombinant antigens and synthetic peptides. *J. Virol. Methods* **38**:175–186.

29. **De Cock, K. M., D. W. Bradley, N. L. Sandford, S. Govindarajan, J. E. Maynard, and A. G. Redeker.** 1987. Epidemic non-A, non-B hepatitis in patients from Pakistan. *Ann. Intern. Med.* **106**:227–230.

30. **Favorov, M. O.** 1996. Unpublished data.

31. **Favorov, M. O., H. A. Fields, M. A. Purdy, T. L. Yashina, A. G. Aleksandrov, M. J. Alter, D. M. Yarasheva, D. W. Bradley, and H. S. Margolis.** 1992. Serologic identification of hepatitis E virus infections in epidemic and endemic settings. *J. Med. Virol.* **36**:246–250.

32. **Favorov, M. O., Y. E. Khudyakov, H. A. Fields, N. S. Khudyakova, N. Padhye, M. J. Alter, E. E. Mast, L. Polish, T. L. Yashina, D. M. Yarasheva, and H. S. Margolis.** 1994. Enzyme immunoassay for the detection of antibody to hepatitis E virus based on synthetic peptides. *J. Virol. Methods* **46**:237–250.

33. **Favorov, M. O., Y. E. Khudyakov, E. E. Mast, T. L. Yashina, C. N. Shapiro, N. S. Khudyakova, D. L. Jue, G. G. Onischenko, H. S. Margolis, and H. A. Fields.** 1996. IgM and IgG antibody to hepatitis E virus detected by enzyme immunoassay based on HEV-specific artificial recombinant mosaic protein. *J. Med. Virol.* **50**:50–58.

34. **Favorov, M. O., P. A. Khukhlovich, G. K. Zairov, and E. K. Listovskaia.** 1986. Clinical-epidemiological characteristics and diagnosis of viral non-A, non-B hepatitis with fecal and oral mechanisms of transmission of the infection. *Vopr. Virusol.* **31**:65–69.

35. **Favorov, M. O., S. N. Kuzin, T. L. Iashina, G. K. Zairov, A. Gurov V, S. Shavakhabov, A. I. Buriev, B. U. Zhantemirov, I. Shakhgildian V, and E. S. Ketiladze.** 1989. Characteristics of viral hepatitis non-A, non-B with a fecal-oral mechanism of transmission of the infection in southern Uzbekistan. *Vopr. Virusol.* **34**:436–442.

36. **Feinstone, S. M., A. Z. Kapikian, and R. H. Purcell.** 1973. Hepatitis A: detection by immune electron microscopy of a virus-like antigen association with acute illness. *Science* **182**:1026–1028.

37. **Goldsmith, R., P. O. Yarbough, G. R. Reyes, K. E. Fry, K. A. Gabor, M. Kamel, S. Zakaria, S. Amer, and Y. Gaffar.** 1992. Enzyme-linked immunosorbent assay for diagnosis of acute sporadic hepatitis E in Egyptian children. *Lancet* **339**:328–331.

38. **Gouvea, V., N. Snellings, S. J. Cohen, R. L. Warren, K. S. A. Myint, M. P. Shrestha, D. W. Vaughn, C. H. Hoke, and B. L. Innis.** 1997. Hepatitis E virus in Nepal: similarities with Burmese and Indian variants. *Virus Res.* **52**:87–96.

39. **Hadler, S. C., H. Webster, J. J. Erben, J. E. Swanson, and J. E. Maynard.** 1980. Hepatitis A in day-care centers: a community-wide assessment. *N. Engl. J. Med.* **302**:1222–1227.

40. **Hillis, A., S. M. Shrestha, and N. K. Saha.** 1973. An epidemic of infectious hepatitis in the Kathmandu Valley. *J. Nepal. Med. Assoc.* **11:**145–151.

41. **Hoke, C. H., L. N. Binn, J. E. Egan, R. F. DeFraites, P. O. MacArthy, B. L. Innis, K. H. Eckels, D. Dubois, E. D'Hondt, K. H. Sjogren, R. Rice, J. C. Sodoff, and W. H. Bancroft.** 1992. Hepatitis A in the US Army: epidemiology and vaccine development. *Vaccine* **10:**575–579.

42. **Hoofnagle, J. H., and A. M. Di Bisceglie.** 1993. Therapy of chronic delta hepatitis: overview, p. 337–344. *In* S. J. Hadziyannis, J. M. Taylor, and F. Bonino (ed.), *Hepatitis Delta Virus. Molecular Biology, Pathogenesis, and Clinical Aspects.* Wiley-Liss, Inc., New York, N.Y.

43. **Iarasheva, D. M., M. O. Favorov, T. L. Iashina, I. V. Shakgil'dian, A. A. Umarova, S. A. Sorokina, K. K. Kamardinov, and V. I. Mavashev.** 1991. The etiological structure of acute viral hepatitis in Tadzhikistan in a period of decreased morbidity. *Vopr. Virusol.* **36:**454–456.

44. **Jothikumar, N., K. Aparna, S. Kamatchiammal, R. Paulmurugan, S. Saravanadeve, and P. Khanna.** 1993. Detection of hepatitis E virus in raw and treated wastewater with the polymerase chain reaction. *Appl. Environ. Microbiol.* **59:**2558–2562.

45. **Kane, M. A., D. W. Bradley, S. M. Shrestha, J. E. Maynard, E. H. Cook, R. P. Mishra, and D. D. Joshi.** 1984. Epidemic non-A, non-B hepatitis in Nepal: recovery of a possible etiologic agent and transmission studies to marmosets. *JAMA* **252:**3140–3145.

46. **Khudyakov, Y. E., M. O. Favorov, N. S. Khudyakova, M. Cong, B. P. Hooloway, N. Padhye, S. B. Lambert, D. L. Jue, and H. A. Fields.** 1994. Artificial mosaic protein (MPr) containing antigenic epitopes of the hepatitis E virus. *J. Virol.* **68:**7067–7074.

47. **Khuroo, M. S.** 1980. Study of an epidemic of non-A, non-B hepatitis: possibility of another human hepatitis virus distinct from post-transfusion non-A, non-B type. *Am. J. Med.* **68:**818–824.

48. **Khuroo, M. S., W. Duermeyer, S. A. Zargar, M. A. Ahanger, and M. A. Shah.** 1983. Acute sporadic non-A, non-B hepatitis in India. *Am. J. Epidemiol.* **118:**360–364.

49. **Khuroo, M. S., S. Kamili, M. Y. Dar, R. Moecklii, and S. Jameel.** 1993. Hepatitis E and long-term antibody status. *Lancet* **341:**1355.

50. **Khuroo, M. S., M. R. Teli, S. Skidmore, M. A. Sofi, and M. I. Khuroo.** 1981. Incidence and severity of viral hepatitis in pregnancy. *Am. J. Med.* **70:**252–255.

51. **Krawczynski, K., and D. W. Bradley.** 1989. Enterically transmitted non-A, non-B hepatitis: identification of virus-associated antigen in experimentally infected cynomolgus macaques. *J. Infect. Dis.* **159:**1042–1049.

52. **Krawczynski, K., K. McCaustland, E. Mast, P. O. Yarbough, M. Purdy, M. O. Favorov, and J. Spelbring.** 1996. Elements of pathogenesis of HEV infection in man and experimentally infected primates, p. 317–328. *In* Y. Buisson, P. Coursaget, and M. Kane (ed.), *Enterically-Transmitted Hepatitis Viruses.* La Simarre, Paris, France.

53. **Levy, B. S., R. E. Fontaine, C. A. Smith, J. Brinda, G. Hirman, D. B. Nelson, P. M. Johnson, and O. Larson.** 1975. A large food-borne outbreak of hepatitis A. *JAMA* **234:**289–294.

54. **Lok, A. S. F., W.-K. Kwan, R. Moeckli, P. O. Yarbough, R. T. Chan, G. R. Reyes, C.-L. Lai, H.-T. Chung, and T. S. T. Lai.** 1992. Seroepidemiological survey of hepatitis E in Hong Kong by recombinant-based enzyme immunoassays. *Lancet* **340:**1205–1208.

55. **Maneerat, Y., E. T. Clayson, K. S. Myint, G. D. Young, and B. L. Innis.** 1996. Experimental infection of the laboratory rat with the hepatitis E virus. *J. Med. Virol.* **48:**121–128.

56. **Margolis, H. S., M. J. Alter, and S. C. Hadler.** 1997. Viral hepatitis, p. 363–418. *In* A. S. Evans, and R. A. Kaslow (ed.), *Viral Infection of Humans: Epidemiology and Control,* 4th ed. Plenum Medical Book Company, New York, N.Y.

57. **Marion, P. L., C. Trepo, K. Matsubara, and P. M. Price.** 1991. Experimental models in hepadnavirus research: report of a workshop, p. 866–874. *In* F. B. Hollinger, S. M. Lemon, and H. S. Margolis (ed.), *Viral Hepatitis and Liver Disease,* The Williams & Wilkins Co., Baltimore, Md.

58. **Mast, E. E., M. J. Alter, P. V. Holland, and R. H. Purcell, for the Hepatitis E Virus Antibody Serum Panel Evaluation Group.** 1998. Evaluation of assays for antibody to hepatitis E virus by a serum panel. *Hepatology* **27:**857–861.

59. **Mast, E. E., K. Kuramoto, M. O. Favorov, V. R. Schening, B. T. Burkholder, C. N. Shapiro, and P. V. Holland.** 1997. Prevalence and risk factors for antibody to hepatitis E virus seroreactivity among blood donors in northern California. *J. Infect. Dis.* **176:**34–40.

60. **McCaustland, K. A., S. Bi, M. A. Purdy, and D. W. Bradley.** 1991. Application of two RNA extraction methods prior to amplification of hepatitis E virus nucleic acid by the polymerase chain reaction. *J. Virol. Methods* **35**:331–342.

61. **Melnick, J. L.** 1957. A water-borne urban epidemic of hepatitis, p. 211–225. *In* F. W. Hartman, G. A. LoGrippo, J. G. Matffer, and J. Barron (ed.), *Hepatitis Frontiers.* Little, Brown & Company, Boston, Mass.

62. **Meng, J., P. Dubreuil, and J. Pillot.** 1997. A new PCR-based seroneutralization assay in cell culture for diagnosis of hepatitis E. *J. Clin. Microbiol.* **35**:1373–1377.

63. **Meng, X.-J., P. G. Halbur, M. S. Shapiro, S. Govindarajan, J. D. Bruna, I. K. Mushahwar, R. H. Purcell, and S. U. Emerson.** 1998. Genetic and experimental evidence for cross-species infection by swine hepatitis E virus. *J. Virol.* **72**:9714–9721.

64. **Meng, X.-J., R. H. Purcell, P. G. Halbur, J. R. Lehman, D. M. Webb, T. S. Tsareva, J. S. Haynes, B. J. Thacker, and S. U. Emerson.** 1997. A novel virus in swine is closely related to the human hepatitis E virus. *Proc. Natl. Acad. Sci. USA* **94**:9860–9865.

65. **Myint, H., M. M. Soe, T. Khin, T. M. Myint, and K. M. Tin.** 1985. A clinical and epidemiological study of an epidemic of non-A, non-B hepatitis in Rangoon. *Am. J. Trop. Med. Hyg.* **34**:1183–1189.

66. **Nainan, O. V., H. S. Margolis, B. H. Robertson, M. Balayan, and M. A. Brinton.** 1991. Sequence analysis of a new hepatitis A virus naturally infecting cynomolgus macaques (Macaca fascicularis). *J. Gen. Virol.* **72**:1685–1689.

67. **Nanda, S. K., I. H. Ansari, S. K. Acharya, S. Jameel, and S. K. Panda.** 1995. Protracted viremia during acute sporadic hepatitis E virus infection. *Gastroenterology* **108**:225–230.

68. **Paul, D. A., M. F. Knigge, A. Ritter, R. Gutierrez, T. Pilot-Matias, K. H. Chau, and G. J. Dawson.** 1994. Determination of hepatitis E virus seroprevalence by using recombinant fusion proteins and synthetic peptides. *J. Infect. Dis.* **169**:801–806.

69. **Paul, K. Y., G. G. Schlauder, H. A. Carpenter, P. J. Murphy, J. E. Rosenblatt, G. J. Dawson, E. E. Mast, K. Krawczynski, and V. Balan.** 1997. Acute hepatitis E by a new isolate acquired in the United States. *Mayo Clin. Proc.* **72**:1133–1136.

70. **Pina, S., J. Jofre, S. U. Emerson, R. H. Purcell, and R. Girones.** 1998. Characterization of a strain of infectious hepatitis E virus isolated from sewerage in an area where hepatitis E is not endemic. *Appl. Environ. Microbiol.* **64**:4485–4488.

71. **Purdy, M., K. McCaustland, K. Krawczynski, M. Beach, J. Spelbring, G. Reyes, and D. Bradley.** 1992. An expressed recombinant HEV protein that protects cynomologus macaques against challenge with wild-type hepatitis E virus, p. 41. *In Immunobiology and Pathogenesis of Persistent Virus Infections.* Elsevier Science Publishers, Amsterdam, The Netherlands.

72. **Purdy, M. A., K. A. McCaustland, K. Krawczynski, A. Tam, M. J. Beach, N. C. Tassopoulos, G. R. Reyes, and D. W. Bradley.** 1992. Expression of a hepatitis E virus (HEV)-*trpE* fusion protein containing epitopes recognized by antibodies in sera from human cases and experimentally infected primates. *Arch. Virol.* **123**:335–349.

73. **Rab, M. A., M. K. Bile, M. M. Mubarik, H. Asghar, Z. Sami, S. Siddiqi, A. S. Dil, M. A. Barzgar, M. A. Chaudry, and M. I. Burney.** 1997. Water-borne hepatitis E virus epidemic in Islamabad, Pakistan: a common source outbreak traced to the malfunction of a modern water treatment plant. *Am. J. Trop. Med. Hyg.* **57**:151–157.

74. **Ray, R., R. Aggarwal, P. N. Salunke, N. N. Mehrotra, G. P. Talwar, and S. R. Naik.** 1991. Hepatitis E virus genome in stools of hepatitis patients during large epidemic in north India. *Lancet* **338**:783–784.

75. **Reyes, G. R., M. A. Purdy, J. P. Kim, D.-C. Luk, L. M. Young, A. W. Tam, and D. W. Bradley.** 1990. Isolation of a cDNA from the virus responsible for enterically transmitted non-A, non-B hepatitis. *Science* **247**:1335–1339.

76. **Rizzetto, M., M. C. Canese, S. Arico, O. Crivelli, C. Trepo, R. Bonino, and G. Verme.** 1977. Immunofluorescence detection of a new antigen-antibody system (δ/anti-δ) associated to the hepatitis B virus in the liver and in the serum of HBsAg carriers. *Gut* **18**:997–1003.

77. **Sarthou, J. L., A. Budkowska, M. D. Sharma, M. Lhuillier, and J. Pillot.** 1976. Characterization of an antigen-antibody system associated with epidemic non-A, non-B hepatitis in West Africa and experimental transmission of an infectious agent to primates. *Ann. Inst. Pasteur Virol.* **137E**:225–232.

78. **Sergeev, N. W., E. A. Paktoris, W. A. Ananev, G. A. Sinajko, A. I. Antinova, and E. P. Semenov.** 1957. General characteristics of Botkin's disease occurring in Kirgiz Republic of USSR in 1955–1956. *Soviet Healthcare Kirgizii* **5:**16–23.

79. **Shakhgildian, I. V., P. A. Khukhlovich, S. N. Kuzin, M. O. Favorov, and A. E. Nedachin.** 1986. Epidemiological characteristics of non-A, non-B hepatitis with a fecal-oral transmission mechanism. *Vopr. Virusol.* **31:**175–179.

80. **Shapiro, C. N., and H. S. Margolis.** 1993. Worldwide epidemiology of hepatitis A virus infection. *J. Hepatol.* **18**(Suppl 2):S11–S14.

81. **Shaw, F. E., Jr., J. H. Sudman, S. M. Smith, D. L. Williams, L. A. Kapell, S. C. Hadler, T. J. Halpin, and J. E. Maynard.** 1986. A community-wide epidemic of hepatitis A in Ohio. *Am. J. Epidemiol.* **123:**1057–1065.

82. **Shi, G. R., S. Q. Li, and L. Qian.** 1987. The epidemiological study on a foodborne outbreak of non-A, non-B hepatitis. *J. Chin. Med. Univ.* **16:**150.

83. **Shrestha, S. M., and D. S. Mala.** 1957. An epidemic of infectious hepatitis in the Kathmandu valley. *J. Nepal. Med. Assoc.* **13:**58.

84. **Smedile, A., M. Rizzetto, K. Denniston, F. Bonino, F. Wells, G. Verme, F. Consolo, B. Hoyer, R. H. Purcell, and J. L. Gerin.** 1986. Type D hepatitis: the clinical significance of hepatitis D virus RNA in serum as detected by a hybridization-based assay. *Hepatology* **6:**1297–1302.

85. **Sreenivasan, M. A., K. Banerjee, P. G. Pandya, R. R. Kotak, P. M. Pandya, N. J. Desai, and L. H. Vaghela.** 1978. Epidemiological investigations of an outbreak of infectious hepatitis in Ahmedabad City during 1975–76. *Indian J. Med. Res.* **67:**197–206.

86. **Tam, A. W., M. M. Smith, M. E. Guerra, C.-C. Huang, D. W. Bradley, K. E. Fry, and G. R. Reyes.** 1991. Hepatitis E virus (HEV): molecular cloning and sequencing of the full-length viral genome. *Virology* **185:**120–131.

87. **Tandon, B. N., Y. K. Joshi, S. K. Jain, B. M. Gandi, L. R. Mathiesen, and H. D. Tandon.** 1982. An epidemic of non-A, non-B hepatitis in north India. *Indian J. Med. Res.* **75:**739–744.

88. **Tavera, C., O. Velazquez, C. Avila, G. Ornelas, C. Alvarez, and J. Sepulveda.** 1987. Enterically transmitted non-A, non-B hepatitis—Mexico. *Morbid. Mortal. Weekly Rep.* **36:**597–602.

89. **Thomas, D. L., P. O. Yarbough, D. Vlahov, S. A. Tsarev, K. E. Nelson, A. J. Saah, and R. H. Purcell.** 1997. Seroreactivity to hepatitis E virus in areas where the disease is not endemic. *J. Clin. Microbiol.* **35:**1244–1247.

90. **Thomas, H. C., R. W. Mahley, S. Badur, K. E. Palaoglu, and T. C. Quinn.** 1993. Epidemiology of hepatitis E virus infection in Turkey. *Lancet* **341:**1561–1562.

91. **Ticehurst, J.** 1991. Identification and characterization of hepatitis E virus, p. 501–513. *In* F. B. Hollinger, S. M. Lemon, and H. S. Margolis (ed.), *Viral Hepatitis and Liver Disease.* The Williams & Wilkins Co., Baltimore, Md.

92. **Ticehurst, J., T. J. Popkin, J. P. Bryan, B. L. Innis, J. F. Duncan, A. Ahmed, M. Iqbal, I. Malik, A. Z. Kapikian, L. J. Legters, and R. H. Purcell.** 1992. Association of hepatitis E virus with an outbreak of hepatitis in Pakistan: serologic responses and pattern of virus excretion. *J. Med. Virol.* **36:**84–92.

93. **Tsarev, S., S. U. Emerson, G. R. Reyes, T. S. Tsareva, L. J. Legters, I. A. Malik, M. Iqbal, and R. H. Purcell.** 1992. Characterization of a prototype strain of hepatitis E virus. *Proc. Natl. Acad. Sci. USA* **89:**559–563.

94. **Tsarev, S. A., S. U. Emerson, M. S. Balayan, J. Ticehurst, and R. H. Purcell.** 1991. Simian hepatitis A virus (HAV) strain AGM-27: comparison of genome structure and growth in cell culture with other HAV strains. *J. Gen. Virol.* **72:**1677–1683.

95. **Tsarev, S. A., T. S. Tsareva, and S. U. Emerson.** 1993. ELISA for antibody to hepatitis E virus (HEV) based on complete open-reading frame-2 protein expressed in insect cells: identification of HEV infection in primates. *J. Infect. Dis.* **168:**369–378.

96. **Tsarev, S. A., T. S. Tsareva, S. U. Emerson, S. Govindarajan, M. Shapiro, J. L. Gerin, and R. H. Purcell.** 1994. Successful passive and active immunization of cynomolgus monkeys against hepatitis E. *Proc. Natl. Acad. Sci. USA* **91:**10198–10202.

97. **Tsarev, S. A., T. S. Tsareva, S. U. Emerson, P. O. Yarbough, L. J. Legters, T. Moskal, and R. H. Purcell.** 1994. Infectivity and titration of a prototype strain of hepatitis E virus in cynomolgus monkeys. *J. Med. Virol.* **43:**135–142.

98. Tsarev, S. A., T. S. Tsareva, S. U. Emerson, S. Govindarajan, M. Shapiro, J. L. Gerin, and R. H. Purcell. 1997. Recombinant vaccine against hepatitis E: dose response and protection against heterologous challenge. *Vaccine* **15:**1834–1838.

99. Uchida, T., K. Suzuki, F. Iida, T. Shidata, M. Araki, M. Ichikawa, T. Rikihisa, K. Mizuno, S. Soe, and K. Win. 1991. Virulence of hepatitis E with serial passage to cynomolgus monkeys and identification of viremia, p. 526–527. *In* F. B. Hollinger, S. M. Lemon, and H. S. Margolis (ed.), *Viral Hepatitis and Liver Disease.* The Williams & Wilkins Co., Baltimore, Md.

100. Usmanov, R. K., M. S. Blayan, O. V. Dvoinikova, D. B. Alymbaeva, N. A. Zamiatina, I. A. Kazachkov, and V. I. Belov. 1994. An experimental infection in lambs by hepatitis E virus. *Vopr. Virusol.* **39:**165–168.

101. Usmanov, R. K., M. O. Favorov, V. I. Vasil'eva, D. S. Aidarbekova, F. R. Karas, T. L. Iashina, R. M. Mineeva, R. G. Aslanian, G. K. Zairov, and D. B. Alymbaeva. 1991. A comparative study of enteral hepatitis E (non-A, non-B) in the valley and mountain areas of Kirghizia. *Vopr. Virusol.* **36:**66–69.

102. vanCuyck-Gandre, H., H. Zhang, S. A. Tsarev, N. Clements, S. Cohen, J. Caudill, Y. Buisson, P. Coursaget, R. L. Warren, and C. F. Longer. 1997. Characterization of hepatitis E virus (HEV) from Algeria and Chad by partial genome sequence. *J. Med. Virol.* **53:**340–347.

103. Velazquez, O., H. C. Stetler, C. Avila, G. Ornelas, C. Alvarez, S. C. Hadler, D. W. Bradley, and J. Sepulveda. 1990. Epidemic transmission of enterically transmitted non-A, non-B hepatitis in Mexico, 1986–1987. *JAMA* **263:**3261–3285.

104. Viswanathan, R. 1957. Infectious hepatitis in Delhi (1955–56): a critical study; epidemiology. *Indian J. Med. Res.* **45**(Suppl.)**:**1–30.

105. Wong, D. C., R. H. Purcell, M. A. Sreenivasan, S. R. Prasad, and K. M. Pavri. 1980. Epidemic and endemic hepatitis in India: evidence for non-A/non-B hepatitis virus etiology. *Lancet* **ii:**876–878.

106. Xia, X. 1991. An epidemiologic survey on a type E hepatitis (HE) outbreak. *Chung Hua Liu Hsing Ping Hsueh Tsa Chih* **12:**257.

107. Yarbough, P. O., A. W. Tam, K. E. Fry, K. Krawczynski, K. A. McCaustland, D. W. Bradley, and G. R. Reyes. 1991. Hepatitis E virus: identification of type-common epitopes. *J. Virol.* **65:**5790–5797.

108. Yin, S., R. H. Purcell, and S. U. Emerson. 1994. A new Chinese isolate of hepatitis E virus: comparison with strains recovered from different geographical regions. *Virus Genes* **92:**23–32.

109. Zafrullah, M., M. H. Ozdener, S. K. Panda, and S. Jameel. 1997. The ORF3 protein of hepatitis E virus is a phosphoprotein that associates with the cytoskeleton. *J. Virol.* **71:**9045–9053.

110. Zhuang, H., W.-Y. Cao, C.-B. Liu, and G.-M. Wang. 1991. Epidemiology of hepatitis E in China. *Gastroenterol. Jpn.* **26:**135–138.

Emerging Infections 3
Edited by W. M. Scheld, W. A. Craig, and J. M. Hughes
© 1999 ASM Press, Washington, D.C.

Chapter 2

Emerging Rickettsioses

Didier Raoult and James G. Olson

Bacteria of the order *Rickettsiales* are gram-negative microorganisms that grow in association with eukaryotic cells. Molecular phylogeny methods, in particular, 16S rRNA analysis, have been useful and have provided a basis for the reclassification of several species. *Coxiella burnetii* and the genus *Bartonella*, including the former *Rochalimaea* spp., have been removed from the order *Rickettsiales*. All rickettsiae belong to the family *Rickettsiaceae*. The genus *Rickettsia* is subdivided into the typhus group, whose members are *Rickettsia typhi* and *Rickettsia prowazekii*; the spotted fever group (SFG), which includes about 20 different species of organisms pathogenic for humans (Table 1); and the scrub typhus group (STG), whose only member is *Orientia tsutsugamushi*, the cause of scrub typhus. The genus *Ehrlichia* includes at least three distinct species that are pathogenic for humans: *Ehrlichia chaffeensis*, *Ehrlichia equi* and *Ehrlichia phagocytophila* (the agents of human granulocytic ehrlichiosis), and *Ehrlichia sennetsu*. Rickettsiae are exclusively intracellular. Rickettsial genomes are small (1.2 to 1.6 Mb) and consist of a single circular chromosome (66). Rickettsiae are associated with arthropods and are transmitted to humans principally by the infected arthropods, but contamination by aerosols of infected insect feces and blood transfusion has also been described. Ixodid or hard ticks are the vectors of SFG rickettsiae and ehrlichiae (except *E. sennetsu*), mites are the vectors of *Rickettsia akari* and *O. tsutsugamushi*, lice are the vectors of *R. prowazekii*, and fleas are the vectors of *R. typhi* and *Rickettsia felis*.

Rickettsioses represent some of the oldest recognized infectious diseases. Epidemic typhus is suspected as the cause of the plague in Athens during the 5th century B.C. and the Black Death in the Middle Ages. It was differentiated from typhoid in the 16th century (34). Some authors suspected an American origin for typhus because of the American sylvatic flying squirrel reservoir (87). The role of the louse was definitely established by Nicolle (86) in 1909. At the beginning of

Didier Raoult • Unité des Rickettsies, Faculté de Médecine, Université de la Méditerranée, CNRS UPRES A 6020, 27, Boulevard Jean Moulin, 13385 Marseille Cedex 05, France. *James G. Olson* • Division of Viral and Rickettsial Diseases, National Center for Infectious Diseases, Centers for Disease Control and Prevention, Mail Stop A-26, 1600 Clifton Rd., Atlanta, GA 30333.

Table 1. Rickettsial diseases

Geographical location(s)	Rickettsia	Disease(s)	Vector(s)	Yr of isolation or discovery
Worldwide	*Rickettsia prowazekii*	Epidemic typhus	*Pediculus humanus corporis*	1916
America	*Rickettsia rickettsii*	RMSF	*Dermacentor andersoni, Dermacentor variabilis*	1919
Worldwide	*Rickettsia typhi*	Murine typhus	*Xenopsylla cheopis*	1920
Old World	*Rickettsia conorii*	MSF	*Rhipicephalus sanguineus*	1932
Worldwide	*Rickettsia akari*	Rickettsialpox	*Allodermanyssus sanguineus*	1946
Siberia, People's Republic of China	*Rickettsia sibirica*	Siberian tick typhus, North Asian tick typhus	*Dermacentor nuttalli, Dermacentor marginatus, Haemaphysalis concinna*	1949
Australia	*Rickettsia australis*	Queensland tick typhus	*Ixodes holocyclus*	1950
Israel, Portugal, Sicily	Israeli tick typhus *Rickettsia*	Israeli spotted fever	*Rhipicephalus sanguineus*	1974
Flinders Island, Australia	*Rickettsia honei*	Flinders Island spotted fever	Unknown	1991
Russia	Astrakhan fever *Rickettsia*	Astrakhan fever	*Rhipicephalus pumilio*	1991
Africa, West Indies	*Rickettsia africae*	African tick-bite fever	*Amblyomma hebraeum, Amblyomma variegatum*	1992
Japan	*Rickettsia japonica*	Japanese or Oriental spotted fever	*Dermacentor taiwanensis, Haemaphysalis flava, Haeamaphysalis formosensi, Haemaphysalis hystricis, Haemaphysalis longicornis, Ixodes ovatus*	1992
United States, Mexico	*Rickettsia felis*	Flea typhus of California	*Ctenocephalides felis*	1994
Europe, People's Republic of China	*Rickettsia mongolotimonae*	Spotted fever	*Haemaphysalis asiaticum*	1996
Europe	*Rickettsia slovaca*	Fever	*Dermacentor marginatus*	1997

the 20th century, Ricketts (64) proved that the wood tick, *Dermacentor andersoni*, was involved in the transmission of the Rocky Mountain spotted fever (RMSF). In 1910, the first cases of Mediterranean spotted fever (MSF) were reported in Tunis, Tunisia (19). The role of *Rhipicephalus sanguineus* was established in 1930. Prior to 1984, only eight rickettsioses were recognized, and in the subsequent 13 years, seven new rickettsial diseases were described (57, 60). The main clinical signs and symptoms of rickettsioses include fever, headache, a rash that is maculopapular or sometimes vesicular, an inoculation eschar, named "tache noire," at the site of the arthropod bite, and local lymphadenopathy. New rickettsial strains and other strains of unknown pathogenicity have been isolated from arthropods, in particular, ticks (60), and their roles as human pathogens have yet to be determined. Animal models do not necessarily predict the pathogenicities of rickettsiae for humans, and all rickettsiae isolated to date must be considered potential pathogens.

DIAGNOSTIC TOOLS FOR THE DIAGNOSIS OF RICKETTSIAL DISEASES

The advent of novel diagnostic tools has dramatically improved the efficiency of diagnosis of rickettsioses and the recognition of new rickettsial species. However, careful clinical examination and epidemiologic investigation of patients is critical. The typical clinical signs exhibited by patients with rickettsiosis are high temperature (39.5 to 40°C), headache, and rash.

Serology

Serological assays are the simplest diagnostic tests to perform. The Weil-Felix test was the first to be used and involves antigens from three *Proteus* strains: *Proteus vulgaris* OX2, *P. vulgaris* OX19, and *Proteus mirabilis* OXK. This test, however, lacks sensitivity and specificity. The most commonly used serological test today is microimmunofluorescence, which is reliable but which cannot be used to differentiate among the SFG rickettsiae responsible for the infection. The Western blot immunoassay (41) can be used to determine which SFG rickettsia caused the infection, provided that acute-phase sera are used. The test detects antibodies to two types of antigens: lipopolysaccharide antigens and two high-molecular-weight protein antigens (rOmpA and rOmpB). These proteins are species specific and provide the basis for the serotyping of rickettsiae (10). Cross-adsorption studies are also useful for the differentiation of different species of SFG rickettsiae as causes of infection, but they are very expensive to perform and are time-consuming. Positive serological test results should be considered only indicative of rickettsial infections. For the definitive diagnosis of a rickettsial infection, the rickettsial pathogens must be demonstrated to be present by culture, microscopic examination, and/or genetic detection techniques. This is particularly important if new syndromes, new manifestations of disease, or new areas where rickettsial infections are occurring are to be described.

Isolation

Rickettsia may be isolated in embryonated eggs, guinea pigs, mice, rats, and voles. Cell culture is the most widely used system for primary isolation. This system differs from that used for viral isolation because antibiotics, with the exception of co-trimoxazole, cannot be used for the isolation of rickettsiae. Raoult and La Scola (41) have used a microculture system, the shell vial assay, to isolate rickettsiae from human blood and other sources. The assay was adapted from a commercially available method for cytomegalovirus culture. It is now performed routinely in our laboratory with heparinized blood, skin biopsy samples, or arthropods. Although this system is useful, about one-third of organisms that are isolated are lost on subsequent passage, and the reasons for this are unknown. The importance of culture should, however, not be underestimated, because the ultimate method for the definitive confirmation of a rickettsial infection is isolation of a rickettsial organism from a patient.

Detection of Rickettsiae

Skin biopsy specimens have been used for the diagnosis of both RMSF and MSF. Samples can be tested fresh or after fixation and embedment in paraffin wax. The hemolymph test enables the demonstration of rickettsia-like organisms in the hemolymphs of live ticks. Rickettsiae may be isolated from hemolymph-positive ticks following surface sterilization. Immunological detection methods have been widely used for the detection of rickettsiae in biopsy specimens and arthropods. *R. typhi* can be demonstrated in infected fleas by an enzyme-linked immunosorbent assay (5). Rickettsiae may be detected by amplification of rickettsial DNA from an array of samples, including blood, skin biopsy specimens, and arthropod tissues, by PCR. The tache noire is the most useful specimen for biopsy and assay (41), and fresh tissues are preferred for PCR. Rickettsial DNA can also be detected in ticks, fleas, and lice by PCR-based amplification methods (5). Detection strategies based on recognition of sequences within the 16S rRNA gene (67) and those encoding a 17-kDa protein citrate synthase (68) and the rOmpB (19) and rOmpA (for SFG rickettsiae) (30) outer membrane proteins have been described. Reaction products must be further analyzed, either by restriction endonuclease analyses or by base sequence determination, for identification of the organism to the species level. Sequencing of the PCR amplification products is a relatively easy method for the precise identification of a new isolate because data banks that contain the sequences of the known species are available.

TICK-TRANSMITTED RICKETTSIOSES

SFG rickettsiae, with the exception of *R. akari*, are closely associated with ticks. They are transmitted transovarially from the mother to the progeny and transtadially from an egg to an adult. The association is probably very stable, and many *Rickettsia* species are strictly associated with one genus of ticks. Most rickettsial species are restricted to a single geographic area. Rickettsiae found in the Americas are different from those found in the Old World. Australia has its own rickettsiae (33).

Mammals play a major role in providing a host for ticks but rarely play a role in the transmission of *Rickettsia* to uninfected ticks, which are mainly infected vertically. Ehrlichiae are a major exception to this rule because there is no evidence of transovarial transmission of *Ehrlichia* spp. from adults to eggs. Therefore, the prevalence of rickettsial diseases is the consequence of complex interactions between humans and the ecosystem. The increase in the prevalence of RMSF and MSF in the 1970s, which was followed by a decrease in the 1980s, has not been explained (85). Possible explanations include climatic variation, spread of ticks, better diagnostic tools, and change of the empiric treatment of community-acquired fever. Until recently, only one pathogenic tick-borne SFG rickettsia was identified in each geographic area, i.e., *Rickettsia ricketsii* for the Americas, *Rickettsia conorii* for Europe, Asia, and Africa, *Rickettsia sibirica* in Siberia, Russia, and *Rickettsia australis* in Australia (20). With the development and use of new tools such as the shell vial assay for culture and PCR and sequencing of specific genes (60), new pathogenic species were identified. *Rickettsia japonica* and *Rickettsia honei* have been reported in islands where spotted fevers were unknown. *Rickettsia africae*, *Rickettsia slovaca*, and *Rickettsia mongolotimonae* have been reported in areas where *R. conorii* was thought to be the only described SFG rickettsia. Moreover, many rickettsiae (Table 1) have been recovered from ticks but have not yet been associated with human infection or disease. These bacteria have long been considered nonpathogenic, but many bacteria previously considered to be nonpathogenic have been shown to cause disease in humans. Examples include *C. burnetii*, *Legionella pneumophila*, and *R. africae*, which were considered to be nonpathogenic (60). We briefly report on the recently described rickettsioses. However, it should be remembered that in addition to rickettsial diseases, ticks transmit other bacterial pathogens, including *Borrelia* spp., *C. burnetii*, and *Francisella tularensis*.

Rickettsia africae

African tick-bite fever has been recognized since the beginning of the 20th century. However, the first documented infection with *R. africae* was reported in Zimbabwe in 1992 (38). In the 1930s, Pijper described a tick-borne disease in South Africa (55). This disease was rural, occurred in cattle and wild animals following tick bites, and was considered to be distinct from MSF, which is caused by *R. conorii*. Later, *R. conorii* was isolated in South Africa (32) and was established as the etiologic agent of tick-bite fever. Kelly and coworkers (39) isolated rickettsiae from *Amblyomma hebraeum* ticks in Zimbabwe in 1990 and showed that it was distinct from *R. conorii* and similar to an isolate from Ethiopian *Amblyomma variegatum* ticks (15). It was highly prevalent in *Amblyomma* ticks, which readily feed on humans. The rickettsial isolate was subsequently characterized as a distinct species and was named *R. africae* (36). Since then, Fournier et al. (29) have confirmed 38 cases among travellers returning from Zimbabwe, Tanzania, or South Africa (29). Parola et al. have recently shown that the disease is also prevalent in Guadeloupe in the Caribbean islands (50) and that *R. africae* widely infects local *Amblyomma* ticks (51). The incubation period is 7 days. The disease is mild and comprises headache, fever, eschar at the tick-bite site, and regional lymphadenopathy. *Amblyomma* ticks are aggressive biters, and groups of several ticks typically attack humans. As a result multiple eschars are common in patients with African tick-bite fever, which is the only tick-transmitted rickettsial disease with multiple eschars. Rash is frequently absent or transient and may be vesicular. Only rickettsialpox and Queensland tick typhus also have vesicular rashes. The prevalence is high in sub-Saharan Africa, where most tick bites in humans are due to *Amblyomma* spp. The seroprevalence of antibodies to SFG rickettsiae is higher in sub-Saharan Africa than elsewhere in the world and parallels the geographic distribution of *Amblyomma* ticks (37, 79). We believe that it is currently the most prevalent of the rickettsioses in the world. As tourism and travel to sub-Saharan Africa increase, it is expected that more cases of African tick-bite fever will be reported. Laboratory confirmation of the diagnosis is provided by isolation of *R. africae* from blood or a skin biopsy, positive result of PCR with a skin lesion specimen, or a positive serology result (microimmunofluorescence). In half of the patients the levels of antibodies to *R. africae* and *R. conorii* are not different, and only cross-absorption can determine the causative organism (29, 41).

Japanese or Oriental Spotted Fever

During the summer of 1984, Mahara (45) observed three patients who presented with a high temperature and a rash. In two patients a tache noire, a black necrotic lesion at the tick-bite site, was noted. The patients' sera tested positive for OX2 by the Weil-Felix test, which was carried out because scrub typhus was suspected. This was confirmed by indirect immunofluorescence with antigens of an SFG rickettsia (82). The causative agent was isolated in 1986 from patients (83) and was named *Rickettsia japonica* (81). This rickettsia has been detected in *Dermacentor taiwanensis* and *Haemaphysalis longicornis*. Since 1984, 140 cases have been reported in Japan (46), where cases are observed from April to October. The disease begins with an abrupt onset of headache, high temperature (39 to 40°C), and chills. A maculopapular rash appears in 2 to 3 days, and a tache noire is frequently observed. Fatal cases of infection have been reported. The story of Japanese spotted fever shows that without a physician's curiosity no new disease would have been found. In fact, in Japan, a country with a strong medical infrastructure, the disease has probably been present for at least 100 years but was only recently described. It was finally detected in a way similar to that in which MSF was detected in 1909, when two successive patients with similar syndromes were observed by the same physician. It also shows that luck could be necessary for the identification of a new disease because sera from these patients were tested by the Weil-Felix test, which is now considered outdated. The test detects antibodies to the three rickettsial groups: the SFG, typhus, and scrub typhus groups. When it was performed because of a suspicion of scrub typhus, it allowed the detection of an SFG rickettsial infection. A more specific test (microimmunofluorescence, for example) for the detection of scrub typhus would have failed to detect a rickettsial disease.

Astrakhan Fever

In Astrakhan, Russia, a febrile rash illness has been reported since 1983 (76). Its etiology was unknown, and it was named Astrakhan fever (75). Tarasevich and others (75) investigated this disease, which was considered locally to be caused by a virus. In fact, if physicians in Astrakhan had been aware of the clinical description of spotted fevers, they could have described the disease clinically as Conor and Bruch (19) had done for MSF. The disease, in fact, is characterized by a high fever, headaches, a papular rash, and a favorable prognosis, with spontaneous remission of signs in 2 to 3 weeks. Serum samples from patients were sent to the Gameleya Institute in Moscow, where the detection of antibodies to SFG rickettsiae indicated that further investigations were required. An eschar is observed in about 20% of the patients. The causative agent has been isolated from patients (23) and from *Rhipicephalus pumilio*, which parasitizes dogs (25). More than 1,000 cases have been recognized, but fatal cases of infection have not been reported.

Flinders Island Spotted Fever

Flinders Island spotted fever was described in 1991 by Stewart, the only physician on Flinders Island, which is between Australia and Tasmania (33). He reported a febrile eruptive disease which occurred in the summer. The rash is maculopapular in most patients. An eschar is noted in 25% of patients, and enlarged local lymph nodes are present in 55% of patients. The patients' sera tested positive by the Weil-Felix test and subsequently by indirect immunofluorescence with antigens of an SFG rickettsia. The causative agent was isolated in 1992 and was named *R. honei* (7). It is closely related to the Thai tick typhus rickettsia (Table 1).

Spotted Fever due to *"Rickettsia mongolotimonae"*

In 1991, a rickettsia was isolated from a *Hyalomma asiaticum* tick collected in Inner Mongolia, People's Republic of China. It was characterized and described as a distinct species of the SFG rickettsiae closely related to but distinct from *R. sibirica* (89). The reservoir of this rickettsia is unknown. A second isolate was obtained from the blood and the skin of a woman from Marseille, France, in 1996 (58). She presented with fever, a discrete rash, and an eschar in her left groin. It was suspected that the patient was bitten by a tick carried by a migratory bird. A second case (unpublished data) occurred in Marseille in 1998 in a 60-year-old man who presented with fever, tache noire, and lymphangitis. *R. mongolotimonae* was isolated from the skin. The name *"R. mongolotimonae"* is suggested to acknowledge the sites (Mongolia and La Timone Hospital, Marseille) where the organism was isolated (30).

Infection due to *Rickettsia slovaca*

Raoult and colleagues (57) reported on the first definitively documented case of infection due to *R. slovaca* in 1997. A woman walked in the woods in November and 1 week later presented with fever, arthralgias, and fatigue. She had removed a tick from her hair. She was hospitalized because of suspicion of Lyme disease and had fever, headache, a necrotic eschar at the site of the tick bite surrounded by an erythematous halo, and four enlarged cervical lymph nodes. The tick was identified as *Dermacentor marginatus*, and from the acute phase to the convalescent phase of illness the patient developed increased levels of antibodies to *R. slovaca*, which was isolated from the tick. *R. slovaca* DNA was also detected in a biopsy specimen taken from the eschar. *R. slovaca* was first isolated in 1968 from *D. marginatus* ticks in Czechoslovakia (62). Subsequently, it has been detected or isolated from this tick species in other European countries including France, Switzerland, Armenia, and Portugal (71). A rickettsial isolate from Pakistan was obtained in 1970 (20). It seems to be very closely related to *R. slovaca* and may be prevalent in central Asia. A suspected case of *R. slovaca* infection was reported in 1980 (48); the patient presented with meningoencephalitis and erythema, and his acute- and convalescent-phase sera showed increased titers of antibodies to *R. slovaca*. We have also recorded two cases from Hungary (reported by A. Lakos), which were very similar to our first case, and a case of meningoencephalitis from France. The prevalence of *R. slovaca* infection has yet to be described. These rickettsiae may follow the distribution of their host, *D. marginatus*, which is found throughout Europe. Patients who have illnesses that resemble Lyme disease but who have no serological evidence of *Borrelia* infection should be tested for antibodies to *R. slovaca* (71). However, this disease may be an entirely new entity because it is not a spotted fever and more resembles Lyme disease than a rickettsial disease. It should be kept in mind that some tick-transmitted rickettsial diseases could be aneruptive. It could be a common disease. In Spain a recent study showed that 20% of tick bites in the province of Castilla y León are caused by *D. marginatus*, of which 31% are infected with a *Rickettsia* sp. In that region the occurrence of *R. slovaca* could be twice as frequent as that of either the Lyme disease spirochete or the MSF rickettsia (69a).

Other Tick-Transmitted Rickettsioses

All rickettsiae isolated from ticks (Table 2) are potential pathogens. It is suspected that the Spanish strain Bar 29 (8) causes an MSF-like disease, which may explain why MSF in Catalonia is resistant to rifampin, an antibiotic that is highly effective against all rickettsia strains apart from members of the *Rickettsia massiliae* group (9, 65). In fact, only a single group of SFG rickettsiae that includes *Rickettsia montanensis*, *R. massiliae*, *Rickettsia rhipicephali*, and *Rickettsia aeschlimannii* is resistant to rifampin. This is due to a mutation in the RNA polymerase gene (unpublished data) specific to this group of rickettsiae. In the area of Barcelona, Spain, Bar 29, an isolate closely related to *R. massiliae*, is the rickettsia most commonly isolated from ticks. Rifampin has also been described as inefficient for treatment of children in Barcelona (9), and this prompted us to test the isolate for its susceptibility to rifampin (65). After recognition of the resistance, they suspected that some cases of MSF in this area could be caused by Bar 29. This is being investigated in Catalonia. Other American rickettsiae such as "*Rickettsia cooleyi*" (12), strain Tillamook, strain Parumapertus, *R. montanensis*, "*Rickettsia amblyommii*," *Rickettsia bellii*, and *Rickettsia canadensis* (20) may subsequently be shown to cause diseases, as has been the case with rickettsiae in Europe (72).

Table 2. Rickettsiae of unknown pathogenicity isolated from ticks

Rickettsia	Tick reservoir(s)	Geographic location(s)
Rickettsia massiliae	*Rhipicephalus sanguineus,* *Rhipicephalus* sp.	France, Greece, Spain, Portugal, Central Africa
Bar 29	*Rhipicephalus sanguineus*	Spain
JC880	*Rhipicephalus sanguineus*	Pakistan
Strain S	*Rhipicephalus sanguineus*	Armenia
Rickettsia rhipicephali	*Rhipicephalus sanguineus,* *Dermacentor andersoni*	United States, France, Portugal, Central Africa
Rickettsia montanensis	*Dermacentor andersoni,* *Dermacentor variabilis*	United States
Rickettsia peacockii	*Dermacentor andersoni*	United States
Rickettsia bellii	*Dermacentor* sp., *Ornithodoros concanensis, Argas cooleyi, Haemaphysalis leporispalustris*	United States
Thai tick typhus *Rickettsia*	Pool *Rhipicephalus* sp. and *Ixodes* spp.	Thailand
Rickettisa helvetica	*Ixodes ricinus*	France, Switzerland
Rickettsia aeschlimannii	*Hyalomma marginatum*	Morocco
"*Rickettsia amblyommii*"	*Amblyomma americanum*	United States
Rickettsia parkeri	*Amblyomma maculatum*	United States
"*Rickettsia texiana*"	*Amblyomma americanum*	United States
Rickettsia canadensis	*Haemophysalis leporispalustris*	United States, Canada
Unnamed *Rickettsia*	*Dermacentor occidentalis, Dermacentor parumapertus, Ixodes pacificus, Amblyomma americanum*	United States
Unnamed *Rickettsia*	*Ixodes ricinus*	Spain
"*Rickettsia cooleyi*"	*Ixodes scapularis*	United States
"*Rickettsia heilongjiangi*"	*Haemaphysalis* sp.	People's Republic of China
Tillamook	*Ixodes pacificus*	United States
Parumapertus	*Dermacentor parumapertus*	United States

Ehrlichioses

In 1986 a patient from Illinois who had recently visited Arkansas was admitted to a hospital with fever and confusion (44). Five days earlier he had experienced fever, malaise, myalgia, and headache. A presumptive diagnosis of RMSF was made on clinical grounds, despite the absence of serological findings, and the patient was initially treated with chloramphenicol and was then treated with doxycycline. The patient fully recovered and was discharged after a 12-week hospitalization. Because serological tests failed to identify the etiology of the illness, laboratory studies continued. Two separate lines of laboratory evidence implicated *Ehrlichia* as the causative agent: microscopic visualization of characteristic inclusions (morulae) in a peripheral blood film and serological evidence of infection with *Ehrlichia canis*. The true cause of this form of ehrlichiosis that predominately infects monocytes, *E. chaffeensis*, was described in 1991 (1). Since then more than 500 laboratory-confirmed cases of monocytic ehrlichiosis have been described in 30 U.S. states. Most cases occur in the southeastern quarter of the United States, especially Missouri, Tennessee, Oklahoma, Texas, Virginia, Arkansas, and Georgia. The vector tick is the Lone Star tick, *Amblyomma americanum* (2), and the vertebrate reservoir is probably the white-tailed deer, *Odocoileus virginianus* (22). There is no evidence of transmission of ehrlichial infections from adult ticks to offspring via the transovarial route.

Nearly 67% of patients report a tick bite, rash occurs in less than 30% of patients, and approximately 90% of cases occur during the late spring and summer (28). Older patients have a higher incidence of disease, which suggests that waning immunity may have an effect on the incidence of infection or disease. The rate of ehrlichiosis in males exceeds that in females by nearly 3:1. These differences are attributed to differences in occupational and recreational exposures. The case fatality rate is 5%.

In 1992 a 78-year-old patient was admitted to a hospital in Duluth, Minn., with fever, headache, myalgia, leukopenia, and pulmonary infiltrates (18). Morulae were observed in granulocytes of the patient's peripheral blood smear, suggesting ehrlichiosis. Acute-phase blood from this and five additional febrile patients who had similar cytoplasmic morulae were prepared for DNA extraction and PCR amplification and sequencing. The results indicated that the *Ehrlichia* that infected these patients was closely related to *E. equi* and *E. phagocytophila*.

Human granulocytic ehrlichiosis (HGE) has caused more than 1,000 laboratory-confirmed cases of ehrlichiosis in the upper Midwest, especially Wisconsin and Minnesota, and in the northeastern United States, especially New York and Connecticut. The vector is the black-legged tick, *Ixodes scapularis*, which is also the vector of *Borrelia burgdorferi*, the agent that causes Lyme disease. The vertebrate reservoir for HGE is the white-footed mouse, *Peromyscus leucopus* (77). The disease is similar in clinical presentation to monocytic ehrlichiosis, and patients with this disease have similar age and gender distributions. The case fatality rate is between 3 and 7%.

Cases of HGE have been confirmed in both Slovenia (43) and Sweden (12a). The etiologic agent in Europe is *E. phagocytophila*, and the vector is *Ixodes ricinus* ticks (54). The incidence of HGE will be confirmed elsewhere in Europe. Studies in Denmark (42) have demonstrated serological evidence of HGE infection among Lyme disease patients with headache, fever, and myalgia, and studies in Switzerland (56) have shown that subjects at risk of tick bite have antibodies to *E. phagocytophila*.

Epidemic (Louse-Borne) Typhus

The human body louse (which lives in clothing) is capable of being a vector for bacteria that cause three diseases: epidemic typhus (which is caused by *R. prowazekii*), trench fever (which is caused by *Bartonella quintana*), and louse-borne relapsing fever (which is caused by *Borrelia recurrentis*). All three have recently reemerged.

The human body louse lives in clothing and is therefore associated with both cold weather and a lack of hygiene. Its prevalence reflects the low socioeconomic status of certain members of society, it is prevalent during war, and it is increasingly found in the poorest populations of developed countries such as France (73), Russia (69), The Netherlands (84), and the United States (35, 40). Because of its ability to spread rapidly within a population, infestations of human body lice threaten the populations of all countries with severe socioeconomic problems (47).

Because human body lice live in clothing, the prevalence of body lice is determined by the weather, humidity, the poverty level, and a lack of hygiene. Consequently, they are more prevalent in colder months, and louse-transmitted diseases, especially epidemic typhus, are more frequently reported during winter and early spring (52). Louse-borne diseases apparently disappeared from developed countries following World War II but remained prevalent in several foci of endemicity. The areas where infestations with body lice remain are those where cold weather requires the wearing of multiple layers of clothes and where poverty results in the lack of several sets of clothing to allow for proper laundering of clothing. The disease primarily occurs in mountainous regions of the intertropical zone, including Ethiopia, Burundi, and Rwanda in Africa (59), the Andes Mountains in South America, and the Himalaya Mountains in Asia (27), where the proportion of people infested with human body lice may be very high (78). The civil war that involved Burundi and Rwanda in Africa and that started in 1993 was associated with a large infestation of lice (3, 4). Under such conditions the rate of louse infestation among the population reached 90 to 100%. An outbreak of typhus started in jails in Burundi in 1996 (4, 61), and a large outbreak of typhus spread to refugee camps in 1997, where nearly all refugees were infested with lice (59). This experience illustrates how rapidly the spread of louse infestations can occur when conditions such as war, cold weather, and a lack of hygiene are prevalent.

Reported body louse infestations are increasing in developed countries as well, primarily among homeless people. Louse infestations have been associated with *B. quintana* infections in the United States (40), France (14, 24), and The Netherlands (84) and in Moscow, Russia (69), where a small outbreak of typhus occurred in December 1997 (74). Wherever human body louse infestations occur, the potential for louse-borne diseases exists. The most successful strategies for elimination of louse infestations involve the raising of living standards. Interventions with insecticides alone have not resulted in long-term solutions. The only way to eradicate lice is to change and launder clothes, thus eliminating the vector lice. Until recently, typhus was considered a disease of the past, and in 1995 it was suspected to be prevalent only in Ethiopia (88). Since the 1980s no cases had been recorded in Eastern Europe, including Russia, or in Rwanda, Burundi, Uganda, and Nigeria, which have been regular foci (53). Few data were obtained from other mountainous tropical countries such as Tibet, Nepal, or Peru, which remain louse infested. Since then typhus has made a dramatic reemergence. A large outbreak was reported in Burundi in 1997 (59). In that outbreak 100,000 persons were estimated to have been infected. Sporadic cases were reported in northern Africa (26). Small outbreaks were observed in Peru in 1998 (unpublished data), and even in developed countries typhus should be considered a serious threat when body louse infestations are prevalent, because of all rickettsiae *R. prowazekii* has the potential to cause the most serious epidemics.

The human body louse acquires *R. prowazekii* after feeding on an infected human, but it does not become infectious until 5 to 7 days later. Transmission of *R. prowazekii* from the louse to humans occurs by contamination of the bite site with louse feces containing rickettsiae or by contamination of conjunctivae or mucous membranes with the crushed bodies or feces of infected lice. Infection through the transmission of aerosols of feces-infected dust has been reported and is the main risk for medical personnel who treat patients with typhus.

Individuals with recrudescent typhus (Brill-Zinsser disease) provide the mechanism for the interepidemic survival of *R. prowazekii* and a means of dissemination of typhus from foci of endemicity to louse-infested populations. If an individual with a recrudescent *R. prowazekii* infection is simultaneously infested with lice, an epidemic focus of *R. prowazekii* can become established. Bozeman et al. (13) were able to isolate *R. prowazekii* from *Glaucomys volans volans*, the eastern flying squirrel, in the United States. Fleas and lice from flying squirrels were also shown to be infected. When rickettsiae are ingested by the louse as part of a blood meal, they infect the midgut epithelial cells of the louse and undergo rapid multiplication. As a result of the extensive growth of *R. prowazekii*, infected epithelial cells enlarge and eventually burst to release the rickettsiae into the gut lumen. Massive quantities of rickettsiae are discharged in the feces and can remain infective for up to 100 days. Infection with *R. prowazekii* leads to the death of the louse.

Typhus begins abruptly. Headache, myalgias, and nonspecific constitutional symptoms such as malaise, anorexia, chills, and fever are common. Most patients complain of fever, chills, myalgias, arthralgias, and anorexia early in the course of their illness. In a recent study in Burundi, a crouching posture due to myalgia and referred to as "sutama" was reported (59). Cough is frequent, as are confusion and stupor. Most patients develop a skin rash that classically begins on the trunk and that spreads to the periphery. The rash may be macular, maculopapular, or petechial, and it may be difficult to detect in dark-colored individuals. Rarely, patients with severe cases of typhus may develop gangrene of the distal extremities, necessitating amputation.

Thrombocytopenia, jaundice, and abnormal liver function tests may occur in patients with severe cases of typhus. Since a single dose of 200 mg of doxycycline will save the patient, any patient with a suspected case of typhus should be treated with doxycycline; a prompt response to this treatment could be indicative of the diagnosis. Recrudescent typhus, or Brill-Zinsser disease, can appear in patients who have recovered from epidemic typhus years after the onset of the first illness (63).

The diagnosis of typhus is usually suggested by the presence of typical clinical findings such as fever, headaches, and skin rash in patients infested with body lice or in persons who are living in crowed, cold, and unhygienic circumstances. Illness often occurs in clusters, but it may also occur in isolation. Epidemic and murine (flea-borne) typhus cannot be differentiated by serology unless Western blotting and/or tests for the cross-adsorption of sera are done (21, 59). A diagnosis of recent epidemic or murine typhus as a result of rickettsial infection can be established by demonstrating a fourfold or greater rise in antibody titer in serum samples collected during the acute and convalescent phases of illness. Techniques that use the PCR technology have been employed to detect the organisms that cause typhus in blood and to detect these organisms in their vectors (16, 59). Lice and blood collected as drops on filter paper have been very useful for the testing of large numbers of survey specimens (31). These two types of specimens are very efficient as samples for use in diagnosis and may be sent to a reference laboratory to confirm the occurrence of typhus without the use of the specific cold chain needed for serum or frozen materials.

Flea-Transmitted Rickettsioses

Flea-borne bacterial diseases include cat-scratch disease, which is caused by *Bartonella henselae*; plague, which is caused by *Yersinia pestis*; and murine typhus, which is caused by *R. typhi*. The spectrum of human disease determined by the newly described species *R. felis* remains to be established. Interestingly, flea-borne diseases have all emerged or reemerged in recent years. *B. henselae* was described by Regnery and coworkers in 1992 (61a). Plague has reemerged mainly in Madagascar and Vietnam (17). The oriental rat flea, *Xenopsylla cheopis*, is the main flea vector of flea-borne bacterial diseases, including rickettsioses. These fleas are associated with Old World commensal rats, and consequently, the disease associated with these fleas is prevalent in harbors and large cities. The cat flea, *Ctenocephalides felis*, is the vector for cat-scratch disease and cat-flea typhus.

Murine typhus is prevalent throughout the tropics and is occasionally reported in the southern United States and Greece (80), Cyprus (unpublished data), Spain (6, 11), Malaysia (49), and Egypt.

Adams et al. reported that a shift in the distribution of human cases of murine typhus had occurred in southern California during the 1970s. Cases were observed more frequently in Orange County (60). It was an atypical area for the occurrence of murine typhus because it is a relatively wealthy suburb without heavy commensal rat infestations. Opossums were frequently observed in places where cases of murine typhus were observed. Opossums have a high seroprevalence of antibody to *R. typhi*, and they were infested with cat fleas (*Ctenocephalides felis*), which were infected with a rickettsia. This rickettsia was first named the ELB agent and then *R. felis* (5).

These findings prompted the search for fleas on cats and dogs and confirmed that these fleas were infected with *R. felis* or *R. typhi*. These insects were collected from cats, opossums, and dogs in California, Texas, and Georgia, demonstrating that the reservoirs now extended from rats to pets, which explains the epidemiologic variations as well as the rural extension of flea-transmitted diseases. Currently, only one documented case of infection, in a patient with fever and a clinical diagnosis of cholecystitis (70), has been reported. A second case was identified in a 34-year-old Mexican woman from Yucatan who presented with fever, meningeal irritation, hearing loss, hemorrhagic conjunctivitis, and epidermal lesions described as furuncles on the arms and chest (90). *R. felis*-specific gene sequences were obtained following amplification of DNA from a skin lesion. However, because the bacteria are widespread in fleas, which readily bite human beings, it is possible that the disease is unrecognized in the southern United States and elsewhere (91). The clinical spectrum of the disease remains to be established. The taxonomic and phylogenic positions of *R. felis* are not clear because no isolates are available for comparative studies. The 16S rRNA sequence analysis of *R. felis* places it outside the typhus group, and its 16S rRNA sequence is closer to that of the SFG of *Rickettsia*. Humans are infected by contamination of disrupted skin or by aerosols containing infected flea feces. Murine typhus is usually a mild disease, and patients present with fever, headache, and a maculopapular rash, which occurs in about half of the patients (60). The mildness of the illness, together with the nonspecific signs and symptoms, leads to the fact that it is almost never recognized. Diagnosis is confirmed by serology, mainly by microimmunofluorescence. *R. felis* and *R. typhi* have closely related lipopolysaccharide antigens, and cross-reactions are common.

CONCLUSIONS

Eleven new rickettsioses have been described since 1974 (Table 3). Examples include Israeli spotted fever (1974), flying squirrel typhus (1976), Japanese or oriental spotted fever (1986), human ehrlichioses (1987 and 1994), Flinders Island spotted fever (1991), Astrakhan fever (1992), cat-flea typhus (1994), African tick-bite fever (1996), and unnamed illnesses caused by *R. mongolotimonae* (1996) and *R. slovaca* (1997). Several (Japanese spotted fever, Astrakhan fever, and Flinders Island spotted fever) were described in countries where no spotted fevers had previously been identified. Most were identified in areas where one or more recognized rickettsial diseases were known to occur. In Africa, where *R. conorii* was a well-known cause of MSF, *R. africae* was found to be a significant cause of tick-

Table 3. New rickettsial pathogens recognized since 1974

Geographic location	Before 1974	By 1998
Europe	*R. prowazekii*	*R. prowazekii*
	R. conorii	*R. conorii*
		R. slovaca
		R. conorii Israel
		R. conorii Astrakhan
		R. mongolotimonae
Asia	*R. prowazekii*	*R. prowazekii*
	R. sibirica	*R. sibirica*
	R. conorii	*R. conorii*
		R. conorii Israel
		R. mongolotimonae
		R. japonica
Africa	*R. prowazekii*	*R. prowazekii*
	R. conorii	*R. conorii*
		R. africae
Americas	*R. rickettsii*	*R. rickettsii*
	R. prowazekii (body louse)	*R. felis*
	R. prowazekii (body louse, flying squirrel)	*R. africae*
Australia	*R. australis*	*R. australis*
		R. honei

transmitted rickettsioses. Similarly, in France, where MSF was also well-known, tick-borne disease caused by *R. mongolotimonae* was documented. Several examples from the United States include cat-flea typhus, which is caused by *R. felis* and which was misdiagnosed as murine typhus; monolytic ehrlichiosis, which is caused by *E. chaffeensis* and which is clinically confused with RMSF; and human granulocytic ehrlichiosis, which is caused by *E. equi* and which was clinically mistaken for monocytic ehrlichiosis. Finally, an entirely new clinical entity, such as the one caused by *R. slovaca*, which results in disease without the typical rash associated with other spotted fevers, was described. The future of such new diseases is unpredictable because rickettsioses have not been systematically studied in such cases. This is an area for future research.

REFERENCES

1. **Anderson, B. E., J. E. Dawson, D. C. Jones, and K. H. Wilson.** 1991. *Ehrlichia chaffeensis*, a new species associated with human ehrlichiosis. *J. Clin. Microbiol.* **29:**2838–2842.
2. **Anderson, B. E., G. S. Kimetha, J. G. Olson, J. E. Childs, J. F. Piesman, C. M. Happ, G. O. Maupin, and B. J. Johnson.** 1993. *Amblyomma americanum:* a potential vector of human ehrlichiosis. *Am. J. Trop. Med. Hyg.* **49:**239–244.
3. **Anonymous.** 1994. Epidemic typhus risk in Rwandan refugee camps. *Weekly Epidemiol. Rec.* **69:** 259.
4. **Anonymous.** 1997. A large outbreak of epidemic louse-borne typhus in Burundi. *WHO Weekly Epidemiol. Rec.* **72:**152–153.
5. **Azad, A. F., S. Radulovic, J. A. Higgins, B. H. Noden, and J. M. Troyer.** 1997. Flea-borne rickettsioses: ecologic considerations. *Emerg. Infect. Dis.* **3:**319–327.
6. **Bacellar, F., I. Lencastre, and A. R. Filipe.** 1998. Is murine typhus re-emerging in Portugal? *Eurosurveillance* **3:**18–20.
7. **Baird, R. W., J. Stenos, R. Stewart, B. Hudson, M. Lloyd, S. Aiuto, and B. Dwyer.** 1996. Genetic variation in Australian spotted fever group rickettsiae. *J. Clin. Microbiol.* **34:**1526–1530.
8. **Beati, L., V. Roux, A. Ortuno, J. Castella, F. Segura Porta, and D. Raoult.** 1996. Phenotypic and genotypic characterization of spotted fever group rickettsiae isolated from catalan *Rhipicephalus sanguineus* ticks. *J. Clin. Microbiol.* **34:**2688–2694.
9. **Bella, F., E. Espejo-Arenas, S. Uriz, J. A. Serrano, M. D. Alegre, and J. Tort.** 1991. Randomized trial of five-day rifampin versus one-day doxycycline therapy for Mediterranean spotted fever. *J. Infect. Dis.* **164:**433–434.
10. **Berbari, E. F., F. R. Cockerill, and J. M. Steckelberg.** 1997. Infective endocarditis due to unusual or fastidious microorganisms. *Mayo Clin. Proc.* **72:**532–542.
11. **Bernabeu-Wittel, M., J. L. Villanueva-Marcos, A. de Alarcon-Gonzalez, and J. Pachon.** 1998. Septic shock and multiorganic failure in murine typhus. *Eur. J. Clin. Microbiol. Infect. Dis.* **17:**131–132.
12. **Billings, A. N., G. J. Teltow, S. C. Weaver, and D. H. Walker.** 1998. Molecular characterization of a novel Rickettsia species from *Ixodes scapularis* in Texas. *Emerg. Infect. Dis.* **4:**305–309.
12a.**Bjoersdorff, A.** Personal communication.
13. **Bozeman, F. M., S. A. Masiello, M. S. Williams, and B. L. Elisberg.** 1975. Epidemic typhus rickettsiae isolated from flying squirrels. *Nature* **255:**545–547.
14. **Brouqui, P., P. Houpikian, H. Tissot-Dupont, P. Toubiana, Y. Obadia, V. Lafay, and D. Raoult.** 1996. Survey of the seroprevalence of *Bartonella quintana* in homeless people. *Clin. Infect. Dis.* **23:**756–759.
15. **Burgdorfer, W., R. A. Ormsbee, M. L. Schmidt, and H. Hoogstraal.** 1973. A search for the epidemic typhus agent in Ethiopian ticks. *Bull. W. H. O.* **48:**563–569.
16. **Carl, M., C. W. Tibbs, M. E. Dobson, S. Paparello, and G. A. Dasch.** 1990. Diagnosis of acute typhus infection using the polymerase chain reaction. *J. Infect. Dis.* **161:**791–793.

17. **Chanteau, S., L. Ratsifasoamanana, B. Rasoamanana, L. Rahalison, J. Randriambelosoa, J. Roux, and D. Rabeson.** 1998. Plague, a reemerging disease in Madagascar. *Emerg. Infect. Dis.* **4:** 101–104.

18. **Chen, S., J. S. Dumler, J. S. Bakken, and D. H. Walker.** 1994. Identification of a granulocytotropic *Ehrlichia* species as the etiologic agent of human disease. *J. Clin. Microbiol.* **32:**589–595.

19. **Conor, A., and A. Bruch.** 1910. Une fièvre éruptive observée en Tunisie. *Bull. Soc. Pathol. Exot. Filial.* **8:**492–496.

20. **Dasch, G. A., and E. Weiss.** 1992. The genera *Rickettsia, Rochalimaea, Ehrlichia, Cowdria,* and *Neorickettsia,* p. 2407–2470. *In* A. Balows, H. G. Trüper, M. Dworkin, W. Harder, and K. Schleifer (ed.), *The Prokaryotes.* Springer-Verlag, New York, N.Y.

21. **Dasch, G. A., and A. Bourgeois.** 1981. Antigens of the typhus group of rickettsiae: importance of species-specific surface protein antigens in eliciting immunity, p. 61–70. *In* W. Burgdorfer and R. L. Anacker (ed.), *Rickettsiae and Rickettsial Diseases.* Academic Press, Inc., New York, N.Y.

22. **Dawson, J. E., D. E. Stallknecht, E. W. Howerth, C. Warner, K. Biggie, W. R. Davidson, J. M. Lockhart, V. F. Nettles, J. G. Olson, and J. E. Childs.** 1994. Susceptibility of white-tailed deer (*Odocoileus virginianus*) to infection with *Ehrlichia chaffeensis,* the etiologic agent of human ehrlichiosis. *J. Clin. Microbiol.* **32:**2725–2728.

23. **Drancourt, M., L. Beati, I. V. Tarasevich, and D. Raoult.** 1992. Astrakhan fever rickettsia is identical to Israeli tick typhus rickettsia, a genotype of the *Rickettsia conorii* complex. *J. Infect. Dis.* **165:**1167–1168.

24. **Drancourt, M., J. L. Mainardi, P. Brouqui, F. Vandenesch, A. Carta, F. Lehnert, J. Etienne, F. Goldstein, J. Acar, and D. Raoult.** 1995. *Bartonella* (*Rochalimaea*) *quintana* endocarditis in three homeless men. *N. Engl. J. Med.* **332:**419–423.

25. **Eremeeva, M. E., L. Beati, V. A. Makarova, N. F. Fetisova, I. V. Tarasevich, N. M. Balayeva, and D. Raoult.** 1994. Astrakhan fever rickettsiae: antigenic and genotypic of isolates obtained from human and *Rhipicephalus pumilio* ticks. *Am. J. Trop. Med. Hyg.* **51:**697–706.

26. **Ernez, M., M. Chakroun, A. Letaief, and L. Jemni.** 1995. Particularités cliniques et biologiques du typhus exanthématique. *Presse Med.* **24:**1358.

27. **Fan, M. Y., D. H. Walker, S. R. Yu, and Q. H. Liu.** 1987. Epidemiology and ecology of rickettsial diseases in the People's Republic of China. *Rev. Infect. Dis.* **9:**823–840.

28. **Fishbein, D. B., J. E. Dawson, and L. E. Robinson.** 1994. Human ehrlichiosis in the United States, 1985 to 1990. *Ann. Intern. Med.* **120:**736–743.

29. **Fournier, P. E., V. Roux, E. Caumes, M. Donzel, and D. Raoult.** 1998. Outbreak of *Rickettsia africae* infections in participants of an adventure race from South Africa. *Clin. Infect. Dis.* **27:** 316–323.

30. **Fournier, P. E., V. Roux, and D. Raoult.** 1998. Phylogenetic analysis of spotted fever group rickettsiae by study of the outer surface protein rOmpA. *Int. J. Syst. Bacteriol.* **48:**839–849.

31. **Gan, E., F. C. Cadigan, Jr., and J. S. Walker.** 1972. Filter paper collection of blood for use in a screening and diagnostic test for scrub typhus using the IFAT. *Trans. R. Soc. Trop. Med. Hyg.* **66:** 588–593.

32. **Gear, J. H. S.** 1938. South African typhus. *S. Afr. J. Med. Sci.* **3:**134–160.

33. **Graves, S. R.** 1998. Rickettsial diseases: the Australian story so far. *Pathology* **30:**147–152.

34. **Hansen, W., and J. Freney.** 1996. Le typhus épidémique, sa transmission et la découverte de l'agent étiologique. *Lyon Pharm.* **47:**130–138.

35. **Jackson, L. A., and D. H. Spach.** 1996. Emergence of *Bartonella quintana* infection among homeless persons. *Emerg. Infect. Dis.* **2:**141–144.

36. **Kelly, P. J., L. Beati, P. R. Mason, L. A. Matthewman, V. Roux, and D. Raoult.** 1996. *Rickettsia africae* sp. nov., the etiological agent of African tick bite fever. *Int. J. Syst. Bacteriol.* **46:**611–614.

37. **Kelly, P. J., P. R. Mason, L. A. Matthewman, and D. Raoult.** 1991. Seroepidemiology of spotted fever group rickettsial infections in human in Zimbabwe. *J. Trop. Med. Hyg.* **94:**304–309.

38. **Kelly, P. J., L. A. Matthewman, L. Beati, D. Raoult, P. Mason, M. Dreary, and R. Makombe.** 1992. African tick-bite fever—a new spotted fever group rickettsiosis under an old name. *Lancet* **340:**982–983.

39. **Kelly, P. J., D. Raoult, and P. R. Mason.** 1991. Isolation of spotted fever group rickettsias from triturated ticks using a modification of the centrifugation-shell vial technique. *Trans. R. Soc. Trop. Med. Hyg.* **85:**397–398.

40. **Koehler, J. E., M. A. Sanchez, C. S. Garrido, M. J. Whitfeld, F. M. Chen, T. G. Berger, M. C. Rodriguez-Barradas, P. E. Leboit, and J. W. Tappero.** 1997. Molecular epidemiology of *Bartonella* infections in patients with bacillary angiomatosis-peliosis. *N. Engl. J. Med.* **337:**1876–1883.

41. **La Scola, B., and D. Raoult.** 1997. Laboratory diagnosis of rickettsioses: current approaches to the diagnosis of old and new rickettsial diseases. *J. Clin. Microbiol.* **35:**2715–2727.

42. **Lebech, A., K. Hansen, P. Pancholi, L. Sloan, J. Magera, and D. Persing.** 1998. Immunoserologic evidence of human granulocytic ehrlichiosis in Danish patients with Lyme neuroborreliosis. *Scand. J. Infect. Dis.* **30:**173–176.

43. **Lotric-Furlan, S., M. Petrovec, T. A. Zupanc, W. L. Nicholson, J. W. Sumner, J. Childs, and F. Strle.** 1998. Human granulocytic ehrlichiosis in Europe: clinical and laboratory findings for four patients from Slovenia. *Clin. Infect. Dis.* **27:**424–428.

44. **Maeda, K., N. Markowitz, R. C. Hawley, M. Ristic, D. Cox, and J. E. McDade.** 1987. Human infection with *Ehrlichia canis*, a leukocytic rickettsia. *N. Engl. J. Med.* **316:**853–856.

45. **Mahara, F.** 1984. Three Weil-Felix reaction OX2 positive cases with skin eruptions and high fever. *JAMA* **68:**4–7.

46. **Mahara, F.** 1997. Japanese spotted fever: report of 31 cases and review of the literature. *Emerg. Infect. Dis.* **3:**105–111.

47. **Maunder, J. W.** 1983. The appreciation of lice. *Proc. R. Inst. Great Britain* **55:**1–31.

48. **Mittermayer, T., R. Brezina, and J. Urvolgyi.** 1980. First report of an infection with *Rickettsia slovaca*. *Folia Parasitol.* **27:**373–376.

49. **Parola, P., D. Vogelaers, C. Roure, F. Janbon, and D. Raoult.** 1998. Murine typhus in travelers returning from Indonesia. *Emerg. Infect. Dis.* **4:**677–680.

50. **Parola, P., J. Jourdan, and D. Raoult.** 1998. Tick-borne infection caused by *Rickettsia africae* in the West Indies. *N. Engl. J. Med.* **338:**1391.

51. **Parola, P., G. Vestris, D. Martinez, B. Brochier, V. Roux, and D. Raoult.** Tick-borne rickettsiosis in Guadeloupe, the French West Indies: isolation of *Rickettsia africae* from *Amblyomma variegatum* ticks and serosurvey in humans, cattle and goats. *Am. J. Trop. Med. Hyg*, in press.

52. **Patterson, K. D.** 1993. Typhus and its control in Russia, 1870–1940. *Med. Hist.* **37:**361–381.

53. **Perine, P. L., B. P. Chandler, D. K. Krause, P. McCardle, S. Awoke, E. Habte-Gabr, C. L. Wisseman, Jr., and J. E. McDade.** 1992. A clinico-epidemiological study of epidemic typhus in Africa. *Clin. Infect. Dis.* **14:**1149–1158.

54. **Petrovec, M., J. W. Sumner, W. L. Nicholson, J. E. Childs, F. Strle, J. Barlič, S. Lotrič-Furlan, and T. Avšič Zupanc.** 1999. Identity of ehrlichial DNA sequences derived from *Ixodes ricinus* ticks with those obtained from patients with human granulocytic ehrlichiosis in Slovenia. *J. Clin. Microbiol.* **37:**209–210.

55. **Pijper, A.** 1936. Etude expérimentale comparée de la fièvre boutonneuse et de la tick-bite-fever. *Arch. Inst. Pasteur Tunis* **25:**388–401.

56. **Pusterla, N., R. Weber, C. Wolfensberger, G. Schar, R. Zbinden, W. Fierz, J. Madigan, J. Dumler, and H. Lutz.** 1998. Serologic evidence of human granulocytic ehrlichiosis in Switzerland. *Eur. J. Clin. Microbiol. Infect. Dis.* **17:**207–209.

57. **Raoult, D., P. Berbis, V. Roux, W. Xu, and M. Maurin.** 1997. A new tick-transmitted disease due to *Rickettsia slovaca*. *Lancet* **350:**112–113.

58. **Raoult, D., P. Brouqui, and V. Roux.** 1996. A new spotted-fever group rickettsiosis. *Lancet* **348:**412.

59. **Raoult, D., J. B. Ndihokubwayo, H. Tissot-Dupont, V. Roux, B. Faugere, R. Abegbinni, and R. J. Birtles.** 1998. Outbreak of epidemic typhus associated with trench fever in Burundi. *Lancet* **352:**353–358.

60. **Raoult, D., and V. Roux.** 1997. Rickettsioses as paradigms of new or emerging infectious diseases. *Clin. Microbiol. Rev.* **10:**694–719.

61. **Raoult, D., V. Roux, J. B. Ndihokubwaho, G. Bise, D. Baudon, G. Martet, and R. J. Birtles.** 1997. Jail fever (epidemic typhus) outbreak in Burundi. *Emerg. Infect. Dis.* **3:**357–360.

61a. Regnery, R. L., B. E. Anderson, J. E. Clarridge III, M. C. Rodriguez-Barradas, D. C. Jones, and J. H. Carr. 1992. Characterization of a novel *Rochalimaea* species, *R. henselae* sp. nov., isolated from blood of a febrile, human immunodeficiency virus-positive patient. *J. Clin. Microbiol.* **30:**265–274.

62. Rehacek, J. 1984. Rickettsia slovaca, the organism and its ecology. *Acta Sci. Nat. Acad. Sci. Bohem. Brno* **18:**1–50.

63. Reilly, P. J., and R. W. Kalinske. 1980. Brill-Zinsser disease in North America. *West. J. Med.* **133:**338–340.

64. Ricketts, H. T. 1991. Some aspects of Rocky Mountain spotted fever as shown by recent investigations. *Rev. Infect. Dis.* **13:**1227–1240.

65. Rolain, J. M., M. Maurin, G. Vestris, and D. Raoult. 1998. In vitro susceptibilities of 27 rickettsiae to 13 antimicrobials. *Antimicrob. Agents Chemother.* **42:**1537–1541.

66. Roux, V., and D. Raoult. 1993. Genotypic identification and phylogenetic analysis of the spotted fever group rickettsiae by pulsed-field gel electrophoresis. *J. Bacteriol.* **175:**4895–4904.

67. Roux, V., and D. Raoult. 1995. Phylogenetic analysis of the genus *Rickettsia* by 16S rDNA sequencing. *Res. Microbiol.* **146:**385–396.

68. Roux, V., E. Rydkina, M. Eremeeva, and D. Raoult. 1997. Citrate synthase gene comparison, a new tool for phylogenetic analysis, and its application for the rickettsiae. *Int. J. Syst. Bacteriol.* **47:**252–261.

69. Rydkina, E. B., V. Roux, E. M. Gagua, A. B. Predtechenski, I. V. Tarasevich, and D. Raoult. 1999. *Bartonella quintana* in body lice collected from homeless persons in Russia. *Emerg. Infect. Dis.* **5:**176–178.

69a. Sanz, R. A. Personal communication.

70. Schriefer, M. E., J. B. J. Sacci, J. S. Dumler, M. G. Bullen, and A. F. Azad. 1994. Identification of a novel rickettsial infection in a patient diagnosed with murine typhus. *J. Clin. Microbiol.* **32:**949–954.

71. Sekeyova, Z., V. Roux, W. Xu, J. Rehacek, and D. Raoult. 1998. *Rickettsia slovaca* sp. nov., a member of the spotted fever group rickettsiae. *Int. J. Syst. Bacteriol.* **48:**1455–1462.

72. Sparrow, H. 1955. Les spirochètes des fièvres récurrentes et le pou (de l'origine des épidémies de récurrente à poux). *Arch. Inst. Pasteur Tunis* **32:**25–49.

73. Stein, A., and D. Raoult. 1995. Return of trench fever. *Lancet* **345:**450–451.

74. Tarasevich, I., E. Rydkina, and D. Raoult. 1998. Epidemic typhus in Russia. *Lancet* **352:**1151.

75. Tarasevich, I. V., V. Makarova, N. F. Fetisova, A. Stepanov, E. Mistkarova, N. M. Balayeva, and D. Raoult. 1991. Astrakhan fever: new spotted fever group rickettsiosis. *Lancet* **337:**172–173.

76. Tarasevich, I. V., V. A. Makarova, N. F. Fetisova, A. V. Stepanov, E. D. Miskarova, and D. Raoult. 1991. Studies of a "new" rickettsiosis "Astrakhan" spotted fever. *Eur. J. Epidemiol.* **7:**294–298.

77. Telford, S. R. I., J. E. Dawson, P. Katavalos, C. K. Warner, C. P. Kolbert, and D. H. Persing. 1996. Perpetuation of the agent of human granulocytic ehrlichiosis in a deer tick-rodent cycle. *Proc. Natl. Acad. Sci. USA* **93:**6209–6214.

78. Tesfayohannes, T. 1989. Prevalence of body lice in elementary school students in three Ethiopian towns at different altitudes. *Ethiop. Med. J.* **27:**201–207.

79. Tissot-Dupont, H., P. Brouqui, B. Faugere, and D. Raoult. 1995. Prevalence of antibodies to *Coxiella burnetii*, *Rickettsia conorii*, and *Rickettsia typhi* in seven African countries. *Clin. Infect. Dis.* **21:**1126–1133.

80. Tselentis, Y., E. Edlinger, G. Alexious, D. Chrysantis, and A. Levendis. 1986. An endemic focus of murine typhus in Europe. *J. Infect.* **13:**91–92. (letter.)

81. Uchida, T. 1993. *Rickettsia japonica*, the etiologic agent of Oriental spotted fever. *Microbiol. Immunol.* **37:**91–102.

82. Uchida, T., F. Tashiro, T. Funato, and Y. Kitamura. 1986. Immunofluorescence test with *Rickettsia montana* for serologic diagnosis of rickettsial infection of the spotted fever group in Shikoku, Japan. *Microbiol. Immunol.* **30:**1061–1066.

83. Uchida, T., F. Tashiro, T. Funato, and Y. Kitamura. 1986. Isolation of a spotted fever group rickettsia from a patient with febrile exanthematous illness in Shikoku, Japan. *Microbiol. Immunol.* **30:**1323–1326.

84. **Van Der Laan, J. R., and R. B. Smit.** 1996. Back again: the clothes louse (*Pediculus humanus var. corporis*). *Ned. Tijdschr. Geneeskd.* **140:**1912–1915.
85. **Walker, D. H., and D. B. Fishbein.** 1991. Epidemiology of rickettsial diseases. *Eur. J. Epidemiol.* **7:**237–245.
86. **Weiss, E.** 1988. History of rickettsiology, p. 15–32. *In* D. H. Walker (ed.), *Biology of Rickettsial Disease.* CRC Press, Inc., Boca Raton, Fla.
87. **Weiss, K.** 1988. The role of rickettsiose in history, p. 1–14. *In* D. H. Walker (ed.), *Biology of Rickettsial Disease.* CRC Press, Inc., Boca Raton, Fla.
88. **World Health Organization.** 1982. Rickettsioses: a continuing disease problem. *Weekly Epidemiol. Rec.* **60:**157–164.
89. **Yu, X., M. Fan, G. Xu, Q. Liu, and D. Raoult.** 1993. Genotypic and antigenic identification of two new strains of spotted fever group rickettsiae isolated from China. *J. Clin. Microbiol.* **31:**83–88.
90. **Zavala-Velazquez, J., J. Ruiz-Soja, B. Jimenez, I. Vado-Solis, J. Zavala-Castro, and D. Walker.** *Rickettsia felis*: the etiologic agent of a case of rickettsiosis in the Yucatan. *In American Society for Tropical Medicine and Hygiene Annual Conference 1998*, in press.
91. **Zavala-Velazquez, J. E., X. J. Yu, and D. H. Walker.** 1996. Unrecognized spotted fever group rickettsiosis masquerading as dengue fever in Mexico. *Am. J. Trop. Med. Hyg.* **55:**157–159.

Emerging Infections 3
Edited by W. M. Scheld, W. A. Craig, and J. M. Hughes
© 1999 ASM Press, Washington, D.C.

Chapter 3

Salmonella Enteritidis and *Salmonella* Typhimurium DT104: Successful Subtypes in the Modern World

Robert V. Tauxe

The nontyphoidal salmonellae are early risers among modern pathogens. A vast range of different salmonella serotypes are rare and sylvatic. They are associated with specific bird or reptile reservoirs, suggesting that they are an ancient lineage that predates the separation of birds from thecodont reptiles. However, a few serotypes have expanded into new niches in the modern world and have posed major challenges to public health. One serotype of salmonella that is adapted to the human reservoir, *Salmonella* Typhi, became an enormous problem in the United States early in the industrial era. The disease that it causes, typhoid fever, has now been controlled by modern water and sewer systems, pasteurization of milk, and shellfish sanitation programs (Fig. 1). Decades later, nontyphoidal salmonella emerged as a common cause of illness. Much of this increase is accounted for by two serotypes, *Salmonella* Enteritidis and *Salmonella* Typhimurium, which now account for nearly half of all cases of salmonellosis in the United States (Table 1) and for 82% of all cases of salmonellosis in a recent global survey (17). These two serotypes have been successful under the same conditions that nearly eliminated *Salmonella* Typhi. Investigations into their ecology and transmission are critically important to devising successful control measures. These strains are also of interest to the clinician because they are the most likely causes of salmonellosis. They also provide object lessons for the evolutionist who wishes to understand the dynamics of successful pathogens in general.

PUBLIC HEALTH SURVEILLANCE AND SUBTYPING

In the United States, the modern era of public health surveillance for salmonella began in 1962, when public health officials from states and the Center for Disease

Robert V. Tauxe • Foodborne and Diarrheal Diseases Branch, Division of Bacterial and Mycotic Diseases, National Center for Infectious Diseases, Centers for Disease Control and Prevention, Mailstop A-38, Atlanta, GA 30333.

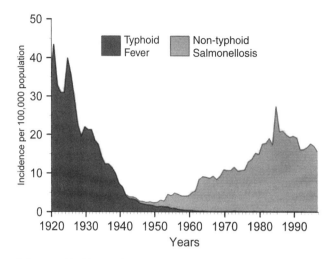

Figure 1. Reported incidence of typhoid fever and nontyphoid salmonellosis, United States, 1920 to 1997.

Control (CDC; now the Centers for Disease Control and Prevention) agreed to begin serotyping clinical isolates of salmonella and reporting the results on a national level (7). Although knowledge of the serotype of a clinical isolate rarely makes a difference in the care of the patient, it has been extremely useful as a public health tool. Tracking of serotypes greatly increases the capacity of surveillance to detect and investigate outbreaks. Serotyping can link cases and clusters

Table 1. Fifteen most common serotypes of *Salmonella* isolated from humans, United States, 1997[a]

Serotype	No. of isolates	% of total
Typhimurium	9,116	26.3
Enteritidis	7,924	22.9
Heidelberg	2,104	6.1
Newport	1,584	4.6
Agona	740	2.1
Montevideo	718	2.1
Thompson	695	2.0
Javiana	675	2.0
Infantis	651	1.9
Hadar	643	1.9
Oranienburg	623	1.8
Braenderup	559	1.6
Muenchen	543	1.6
Saintpaul	436	1.3
Typhi	349	1.0
Other	7,248	20.9
Total	34,608	100

[a]Data are from the National *Salmonella* Surveillance System (8).

that are scattered over wide areas, indicating a relationship that would otherwise be obscured by the noise of many other unrelated cases.

As for most gram-negative bacilli, serotyping depends on O and H antigens (23). The lipopolysaccharide (LPS) O antigens are 62 in number and are used to define serogroups. The H antigens are flagellar protein antigens. Salmonellae have the unusual ability to produce a second suite of flagellae if the first is coated with antibodies; the appearance of the 53 flagellar antigens as either primary or backup flagellar suites allows the serogroups to be divided into more than 2,500 described serotypes.

It is often epidemiologically useful to be able to subtype isolates within a serotype, especially for those of the common serotypes. Several methods have been used for this purpose. Phage typing is the oldest and most formalized of these. The resistance of salmonella strains to a panel of bacteriophages is a relatively stable trait that largely depends on the presence of lysogenized competing phages in the bacterial strain. Originally developed as a susceptibility test to guide the choice of lytic bacteriophages to be used for treatment of infection, it has been preserved as a useful typing system. Systems maintained by the Public Health Laboratory Service in the United Kingdom provide defined numbered types for Typhimurium and Enteritidis (1, 43).

Patterns of antimicrobial resistance to a panel of antimicrobial agents can also be useful for the monitoring of particular strains. This reflects the presence of transmissible plasmids or other mobile genetic elements in the *Salmonella* population.

Most recently, the application of pulsed-field gel electrophoresis (PFGE) has allowed the further subtyping of strains, even within single phage types (4). The CDC national subtyping network for food-borne bacteria, called PulseNet, is based on standardized PFGE and permits the rapid screening of isolates of a given serotype for an individual strain of interest.

SALMONELLA ENTERITIDIS

Salmonella Enteritidis was among the first salmonellae to be identified. It was isolated by Gaertner from the spleen of a young man who died after eating raw steak from a cow that died of septicemia (20). Gaertner's bacillus, or *Bacillus enteritidis*, as it was known in the first decades of microbiology, caused outbreaks of food-borne illness in Europe related to the consumption of undercooked duck eggs, which led to the demise of the duck egg as a popular food. In recent years, this serotype has become dramatically more common and is now the most common serotype worldwide (17, 32). In the United States, it represented 5% of all human cases of salmonellosis in the 1970s, but that proportion has increased to nearly 25% in recent years (8, 36) (Fig. 2). In 1997, 7,924 cases were reported, for a reported national incidence of 3 per 100,000 (8). This increase began in the extreme Northeast in 1979 and slowly expanded across the United States, reaching the Pacific Coast in 1993 and Hawaii in 1996 (Fig. 3).

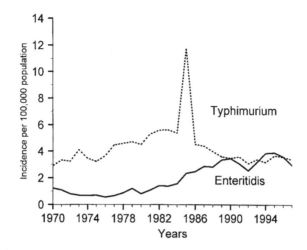

Figure 2. Reported rate of isolation of *Salmonella* Enteritidis and *Salmonella* Typhimurium, by year, United States, 1970 to 1997.

Epidemiology and Biology of Transmission

In the United States, investigations of *Salmonella* Enteritidis outbreaks and of sporadic cases of *Salmonella* Enteritidis infections have repeatedly identified the same dominant food source, the hen's egg. In a series of 660 *Salmonella* Enteritidis outbreak investigations reported from 1986 through 1996, 293 or 44% of the investigations led to the identification of a specific food vehicle. Of these foods, 233 or 79% included shell eggs as the likely source of contamination (2, 24). Similarly, three case-control studies of sporadic cases identified shell eggs as the most common exposure (16, 25, 26). Thus, the slow epidemic wave of human illness is the visible shadow of a silent epizootic wave among the nation's layer flocks. A 1991

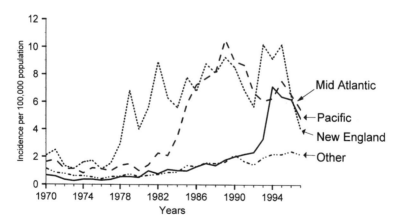

Figure 3. Reported rate of isolation of *Salmonella* Enteritidis by region, United States, 1970 to 1997.

survey of aged hens estimated that 45% of egg-laying flocks in the Northeast and 24% of egg-laying flocks in the West had infected birds, with a national flock prevalence of *Salmonella* Enteritidis infection of 22% (11). In a similar survey conducted in 1995, the prevalence had increased in most parts of the country, and the overall flock prevalence was estimated to be 45%.

This epidemic is the result of the extraordinary biology of *Salmonella* Enteritidis in the avian host. The locus of long-term infection in the hen is periovarian tissue, which provides the opportunity for the bacteria occasionally to infect the yolk membrane of an egg as it forms (5). As an evolutionary strategy, it is brilliant: the bacteria are then sealed in by the albumin and the shell and have access to the chick embryo and her ovaries as they form. As a public health problem, it is catastrophic: sealed inside the intact egg, the bacteria may penetrate the yolk membrane after several weeks and grow to high counts in the nutrient-rich yolk or in the many delicacies that humans contrive to make with raw or lightly cooked eggs. The fact that many traditional dishes of Western Europe require a sterile hen's egg is perhaps indirect evidence that this phenomenon is new to the domesticated hen. However, the strategy itself is likely to be extremely old: other salmonellae are passed transovarially in a variety of birds and reptiles, and one may speculate that the capacity to do so may have evolved long ago. If this capacity has a long evolutionary history, it is not surprising that it is complex and refined and can occur without causing major pathology to the host.

Beyond the egg, *Salmonella* Enteritidis also has a reservoir in the broiler chickens raised for meat, a different industry based on the same bird used as a source of eggs. In Europe, the emergence of *Salmonella* Enteritidis was essentially simultaneous in both egg-laying and broiler flocks, and epidemiologic investigations in Europe have documented the importance of both poultry meat and eggs as sources (12). In a recent case-control study in the United States, consumption of poultry meat was also a risk factor for *Salmonella* Enteritidis infection, suggesting that this transition may be happening in the United States as well (21). Mice may play an important role in the barnyard ecosystem, serving as the intermediate host that can pass *Salmonella* Enteritidis from one chicken flock to the next group of chicks entering the henhouse.

Subtypes of *Salmonella* Enteritidis

Within *Salmonella* Enteritidis, phage typing defines a handful of dominant subtypes, each of which tends to be remarkably homogeneous (31). These different phage types have some geographic specificity. The strains that caused the European epidemic were initially phage type 8, but these were largely replaced by phage type 4 strains; phage type 1 strains were most frequently encountered in Eastern Europe before the fall of the Berlin Wall in 1989 and have appeared in Western Europe since then. In the United States, the northeastern focus was polyclonal from the beginning, being caused by phage type 8, 13a, and 14b strains. Of these, only phage type 8 strains migrated to the Midwest. The strains of *Salmonella* Enteritidis that suddenly appeared in California were phage type 4 strains indistinguishable from those present in Latin America or Western Europe. Despite this geographic variability, the various phage types appear to have similar epidemiologic and clinical characteristics (Table 2). The noteworthy difference in the epidemiology of *Salmonella* Enteritidis between Europe and the United States is the appearance of *Salmonella* Enteritidis in broiler flocks in Europe. Whether this is due to the capacity of phage type 4 itself or to some differences in environmental conditions remains to be determined.

The success of *Salmonella* Enteritidis in association with a specific tissue tropism in one species of bird remains unexplained. One likely possibility is that these strains have acquired a specific virulence factor that makes transovarian transmission likely. If such a factor exists, it is likely to be genetically mobile, because it appeared in several different subtypes of *Salmonella* Enteritidis at once. However, the nature of such a factor remains elusive. One interesting line of evidence comes from examination of strains that vary in their ability to colonize the ovary of an intact hen after oral feeding (28). This research suggests that the structure of the O polysaccharide that is expressed may help determine the virulence. Curiously, the LPS chains that the most virulent strains have resemble in structure as well as in antigenicity the O chains of *Salmonella* Typhi, which, like *Salmonella* Enteritidis, is also a serogroup D *Salmonella* and thus has the same LPS antigens as *Salmonella* Enteritidis.

A second interesting set of observations is that *Salmonella* Enteritidis strains that are most invasive in hens and mice also share the ability to adapt rapidly to a variety of environmental stresses, including heat, acidity, drying, and exposure to hydrogen peroxide (18, 19). This suggests that these invasive strains have a suite of characteristics that would help bacteria survive environmental passage outside the hen host; unfortunately, it also describes organisms that thrive in hollandaise sauce heated gently over a spirit warmer.

A third possibility is that a breed of egg-laying hen that fortuitously was more susceptible to ovarian infection became commercially popular.

It is noteworthy that, in general, *Salmonella* Enteritidis remains susceptible to a variety of antimicrobial agents. There are several possible explanations for this. The egg-laying hen is rarely treated with antimicrobial agents because the drugs would appear in the eggs, so this animal reservoir is not likely to impose much selective pressure favoring emergence of resistance. Location in deep tissue, away from the teeming gut flora, may decrease the opportunity for gene exchange. One

Table 2. Comparison of clinical and epidemiologic characteristics among outbreaks caused by different phage types of *Salmonella* Enteritidis, United States, 1985 to 1997

Phage type	No. of outbreaks	Mean no. of cases/outbreak	% Patients hospitalized	Fatality rate (%)	% Oubreaks with egg vehicle	% Outbreaks in California
8	183	38	9	0.3	90	1
13a	86	26	12	0.2	84	7
4	32	40	10	0.1	90	84
14b	9	30	4	0	80	0

might also speculate that *Salmonella* Enteritidis strains are less capable of absorbing and integrating resistance genes than are other strains of salmonellae.

Control and Prevention

The substantial body of knowledge about the ecology of *Salmonella* Enteritidis is now being translated into practical control measures all along the way from the laying hen to the poised spoon. Extensive testing has eliminated *Salmonella* Enteritidis from the breeder flocks that provide young chicks to the egg industry. The feedstuffs have been extensively evaluated, and although they are frequently contaminated with other serotypes, *Salmonella* Enteritidis contamination is extremely rare. A growing industry-supported program of on-farm hygiene that includes rodent control as well as cleaning and disinfection between one flock and the next may be having an impact. These measures were first developed and implemented in Pennsylvania, the chief egg supplier to the mid-Atlantic region (34). The decrease in the rate of isolation of *Salmonella* Enteritidis seen in that region began shortly after the launch of the Pennsylvania Egg Quality Assurance Program in 1991 (Fig. 3). Bulk liquid eggs can be pasteurized, like milk. The growing use of pasteurized egg product in the kitchens of institutions with high-risk individuals such as nursing homes and hospitals as well as in many restaurants is a simple way to prevent needless outbreaks and deaths. Thanks to new education efforts and new regulations, eggs are now more likely to be refrigerated from farm to kitchen and are less likely to be eaten raw. Further improvement may be possible by use of live bacterial competitive exclusion products to treat newly hatched chicks (10). A technology that pasteurizes eggs in the shell has been developed, and if it can be made commercially viable, it may offer the means of virtually eliminating this infection in the United States.

The emergence of *Salmonella* Enteritidis provides several lessons. The pandemic is identifiable only in those countries that conduct routine serotyping as part of public health surveillance. Because specific control measures are available and appear to be having some impact, the cost of not doing serotyping in terms of illness and lives lost is likely to far outweigh the cost of public health surveillance and serotyping. As control measures in the United States become more widely adopted, and particularly if a definitive in-shell pasteurization step is commercialized, *Salmonella* Enteritidis infection will principally become a disease of travelers to other countries. Concern about the impact that this disease could have on tourism could spur developing countries to begin serotype-specific surveillance and prevention activities for salmonellae.

SALMONELLA TYPHIMURIUM AND DEFINED TYPE 104

Salmonella Typhimurium was also among the first salmonellae to be described, following a devastating outbreak among mice at a research animal facility (22). *Salmonella* Typhimurium has been among the most common of serotypes everywhere ever since serotyping began. This serotype tends to be highly polyclonal, and in those few locations where subtyping beyond the level of serotype has been routine, successive waves of subtypes have been observed. In the United States, the first tool systematically used for the subtyping of *Salmonella* Typhimurium was the antibiogram, starting in 1980 with surveys conducted every 5 years and, since 1996, conducted continuously as part of routine national surveillance. In those surveys, a formerly rare antibiotic resistance profile was noted to emerge between the 1990 and 1995 surveys (14). This was resistance to five antimicrobial agents: ampicillin, chloramphenicol, streptomycin, sulfamethoxazole, and tetracycline (ACSSuT).

The rate of occurrence of this resistance profile among all *Salmonella* Typhimurium isolates jumped from 7% in 1990 to 19% in 1995 and has continued to increase since then (Fig. 4). In 1997, this profile was present in 35.3% of *Salmonella* Typhimurium strains isolated from humans (8a). Because *Salmonella* Typhimurium itself represented 26.3% of isolates from humans, this subtype accounted for 9% of all cases of human salmonellosis reported in the country that year.

In the United Kingdom, routine phage typing conducted since 1960 identified a similar phenomenon (41). A dramatic surge in a previously uncommon phage type, defined type 104 (DT104), was observed in the early 1990s at the same time that strains became resistant to ACSSuT. Expansion of phage typing efforts at CDC and exchange of isolates rapidly revealed that the same strains were rapidly emerging in both countries. Similar explosive increases in pentadrug-resistant DT104 are also occurring in other countries in Europe and North America.

One remarkable feature of this expansion is that it did not lead to a proportionate increase in the total number of *Salmonella* Typhimurium isolates reported. The overall rate of isolation of *Salmonella* Typhimurium in the United States in 1990 was 3.5 per 100,000, and in 1997 it was 3.4 per 100,000 (Fig. 2). It is as though

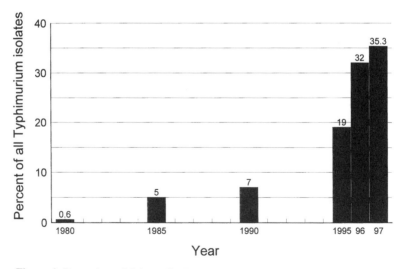

Figure 4. Proportion of *Salmonella* Typhimurium isolates that have the ACSSuT resistance pattern, United States, 1980 to 1997.

the expansion of DT104 has come at the expense of the rate of occurrence of other strains.

A second remarkable epidemiologic feature of this expansion has been the paucity of common-source outbreaks, even as the incidence of sporadic cases of DT104 infection increases. As of the beginning of 1999, only five such outbreaks had been identified in the United States since 1994 (Table 3), despite enhanced surveillance and a concerted effort to phage type strains isolated in any *Salmonella* Typhimurium outbreak. In contrast, at least 245 outbreaks have been reported to be caused by *Salmonella* Enteritidis in the same 5-year time span. Like *Salmonella* Enteritidis, DT104 has a clearly defined animal reservoir (see below), but unlike *Salmonella* Enteritidis, the typical food vehicles that transmit it to humans have yet to be clearly defined. This lack of outbreaks is not explained but suggests that the sources of these infections must have only low-level contamination to begin with. If there is a food vehicle for DT104, it must not be handled in such a way as to permit the rapid bacterial multiplication that leads to a local outbreak. The stealthy nature of this epidemic means that without routine use of methods for the subtyping of strains within a serotype, the presence of this strain may escape notice by public health authorities. As a result, the global extent of the DT104 epidemic is unclear.

A third important epidemiologic feature is that the pentadrug-resistant DT104 phenomenon is not monoclonal. Outbreaks in the United States have been caused by DT104 *Salmonella* Typhimurium strains both with and without the Copenhagen variant antigen (9). A survey of *Salmonella* Typhimurium strains collected in the United States in 1996 and 1997 found that the pentadrug-resistant strains actually represent a cluster of strains with related phage resistance patterns, including DT104, DT104a, DT104b, and U302, a pattern that has not been formally named (Table 4). A similar diversity in PFGE types exists within this group of strains, suggesting that they are related but not identical (8a). Thus, the epidemic is more accurately described as being due to a cluster of related strains. Isolated strains of a few other serotypes also exhibit the same pentadrug resistance pattern, the genetics of which remain to be characterized. Among DT104 strains about 2% remain

Table 3. Outbreaks of *Salmonella* Typhimurium DT104 infections in the United States, 1996 to 1997

Outbreak no.	State	Date	Vehicle of transmission	Reference
1	Nebraska	1996	Not identified	3
2	Washington	1997	Mexican-style soft cheese made from raw milk	40
3	California	1997	Mexican-style soft cheese made from raw milk	9
4	California	1997	Mexican-style soft cheese made from raw milk	9
5	Vermont	1997	Contact with ill animals, consumption of raw milk	13

Table 4. Distribution of ACSSuT resistance by phage type among 504 *Salmonella* Typhimurium strains collected in the United States in 1996 and 1997

Phage type	No. tested	% with ACSSuT resistance
DT104	100	83
DT104b	33	100
10	16	0
U302	16	56
120	12	67
DT104a	11	82
18 other types	36	0
Nontypeable	280	4

pansusceptible, and the majority are pentadrug resistant, suggesting that pentadrug resistance was acquired in a single step (8a).

Genetics of Resistance

The genetic structure of the resistance genes of DT104 is beginning to be mapped (30, 33). All five genes are chromosomally located. Two adjacent type 1 integrons carry the genes for ampicillin resistance and for streptomycin and sulfadiazine resistance. The chloramphenicol and tetracycline resistance genes appear to be near the integrons, forming a genetic "island" of resistance. The size of this island is not larger than 40 kb. This was recently demonstrated by a phage transfer experiment in which an exogenous phage capable of carrying no more than 40 kb was used to transfer the entire pentadrug resistance to susceptible strains (35). The same researchers also demonstrated that DT104 strains harbor a prophage which can transduce the entire portion of the genome encoding pentadrug resistance to nonresistant DT104 recipient strains. These observations suggest that the DT104 pandemic may actually represent the emergence and epidemic spread of a phage-mediated resistance island among specific strains of *Salmonella* Typhimurium susceptible to that phage. If so, understanding of the dynamics of release, environmental survival, resistance to, and uptake of the phage may be critical to future efforts to control the epidemic.

The DT104 complex of strains has continued to acquire further resistance beyond the resistance to the five drugs mentioned above in both the United States and the United Kingdom. For example, in the United States in 1996, and in 1997, 21% of DT104 strains exhibited resistance to more than five antimicrobial agents. The most impressive pattern was ACSSuT resistance plus resistance to clavulanic acid, cephalothin, and ceftiofur (a broad-spectrum veterinary cephalosporin that resembles ceftriaxone) (8a). In the United Kingdom, the appearance of an intermediate level of fluoroquinolone resistance (MIC ≥ 0.25 μg of ciprofloxacin per ml) has been of particular concern. This resistance was first identified in 1992 and by 1996 was detected in 14% of DT104 strains isolated from humans (37). In that year, trimethoprim resistance was documented in 24% of the DT104 strains, and 1% of the strains were resistant to both trimethoprim and ciprofloxacin. This resistance is independent of the presence of the genetic island, although it is chromosomal for ciprofloxacin resistance and plasmid borne for trimethoprim resistance (37). The appearance of fluoroquinolone resistance followed the 1992 licensure and subsequent widespread use of the fluoroquinolone enrofloxacin in cattle and poultry in the United Kingdom (37). No similar strains have been identified in the United States, although the approval of sarafloxacin for use in poultry in 1997 and cattle in 1998 is noteworthy.

Animal Reservoir and Transmission to Humans

Coincident with the emergence of DT104 among humans, DT104 has appeared as a cause of epizootic gastroenteritis and fatal bacteremia among the nation's dairy herds. In sharp contrast to *Salmonella* Enteritidis, which spreads silently through the animal reservoir, DT104 is causing serious outbreaks and losses in affected herds (6, 41). Although the mechanisms of spread among cattle remain largely undocumented, important factors may include the common though clearly hazardous practice of feeding raw milk from sick dairy animals to young calves, the treatment of healthy animals with antimicrobial agents in a prophylactic mode, and the practice of housing ill animals with those that are giving birth. In the United Kingdom, DT104 first emerged among bovines and then spread rapidly to affect pigs, poultry, and household pets (41, 42). In the United States, it remains restricted largely to bovines.

The precise vehicles of transmission to humans remain undefined, although they are likely to be related to the bovine epizootic. Of the five outbreaks identified in the United States, four had sources that were determined to be clearly related to the bovine reservoir (Table 3). The first outbreak occurred among a group of schoolchildren in a rural area in a setting with multiple possible although unconfirmed sources (3). The next three outbreaks were all traced to consumption of fresh Mexican-style soft cheese made from unpasteurized milk (9, 40). The most recent outbreak occurred among dairy farmworkers who were both exposed to ill animals and drank milk raw from that herd (13). Outbreaks in the United Kingdom have been traced to a broad range of prepared foods, suggesting that in-kitchen cross contamination may be an important factor (42). A case-control study in the United Kingdom identified several independent risk factors, including consumption of pork sausages or chicken from a restaurant, chicken from a local butcher, or a specific brand of meat paste, as well as contact with ill animals (27). In the United States, a small case-control study conducted in 1996 and 1997 did not identify a particular food vehicle, which might indicate that the contamination is low level, that it is of multiple foods, or that cross contamination is common (15). This investigation also showed that 34% of patients but only 13% of controls reported taking in the 4 weeks before the onset of illness an antimicrobial agent to which the strain is resistant. This strongly suggests that in many patients intercurrent antibiotic treatment changed a silent and transient carriage into overt and often serious illness. This may mean that most exposures are to extremely low doses and affect individuals at below the threshold of clinical illness unless the balance of the gut flora is altered by antimicrobial treatment. It also means that multidrug-resistant DT104 should be considered in the differential along with *Clostridium difficile* when a patient suddenly develops severe diarrhea in the setting of antibiotic treatment.

Clinical Manifestations

The clinical features of DT104 infections are similar to those of nontyphoid salmonellosis in general. Most patients develop acute gastroenteritis, often with fever; some go on to develop bacteremia and life-threatening illness. As noted above, almost half of the patients have recently taken antibiotics for some other reason. Several preliminary observations suggest that DT104 may be more virulent than other strains of salmonella. In the United States, the proportion of reported isolates which come from blood compared to the total number of reported isolates is 7.8% for DT104, whereas it is only 2.8% for other *Salmonella* Typhimurium isolates and 4% for salmonellae in general (8a). This does not seem to be the case in the United Kingdom, where bacteremia caused by DT104 is no more common than bacteremia caused by other *Salmonella* Typhimurium strains (38). In the United Kingdom, it has been observed that the proportion of patients who die is higher for those infected with DT104 than for those infected with other *Salmonella* Typhimurium strains (27). This does not appear to be the case in the United States, where there is no apparent increase in the rate of mortality related to DT104 (8a). Whether this phenomenon might be related to the emergence of intermediate fluoroquinolone resistance in the United Kingdom is a matter for further investigation.

Other Pentadrug-Resistant *Salmonella* Typhimurium Strains

The DT104 cluster is not the only highly resistant cluster of *Salmonella* Typhimurium strains in circulation. CDC recently identified a distinct pentadrug-resistant *Salmonella* Typhimurium strain which has many epidemiologic similarities to DT104 but which is resistant to ampicillin, kanamycin, streptomycin, sulfamethoxazole, and tetracycline (in which kanamycin resistance takes the place of chloramphenicol resistance in the group of drugs [ACSSuT] to which DT104 is resistant) (8a). Some of these strains are also resistant to broad-spectrum cephalosporins and specifically to ceftriaxone. These strains all exhibit a single phage resistance pattern which does not conform to described patterns and which does not appear to exist among strains in the United Kingdom. In 1998, a cluster of human illness caused by this strain was observed in Ohio. An epidemiologic investigation documented that similar strains were causing illness in cattle and horses and that human illness was typically associated with contact with ill animals as well as the preceding use of antibiotics. The genetic structure of resistance in this strain remains undefined. The ceftriaxone resistance is noteworthy and may be related to the use of the related agent ceftiofur among cattle and other large animals.

Investigators in Italy recently described a dramatically resistant cluster of *Salmonella* Typhimurium strains isolated from children in Tirana, Albania (39). These strains are nontypeable by phage typing; that is, they are resistant to lysis by the standard set of typing phages. They are also remarkably resistant to antimicrobial agents. All of these strains possess resistance to ampicillin, chloramphenicol, kanamycin, streptomycin, sulfamethoxazole, tetracycline, and trimethoprim, and in addition, some strains were resistant to gentamicin and nalidixic acid. Many of these resistance genes reside in three separate class 1 integrons, which are carried by conjugative plasmids. This may represent the assembly of a new genetic island in plasmids that can easily collect integrons in a state before they become fixed in the chromosome. The circumstances under which these strains evolved are unclear.

The emergence of DT104 is most likely to be the result of an epidemic of a phage-borne island of resistance genes in strains circulating among animal herds and people. The spread of this multidrug-resistant cluster of strains is a growing challenge to both human and animal health on at least two continents. The sources of the resistance genes and of the island itself are unknown and may lie outside salmonellae. The possibility that virulence genes may have accumulated in this genetic hot spot merits further research. Equipped with these genes, DT104 thrives in environments where antibiotics are used and now complicates the routine use of antibiotics for any purpose in human and animal medicine. The progressive acquisition of further resistance in the United Kingdom, propelled by efforts to treat the infection in animals, highlights the need for prudence in antibiotic use in the animal sector. The link between overt human infection and the use of antibiotics for other reasons is analogous to the problem of *C. difficile* and highlights the need to reduce unnecessary antimicrobial use of any sort in humans as well.

CONCLUSIONS

One may wonder whether, if the particular characteristics that make these pathogens successful are mobile, they might someday recombine in the same organism. If they did, would a larger epidemic ensue? Already, strains of *Salmonella* Enteritidis that have the ACSSuT pentadrug resistance pattern in association with integrons have been described (29). The reverse has also been demonstrated, because strains of DT104 have recently been shown to have the capacity to infect intact hens' egg following oral ingestion (44). The potential for further emergence may just depend now on the introduction of the right strain into the right reservoir and the impact of ongoing selective pressures.

Prevention of *Salmonella* Enteritidis and DT104 infections in humans depends on interruption of their flow from farm reservoirs to human foods. In the case of *Salmonella* Enteritidis, more than a decade of intensive investigation has led to a multistage control strategy. Improvements in layer-flock management, better egg handling during transport, storage, and cooking, and the growing use of pasteurized eggs are bringing the epidemic under control. The challenge of egg-associated salmonellae may ultimately be prevented by routine in-shell pasteurization. Far less information is available for DT104, so that it remains unclear which specific food vehicle could be targeted. Reduction of cross contamination in institutional and home kitchens may help. The few outbreaks that have occurred demonstrate that prevention education focused on the risk of ingestion of raw milk and cheeses made from raw milk may at least prevent future outbreaks.

The public health challenge by both pathogens described in this chapter illustrates the intimate connection between the microbial ecology of food animals and the health of the consuming public. Meeting this challenge offers broad scope for basic and applied research that may prove to be generally useful in the effort to control and prevent emerging food-borne infections around the world. Useful animal models, using the egg and the mouse, can be utilized to investigate invasion, resistance, phage-mediated gene transfer, and the potential for rapid bacterial adaptation. The pandemic emergence of these two successful subtypes of salmonellae illustrate how they thrive in the food animal reservoirs and infect the public. One uses a tissue tropism to exploit a clever ecologic niche and to insert itself into a food that was previously thought to be pathogen free, the hen's egg. The second has adapted to modern antibiotic-intensive agriculture by becoming highly resistant to the agents commonly used in agriculture. One is dramatic: pandemic *Salmonella* Enteritidis heralds its presence with large common-source outbreaks that are related to eggs. DT104 appears more stealthily, and without advanced surveillance tools it may not even be suspected. Detection and investigation of these emergent food-borne diseases depend on a public health infrastructure that includes both serotyping and further subtyping as part of routine surveillance. The ultimate origins of these strains and of the mobile elements that may be the source of their pandemic potential are unknown. Global surveillance for *Salmonella*, including serotyping and standardized subtyping, would be an important advance in defining the extent of these pandemics, directing control measures against them, and providing earlier warning of the next pandemic wave.

REFERENCES

1. **Anderson, E. S., L. R. Ward, M. J. de Saxe, and J. D. H. de Sa.** 1977. Bacteriophage-typing designations of *Salmonella typhimurium. J. Hyg. Camb.* **78:**297–300.
2. **Angulo, F. J., and D. L. Swerdlow.** 1999. Epidemiology of human *Salmonella enterica* serovar Enteritidis infections in the United States, p. 33–41. *In* A. M. Saeed, R. K. Gast, M. E. Potter, and P. G. Wall (ed.), Salmonella enterica *Serovar Enteritidis in Humans and Animals: Epidemiology, Pathogenesis, and Control.* Iowa State University Press, Ames.
3. **Anonymous.** 1997. Multi-drug resistant *Salmonella* serotype Typhimurium—United States, 1996. *Morbid. Mortal. Weekly Rep.* **46:**308–310.
4. **Barrett, T. J.** 1997. Molecular fingerprinting of foodborne pathogenic bacteria: an introduction to methods, uses and problems, p. 249–263. *In* S. M. Gendel (ed.), *Food Microbiological Analyses: New Technologies.* Marcel Dekker, Inc., New York, N.Y.
5. **Benson, C. E., and L. H. Keller.** 1999. Characterization of chicken ovarian infection with *Salmonella enterica* serovar Enteritidis, p. 213–219. *In* A. M. Saeed, R. K. Gast, M. E. Potter, and P. G. Wall (ed.), Salmonella enterica *Serovar Enteritidis in Humans and Animals: Epidemiology, Pathogenesis, and Control.* Iowa State University Press, Ames.
6. **Besser, T. E., C. G. Gay, J. M. Gay, D. D. Hancock, D. Rice, L. C. Pritchett, et al.** 1997. Salmonellosis associated with *S. typhimurium* DT104 in the USA. *Vet. Rec.* **140:**75.
7. **Brachman, P. S., and M. S. Goldsby.** 1965. Salmonella surveillance program in the United States. *In Proceedings of the National Conference on Salmonellosis*, Public Health Service Publication 1262. U.S. Government Printing Office, Washington, D.C.
8. **Centers for Disease Control and Prevention.** 1999. *1997 Salmonella Surveillance—Annual Tabulation.* Centers for Disease Control and Prevention, Atlanta, Ga.
8a. **Centers for Disease Control and Prevention.** Unpublished data.
9. **Cody, S. H., S. L. Abbott, A. A. Marfin, B. Schulz, P. Wagner, K. Robbins, J. C. Mohle-Boetani, and D. Vugia.** 1999. Two outbreaks of *Salmonella* serotype Typhimurium DT104 infections linked to raw milk cheese in Northern California. *JAMA* **281:**1805–1810.
10. **Corrier, D. E., and D. J. Nisbet.** 1999. Competitive exclusion in the control of *Salmonella enterica* serovar Enteritidis infection in laying poultry, p. 391–396. *In* A. M. Saeed, R. K. Gast, M. E. Potter,

and P. G. Wall (ed.), Salmonella enterica *Serovar Enteritidis in Humans and Animals: Epidemiology, Pathogenesis, and Control.* Iowa State University Press, Ames.

11. **Ebel, E. D., A. T. Hogue, and W. D. Schlosser.** 1999. Prevalence of *Salmonella enterica* serovar Enteritidis in unpasteurized liquid eggs and aged laying hens at slaughter: implications on epidemiology and control of the disease, p. 341–351. *In* A. M. Saeed, R. K. Gast, M. E. Potter, and P. G. Wall (ed.), Salmonella enterica *Serovar Enteritidis in Humans and Animals: Epidemiology, Pathogenesis, and Control.* Iowa State University Press, Ames.

12. **Evans, S. J., R. H. Davies, and C. Wray.** 1999. Epidemiology of *Salmonella enterica* serovar Enteritidis infection in British poultry flocks, p. 313–323. *In* A. M. Saeed, R. K. Gast, M. E. Potter, and P. G. Wall (ed.), Salmonella enterica *Serovar Enteritidis in Humans and Animals: Epidemiology, Pathogenesis, and Control.* Iowa State University Press, Ames.

13. **Friedman, C. R., R. C. Brady, M. J. Celotti, S. E. Schoenfeld, R. H. Johnson, P. D. Galbraith, J. K. Carney, K. Robbins, and L. Slutsker.** 1998. An outbreak of multidrug-resistant *Salmonella* serotype Typhimurium Definitive Type 104 (DT104) infection in humans and cattle in Vermont, Abstr. p. 68. *In Program and Abstracts of the International Conference on Emerging Infectious Diseases,* Centers for Disease Control and Prevention, Atlanta, Ga.

14. **Glynn, M. K., C. Bopp, W. Dewitt, P. Dabney, M. Mokhtar, and F. J. Angulo.** 1998. Emergence of multi-drug resistant *Salmonella enterica* serotype Typhimurium infections in the United States. *N. Engl. J. Med.* **338:**1333–1338.

15. **Glynn, M. K., S. Reddy, T. Fiorentino, B. Shiferaw, D. Vugia, M. Bardsley, J. Bender, F. Angulo, and the FoodNet Working Group.** 1998. Antimicrobial agent use increases infections with resistant bacteria: a FoodNet case-control study of sporadic multiresistant *Salmonella* Typhimurium DT104 infections, 1996–97, abstr. 52. *In Abstracts of the 36th Annual Meeting of the Infectious Diseases Society of America.* Infectious Diseases Society of America, Alexandria, Va.

16. **Hedberg, C. W., M. J. David, K. E. White, et al.** 1993. Role of egg consumption in sporadic Salmonella enteritidis and Salmonella typhimurium infections in Minnesota. *J. Infect. Dis.* **167:**107–111.

17. **Herikstad, H., Y. Motarjemi, and R. V. Tauxe.** *Salmonella* surveillance practices: a global survey. *J. Infect. Dis,* in press.

18. **Humphrey, T. J., E. Slater, K. McAlpine, R. J. Rowbury, and R. J. Gilbert.** 1995. *Salmonella enteritidis* phage type 4 isolates more tolerant of heat, acid or hydrogen peroxide also survive longer on surfaces. *Appl. Environ. Microbiol.* **61:**3161–3164.

19. **Humphrey, T. J., A. Williams, K. McAlpine, M. S. Lever, J. Guard-Petter, and J. M. Cox.** 1996. Isolates of *Salmonella enterica* Enteritidis PT4 with enhanced heat and acid tolerance are more virulent in mice and more invasive in chickens. *Epidemiol. Infect.* **117:**79–88.

20. **Karlinski, J.** 1889. Zur Kenntnis des Bacillus enteritidis Gaertner. *Zentbl. Bakteriol. Parasitenkd. Infektionskr. Hyg. Abt. 1 Orig.* **6:**289–292.

21. **Kimura, A., S. Reddy, R. Marcus, P. Cieslak, J. Mohle-Boetani, H. Kassenborg, S. Segler, D. Swerdlow, and the FoodNet Working Group.** 1998. Chicken, a newly identified risk factor for sporadic *Salmonella* Enteritidis infections in the United States: a case-control study in FoodNet sites, abstr. 540 Fr. *In Abstracts of the 36th Infectious Diseases Society of America Annual Meeting.* Infectious Diseases Society of America, Alexandria, Va.

22. **Loeffler, F.** 1892. Ueber Epidemieen unter den im hygienischen Institute zu Greifswald gehaltenen Maeusen und ueber die Bekaempfung der Feldmausplage. *Zentbl. Bakteriol. Parasitenkd. Infektionskr. Hyg. Abt. 1 Orig.* **12:**1–17.

23. **McWhorter-Murlin, A. C., and F. W. Hickman-Brenner.** 1994. *Identification and Serotyping of Salmonella and an Update of the Kauffman-White Scheme.* Centers for Disease Control and Prevention, Atlanta, Ga.

24. **Mishu, B., J. Koehler, L. A. Lee, D. C. Rodrigue, F. H. Brenner, P. Blake, and R. V. Tauxe.** 1994. Outbreaks of Salmonella enteritidis infections in the United States, 1985–1991. *J. Infect. Dis.* **169:**547–552.

25. **Morse, D. L., G. S. Birkhead, J. Guardino, S. F. Kondracke, and J. J. Guzewich.** 1994. Outbreak and sporadic egg-associated cases of *Salmonella enteritidis*: New York experience. *Am. J. Public Health* **84:**859–860.

26. **Passaro, D. J., R. Reporter, L. Mascola, L. Kilman, G. B. Malcolm, J. Rolka, S. B. Werner, and D. J. Vugia.** 1996. Epidemic *Salmonella enteritidis* infection in Los Angeles County, California: the predominance of phage type 4. *West J. Med.* **165:**126–130.

27. **Poppe, C., N. Smart, R. Khakhria, W. Johnson, J. Spika, and J. Prescott.** 1998. *Salmonella typhimurium* DT104: a virulent and drug resistant pathogen. *Can. Vet. J.* **39:**559–565.

28. **Rahman, M. M., J. Guard-Petter, and R. W. Carlson.** 1997. A virulent isolate of *Salmonella enteritidis* produces a *Salmonella typhi*-like lipopolysaccharide. *J. Bacteriol.* **179:**2126–2131.

29. **Rankin, S. C., and M. J. Coyne.** 1998. Multiple antibiotic resistance in *Salmonella enterica* serotype enteritidis. *Lancet* **351:**1740.

30. **Ridley, A., and E. J. Threlfall.** 1998. Molecular epidemiology of antibiotic resistance genes in multiresistant epidemic *Salmonella typhimurium* DT104. *Microb. Drug Resist.* **4:**113–118.

31. **Rodrigue, D. C., D. N. Cameron, N. D. Puhr, F. W. Brenner, M. E. St. Louis, I. K. Wachsmuth, and R. V. Tauxe.** 1992. Comparison of plasmid profiles, phage types, and antimicrobial resistance patterns of *Salmonella enteritidis* isolates in the United States. *J. Clin. Microbiol.* **30:**854–857.

32. **Rodrigue, D. C., R. V. Tauxe, and B. Rowe.** 1990. International increase in Salmonella enteritidis: a new pandemic? *Epidemiol. Infect.* **105:**21–27.

33. **Sandvang, D., F. M. Aarestrup, and L. B. Jensen.** 1997. Characterisation of integrons and antibiotic resistance genes in Danish multiresistant *Salmonella enterica* Typhimurium DT104. *FEMS Microbiol. Lett.* **157:**177–181.

34. **Schlosser, W. D., D. J. Henzler, J. Mason, D. Kradel, L. Shipman, S. Trock, S. H. Hurd, A. T. Hogue, W. Sischo, and E. D. Ebel.** 1999. The *Salmonella enterica* serovar Enteritidis pilot project, p. 353–365. *In* A. M. Saeed, R. K. Gast, M. E. Potter, and P. G. Wall (ed.), *Salmonella enterica Serovar Enteritidis in Humans and Animals: Epidemiology, Pathogenesis, and Control.* Iowa State University Press, Ames.

35. **Schmeiger, H., and P. Schicklmaier.** 1999. Transduction of multiple drug resistance of *Salmonella enterica* serovar *typhimurium* DT104. *FEMS Microbiol. Lett.* **170:**251–256.

36. **St. Louis, M. E., D. L. Morse, M. E. Potter, T. M. DeMelfi, J. J. Guzewich, R. V. Tauxe, and P. A. Blake.** 1988. The emergence of grade A eggs as a major source of Salmonella enteritidis infections. New implications for the control of salmonellosis. *JAMA* **259:**2103–2107.

37. **Threlfall, E. J., L. R. Ward, and B. Rowe.** 1997. Increasing incidence of resistance to trimethoprim and ciprofloxacin in epidemic *Salmonella typhimurium* DT104 in England and Wales. *EuroSurv* **2**(11)**:**16–21.

38. **Threlfall, E. J., L. R. Ward, and B. Rowe.** 1998. Multiresistant *Salmonella typhimurium* DT104 and salmonella bacteremia. *Lancet* **352:**287–288.

39. **Tosini, F., P. Visca, I. Luzzi, A. M. Dionisi, C. Pezzella, A. Petrucca, and A. Caratolli.** 1998. Class I integron-borne multiple-antibiotic resistance carried by IncFI and IncL/M plasmids in *Salmonella enterica* serotype Typhimurium. *Antimicrob. Agents Chemother.* **42:**3053–3058.

40. **Villar, R. G., M. D. Macek, S. Simons, P. S. Hayes, M. J. Goldoft, J. H. Lewis, L. L. Rowan, D. Hursh, M. Patnode, and P. Mead.** 1999. Investigation of multidrug-resistant *Salmonella* serotype Typhimurium DT104 infections linked to raw-milk cheese in Washington State. *JAMA* **281:**1805–1810.

41. **Wall, P. G., D. Morgan, K. Lamden, M. Ryan, M. Griffin, E. J. Threlfall, L. R. Ward, and B. Rowe.** 1994. A case control study of infection with an epidemic strain of multiresistant *Salmonella typhimurium* DT104 in England and Wales. *Communic. Dis. Rep.* **4:**R130–R135.

42. **Wall, P. G., D. Ross, P. van Someren, L. R. Ward, J. Threlfall, and B. Rowe.** 1997. Features of the epidemiology of multidrug resistant *Salmonella typhimurium* DT104 in England and Wales, p. 565–567. *In* P. Colin, J. M. Le Goux, and G. Clement (ed.), *Salmonella and Salmonellosis '97—Proceedings.* Zoopole, Ploufragan, France.

43. **Ward, L. R., J. D. H. de Sa, and B. Rowe.** 1994. A phage typing scheme for *Salmonella enteritidis. Epidemiol. Infect.* **112:**25–31.

44. **Williams, A., A. C. Davies, J. Wilson, P. D. Marsh, S. Leach, and T. J. Humphrey.** 1998. Contamination of intact eggs by *Salmonella typhimurium* DT104. *Vet. Rec.* **143:**562–563.

Emerging Infections 3
Edited by W. M. Scheld, W. A. Craig, and J. M. Hughes
© 1999 ASM Press, Washington, D.C.

Chapter 4

Streptococcus iniae: an Emerging Pathogen in the Aquaculture Industry

D. E. Low, E. Liu, J. Fuller, and A. McGeer

Zoonoses are diseases transmissible from animals to humans, and more than 150 recognized zoonoses are known to exist. Prevention of human disease requires knowledge of the reservoirs of these pathogens and their epidemiologies. Zoonotic diseases are typically endemic and occur in natural foci. However, ecologic changes and climatic events can promote expansion of the host and geographic ranges of epidemics. For practical reasons, surveillance of zoonotic agents too often relies on the identification of disease caused by those agents in humans. Surveillance of zoonotic agents in natural hosts may be difficult because of the ecologic complexities of zoonoses (5).

In the past few years, the recognition of new infectious diseases has increased globally. The majority of these have involved zoonotic infectious agents; that is, they have involved the transmission of the etiologic agent to humans from a reservoir in animals or arthropods without the establishment of a life cycle in humans. In only a few cases, a new life cycle in humans that no longer requires an animal reservoir has been established (21).

The emergence or reemergence of zoonotic pathogens is unpredictable. A pathogen may become epidemic for a limited time as the result of a temporary ecologic or climatic change or may become established as the cause of a new epidemic. No one could have predicted the emergence of the bovine spongiform encephalopathy prion in cattle and humans in the United Kingdom or the cluster of Sin Nombre virus infections in the Four Corners area of the United States that resulted in the identification of Sin Nombre virus as the cause of hantavirus pulmonary syndrome (21).

Factors that contribute to the emergence of zoonotic diseases include ecologic changes, such as those due to agricultural or economic development or to anomalies in climate; human demographic and behavioral changes; new technology and industry; microbial adaptation and change; and breakdown of the public health in-

D. E. Low, E. Liu, J. Fuller, and A. McGeer • Department of Microbiology, Mount Sinai Hospital, 600 University Avenue, Toronto, Ontario, Canada M5G 1X5.

frastructure (20). Human and livestock populations have continued to grow, bringing increasing numbers of people and animals into close contact; high-intensity raising of livestock has resulted in changes in types of feed and activities that may alter the ecology of animal pathogens; transportation has advanced, making it possible to circumnavigate the globe in less time than the incubation periods of most infectious agents; and human activities continue to alter global wildlife and plant populations (21).

The aquaculture industry, which is increasingly being developed, has not yet been recognized to result in significant human disease. However, during the winter of 1995 and 1996, four patients in Toronto, Ontario, Canada, were diagnosed with acute cellulitis due to *Streptococcus iniae*, a previously unreported occurrence (9, 14). Common to these patients was the handling of fresh, store-bought, aquacultured tilapia (*Oreochromis* spp.) prior to the onset of disease. This resulted in an investigation of the etiology, epidemiology, and pathogenesis of this new zoonotic disease.

BACKGROUND

Aquaculture

Aquaculture is one of the fastest-growing food-producing sectors, providing an acceptable supplement to and substitute for wild fish and plants. In 1996, total world production of finfish and shellfish reached 120 million metric tons. Cultured fish accounted for 22% of this total in 1996, whereas it accounted for 13% in 1990. The total production of cultured finfish, shellfish, and aquatic plants of 34 million metric tons in 1996 represented an increase of 11.0% over that in 1995. Much of the reported increase originated from developing countries, in particular, the People's Republic of China. Asia accounted for 91% of the world's reported tonnage. Europe was the second largest contributor, with 4.7% of world production (28).

Aquaculture is also a steadily growing sector in North America. Between 1984 and 1995, production increased by 44%, from 334,000 to 480,000 metric tons. Total production in 1995 increased by 7.1% over that in 1994. Aquaculture in North America involves diverse farming systems in diverse areas. The industry is facing challenges from environmental groups. The criticisms concern contamination of the environment by aquaculture systems through unwanted obstructions to coastal navigation, unsightly cages or pens, aquaculture effluents such as excess food and chemotherapeutics, and the use of nonnative species or native species that are either domesticated or genetically different from wild stocks (28).

Tilapia

Tilapia are members of the cichlid group of fish (Fig. 1). Cichlids are spiny-rayed freshwater fish that are found in a vast assortment of colors, forms, and habitats. They are indigenous to warm-water rivers and lakes in Africa, Madagascar, southern India, Sri Lanka, and South and Central America. Only one species, the Texas cichlid, is native to North America (33).

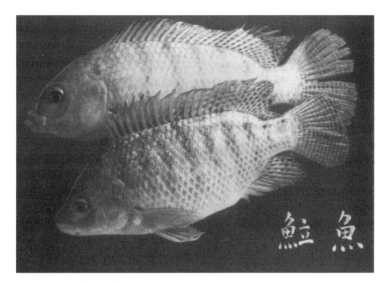

Figure 1. Tilapia (*Oreochromis* species), also known as St. Peter's fish or Hawaiian sunfish.

Tilapia are one of the major groups of food fishes around the world, especially in tropical and semitropical areas, and have been both captured and cultivated for thousands of years. Pictures or carvings appear on artifacts and monoliths in Egyptian tombs as far back as 2,000 BC. Tilapia are now farmed in at least 75 countries and are known as St. Peter's fish, Hawaiian sunfish, golden perch, cherry snapper, aquatic chicken, etc. (26). The total world landings for tilapia from capture and culture increased from 515,000 metric tons in 1984 to 1.16 million metric tons in 1995. In recent years, this increase has been fueled by an expansion of aquaculture. Between 1984 and 1995, the contribution of cultured tilapia to total tilapia production increased from 38 to 57% (29).

Global production was greatly influenced by rapid expansion of Nile and Mozambique tilapia culture in China, the Philippines, Thailand, Indonesia, and Egypt. Nile tilapia dominates global tilapia culture, with its share of total tilapia production increasing from 33% in 1984 to 72% in 1995. The People's Republic of China accounts for 48% of total global tilapia culture (28).

Aquaculture-Associated Infectious Diseases

The principal biological agents that cause food-borne disease are bacteria, viruses, and parasites (30). Parasite-related food safety concerns in aquaculture are limited to a few helminth species, and the hazards are largely focused on communities where consumption of raw or inadequately cooked fish is a cultural habit (39). The main human diseases caused by fish-borne parasites are trematodiasis, cestodiasis, and nematodiasis. Trematodes are by far the most important food safety hazard linked with fish and fishery products. The most important trematodes, so far as numbers of people affected are concerned, are species of the genera *Clon-*

orchis, *Opisthorchis*, and *Paragonimus*. There is a lack of specific and quantitative information about the extent of the hazard in farmed fish, but parasites are found in farmed fish, and there is some epidemiologic evidence of the transmission of trematode parasites from farmed fish. Humans are at a higher risk of becoming infected with bacterial or viral pathogens from molluscs than from crustaceans and finfish. The greatest numbers of seafood-associated illnesses are from the consumption of raw molluscs harvested in waters contaminated with raw or poorly treated human sewage (1, 11). Although viral diseases such as gastroenteritis and hepatitis A may be associated with the consumption of finfish and crustaceans, viruses that cause disease in fish are not pathogenic for humans.

The level of contamination of aquaculture products with pathogenic bacteria depends on the environment and the bacteriological quality of the water where the fish are cultured. Two broad groups of bacteria of public health significance may contaminate products of aquaculture: those naturally present in the environment (e.g., *Aeromonas hydrophila*, *Clostridium botulinum*, *Vibrio parahaemolyticus*, *Vibrio cholerae*, *Vibrio vulnificus*, and *Listeria monocytogenes*) and those introduced through environmental contamination with domestic animal excreta and/or human wastes (e.g., members of the family *Enterobacteriaceae*, such as *Salmonella* spp., *Shigella* spp., and *Escherichia coli*, and hepatitis A virus) (13).

It should be noted that nonindigenous bacteria of fecal origin could be introduced into aquaculture ponds via contamination by birds and wild animals associated with farm waters. Enteric organisms and viruses die off rapidly in water, but significant numbers of organisms may remain on the skin and in the guts of fish and can pose a health risk to human consumers of those fish. Adequate cooking (i.e., the thermal center of the product should reach 70°C) before consumption will eliminate the risk.

Streptococcus iniae

S. iniae was first reported in 1976 to cause subcutaneous abscesses in Amazon freshwater dolphins (*Inia geoffrensis*) at aquariums in San Francisco and New York (24, 25). Identifiable (25, 32) characteristics of *S. iniae* are a beta-hemolytic reaction on Trypticase soy agar with 5% sheep blood; nongroupability with Lancefield group A through V antisera; vancomycin susceptibility; no gas production; nonmotility; positive results by the CAMP, pyrrolidonyl arylamidase, and leucine aminopeptidase tests; and negative results by bile-esculin, Voges-Proskauer, and hippurate tests (23, 24, 30). Most strains grow at 10°C but not at 45°C, and most do not grow in 6.5% sodium chloride. Molecular techniques have been developed to aid in the identification of this species (4, 10). Berridge et al. (4) constructed, from a 524-bp consensus sequence of the *S. iniae* 16S-23S ribosomal DNA intergenic spacer, a set of nested oligonucleotide PCR primers that specifically amplified a 373-bp subunit from a variety of clinical isolates from farmed fish and human patients. Goh et al. (10), using the chaperonin 60 (Cpn60) gene identification method, correctly identified each of 12 *S. iniae*-infected samples among 34 samples from animal and human clinical sources containing aerobic gram-positive isolates.

Since the early 1980s, epizootic meningoencephalitis caused by streptococci has been recognized as an important cause of morbidity and mortality in ponds containing cultured fish (7, 8, 14, 15, 23, 31). Infected fish become lethargic, swim erratically, and show dorsal rigidity, and death occurs within several days. Pathologic studies show extensive involvement of the central nervous system (14). Several bacteria have been shown to cause epidemics of meningoencephalitis, including *S. iniae*, *Streptococcus agalactiae* (7, 35), and *Lactococcus garvieae* (17). Outbreaks due to *S. iniae* described in Japan, Taiwan, Israel, and the United States have affected tilapia (*Oreochromis* species), yellowtail (*Serida quinqueradiata*), rainbow trout, and coho salmon (7–9, 14–16, 23, 31, 34). *S. iniae* may colonize the surfaces of fish without causing disease, but it has also been associated with epidemics in which 30 to 50% of fish in affected fishponds die (7). Since 1979, fish farms in various districts of Japan, where aquaculture is a prolific industry, have suffered serious economic losses from large-scale epizootics of streptococcal disease, caused mainly by *S. iniae* (15). In Israeli aquaculture farms, streptococcal infection was first recognized in 1984. The disease affects both of the major fish species cultured in Israel, tilapia and trout (7). *S. iniae* has also been reported to be the causative agent of ongoing infection and excess mortality of tilapia in Texas aquaculture farms (23).

STREPTOCOCCUS INIAE AS A ZOONOTIC PATHOGEN

The Toronto Experience

A Cluster of Cases

Weinstein et al. (37) reported on an initial cluster of cases of *S. iniae* cellulitis in Toronto in 1995 and 1996 (2). On 15 December 1995, a 64-year-old Chinese female who had previously been in good health presented to a community hospital in Toronto with cellulitis of the hand. The patient gave a history of a puncture wound to the same hand that she had received 1 day previously while preparing fresh whole tilapia for cooking. The tilapia, which had been bred in an aquaculture farm, had been purchased live from a local supermarket just prior to the injury. On 18 December 1995, a 74-year-old Chinese female who had previously been in good health presented to the same hospital with a 24-hour history of cellulitis and lymphangitis of the hand, which on 15 December she had lacerated with a knife that she was using to prepare an unidentified fresh whole fish for dinner. On 20 December 1995, a 40-year-old Chinese female who had previously been in good health presented to the same hospital with cellulitis of the hand following a puncture due to the dorsal fin of a fresh whole tilapia, which she had been preparing for dinner.

All three patients had purchased the live fish from aquariums in different local supermarkets, and the aquariums were supplied with fish from American aquaculture farms. All three patients were admitted to a hospital, and cultures of their blood grew gram-positive cocci that were initially identified with the Vitek GPI card (bioMerieux Vitek, Hazelwood, Mo.) as *Streptococcus uberis*, but they were subsequently identified by the National Center for Streptococcus, Edmonton, Alberta, Canada, and the Centers for Disease Control and Prevention (CDC), Atlanta, Ga., as *S. iniae*. At the time *S. iniae* was not in the Vitek database. The patients were treated parenterally with β-lactam antibiotics and had uncomplicated recoveries.

The fourth case of *S. iniae* cellulitis occurred in a 77-year-old Chinese male who had a history of diabetes mellitus, osteoarthritis, rheumatic heart disease, and chronic renal failure. On 1 February 1996, he presented to the same hospital to which the other patients presented. He had a 1-week history of a painful right knee associated with fever and sweats. On 20 January he had been given a fresh whole tilapia, which he prepared for dinner that evening. There was no history of trauma or cellulitis. On examination, the knee was inflamed and a new cardiac murmur was noted. While in the emergency department, he had a respiratory arrest and was admitted to the intensive care unit and started on empiric antimicrobial therapy. Cultures of blood taken at the time of admission grew what was subsequently identified as *S. iniae*. Twelve hours after admission and the institution of antimicrobials, a lumbar puncture was performed and an aspirate of the right knee was obtained. Laboratory results were consistent with meningitis and septic arthritis, but cultures were negative. This patient met the Duke criteria for infective endocarditis (6). He eventually recovered without sequelae.

The Investigation

Following identification of the four cases of cellulitis described above, investigators in Toronto initiated retrospective and prospective surveillance to identify additional cases (38). Toronto area hospital infection control practitioners reviewed their medical records to identify all patients hospitalized with upper-limb cellulitis between 1 October 1995 and 31 March 1996. The patients were excluded if they had a predisposing condition that would have been a cause of cellulitis (e.g., intravenous lines in place, burns, chronic skin diseases, or lymphedema) or if an etiologic agent other than *S. uberis*, *S. iniae*, or an unidentified streptococcal species was identified from cultures of blood. Once identified, the patients were interviewed by using a standardized questionnaire to obtain clinical and epidemiologic data. From 1 April to 31 December 1996, emergency departments in Toronto were asked to prospectively identify patients presenting with acute upper-limb cellulitis. Patients with confirmed cases of invasive disease were those for whom *S. iniae* was isolated from any sterile body site. A suspect case was one where an individual had a diagnosis of upper-limb cellulitis and had a positive history of handling fresh whole fish within 72 h before the onset of signs and symptoms.

Between December 1995 and December 1996, a total of nine additional patients with bacteremic *S. iniae* infections were identified (patients 1 to 9, Table 1). The median age was 69 years (mean age, 67.0 years; age range, 40 to 80 years) and the female-to-male ratio was 2:1. All of the patients with confirmed cases of infection were of Asian descent: eight Chinese and one Korean. All patients had reported that they had prepared whole, raw fish, and eight patients recalled that they had injured their hands by puncturing the skin with the dorsal fin, a fish bone, or a knife used for cleaning and scaling. None of the patients had prior breaks in the skin. Six patients were able to identify tilapia as the fish that they had been

Table 1. Demographic characteristics of patients with culture-confirmed cases of invasive *S. iniae* infection[a]

Patient no.	Age (yr)	Sex[b]	Date of culture (mo/day/yr)	Underlying illness	Type of infection – Primary	Type of infection – Secondary	Type of fish	Treatment – Antibiotic(s)	Treatment – Duration (days)
1	74	F	12/19/1995	None	Cellulitis of hand	None	Unknown	Penicillin	10
2	64	F	12/16/1995	None	Cellulitis of hand	None	Tilapia	Penicillin	10
3	40	F	12/22/1995	Rheumatic heart disease	Cellulitis of hand	None	Tilapia	Penicillin, cloxacillin	10
4	77	M	01/02/1996	Rheumatic heart disease, chronic renal failure, diabetes, osteoarthritis	Unknown	Endocarditis, meningitis, arthritis	Tilapia	Erythromycin, cefuroxime	35
5	80	M	4/17/1996	Diabetes, osteoarthritis	Cellulitis of hand	None	Unknown	Ampicillin	10
6	69	F	2/29/1996	None	Cellulitis of hand	None	Unknown	Cloxacillin	10
7	70	F	8/20/1996	Diabetes	Cellulitis of hand	Cellulitis of leg	Tilapia	Ampicillin, cephalexin	10
8	71	M	8/29/1996	None	Cellulitis of hand	None	Tilapia	Penicillin	10
9	58	F	12/6/1996	None	Cellulitis of hand	None	Tilapia	Penicillin	10
10	79	M	8/1994	Unknown	Unknown	Arthritis of knee	Unknown	Cloxacillin	Unknown
11	Unknown	Unknown	1991	Unknown	Cellulitis	None	Unknown	Unknown	Unknown

[a]Reprinted from reference 38 with permission from M. Weinstein and the *New England Journal of Medicine.*
[b]F, female; M, male.

preparing, but three patients were not certain of the fish species. The MICs for all clinical isolates tested were ≤0.25 mg/liter for penicillin, cefazolin, ceftriaxone, erythromycin, clindamycin, and trimethoprim-sulfamethoxazole, 0.5 mg/liter for ciprofloxacin, and 16 mg/liter for gentamicin.

Cellulitis of the hand was present in eight of the nine patients with confirmed cases of infection. All had fever and lymphangitis that originated from the site of injury. The onset of cellulitis occurred 16 to 24 h after injury. In no case was there evidence of skin necrosis or bulla formation. Leukocyte counts were elevated (range, 12,900 to 33,400 per mm^3) with neutrophil predominance and left shifts. All patients were admitted to a hospital, were given parenteral antibiotics, and responded within 2 to 4 days. Eleven patients with suspect cases of *S. iniae* infection were identified. The median age of the patients with suspect cases of infection was 46 years (mean age, 50 years; age range, 36 to 68 years), and the female-to-male ratio was 1:1. All patients with suspect cases of infection were of Asian origin. All reported that they had injured themselves while handling whole or partially prepared fresh fish. Nine reported that the fish was tilapia, one reported that the fish was bass, and one did not know the type of fish. One patient with a suspect case of *S. iniae* infection had purchased a tilapia from the same retail store and on the same day that the patient with a confirmed case of infection had purchased tilapia.

Pulsed-field gel electrophoresis (PFGE) with *Sma*I was performed with the *S. iniae* isolates from these 10 patients: all isolates had identical patterns (pattern A) (Fig. 2).

Additional Cases of *S. iniae* Infection

Because more than half of hospital microbiology laboratories in the Toronto area routinely refer all isolates of viridans group streptococci to reference laboratories for species identification, the records of CDC, the Public Health Laboratory of Ontario, Toronto, and the National Center for Streptococcus, Edmonton, were reviewed to determine whether *S. iniae* had previously been identified. In addition, in order to determine if cases of cellulitis had occurred in workers whose jobs included the processing of whole fish, injury claims made over the previous 5 years to the Workers Compensation Board of Ontario were reviewed.

The Workers Compensation Board claims failed to identify any individuals with suspect cases of infection. The review of the microbiology laboratory database at CDC revealed two additional patients from whom *S. iniae* was isolated. One patient (Table 1, patient 10) was employed as a cook in Ottawa, Ontario, Canada, and was bacteremic, and the other patient (Table 1, patient 11) was from Texas and *S. iniae* was isolated from synovial fluid from his knee. When isolates from these two patients were analyzed by PFGE with *Sma*I digestion, the patterns obtained (pattern A′) were indistinguishable and had a one-band shift relative to the patterns for the other isolates from patients (Fig. 2).

Isolation of *S. iniae* from Aquacultured Fish

In the initial investigation, samples for culture were obtained from the surfaces of aquacultured fish purchased in retail stores in the greater Toronto area and Van-

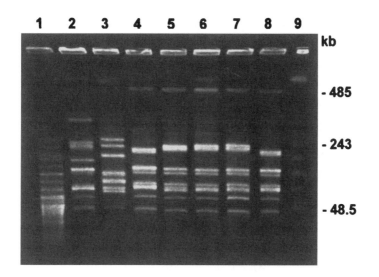

Figure 2. PFGE analysis of *S. iniae* strains after digestion of chromosomal DNA with *Sma*I. Lane 8, pattern A seen for all isolates from patients in the greater Toronto area with clinical cases of infection; Lanes 5 (tilapia brain, Texas, 1993), 6 (patient 11, Texas, 1991), and 7 (patient 10, Ottawa, 1994) have a single band shift (pattern A'). Lane 4, sample from a fish from a Toronto retail store with pattern A. Lanes 1 (ATCC 29177), 2 (ATCC 29178), and 3 (*S. iniae* from a Toronto retail store) all have unrelated PFGE patterns. Lane 9, bacteriophage lambda ladder molecular size standard. (Reprinted from reference 38 with permission from M. Weinstein and the *New England Journal of Medicine*.)

couver, British Columbia, Canada (courtesy of N. Press and E. A. Bryce, Vancouver Hospital Health Science Center, Vancouver). Eleven isolates were obtained from the brains of tilapia involved in epizootics that occurred in 1993 in Texas and Virginia (CDC and courtesy of P. Frelier, Texas A&M University). Type strains of *S. iniae*, strains ATCC 29177 and ATCC 29178 (American Type Culture Collection, Manassas, Va.), were used as controls. Additional *S. iniae* isolates included 11 isolates from cultures of specimens from live fish obtained from retail stores and 27 isolates from cultures of specimens from tilapia from fish suppliers.

Strains from the brains of tilapia with meningoencephalitis had either PFGE pattern A (1 isolate) or PFGE pattern A' (10 isolates) (Fig. 2). Isolates in two cultures of specimens from different Toronto retail fish stores, all four isolates from tilapia identified in Vancouver, and four of the isolates from two of the seven American fish farms sampled were found to have pattern A. The remaining strains, including the type strains from the American Type Culture Collection, had 19 different unrelated patterns.

In a subsequent study designed to characterize the frequency of occurrence and patterns of *S. iniae* strains found on fish in retail stores, Liu et al. (19) purchased fish from a random selection of retail stores throughout Toronto. A total of 66 fresh whole fish (31 tilapia, 11 bass, 5 catfish, 4 each of cod and trout, and 11 other species) were purchased from 19 fish retailers. Twenty-one had previously been killed and were being kept on ice. Forty-five were alive at the time of purchase. Five surface swab specimens were taken from each fish on the day of purchase, after the fish had been stored at 4°C for 48 h, and after the fish had been stored for an additional 24 h at −10°C. A total of 330 isolates of *S. iniae* were cultured from 42 of the 66 (64%) fish purchased from 8 of 19 retailers. Fish that were positive and fish that were negative for *S. iniae* were purchased from the same retailers. There were no significant differences in the rates of colonization between tilapia and nontilapia. There was a significant difference between the rates of *S. iniae* colonization of fish killed prior to purchase and stored on ice and fish killed at the time of purchase (7 of 21 versus 35 of 45, respectively; $P < 0.001$). Storage of the samples at 4°C for 48 h did not reduce the amount of *S. iniae* isolated; however, freezing reduced the amount by about 50%. PFGE analyses of these isolates identified patterns, but none of these patterns were related to the patterns for *S. iniae* strains isolated from humans or fish with disease.

Further Epidemiologic Investigation

In an attempt to better understand why all 9 patients with confirmed cases of infection and 11 of 12 patients with suspected cases of infection reported on by Weinstein et al. (38) were of Asian origin, Liu et al. (19) carried out a prospective study in Toronto regarding the type of fish purchased by consumers, the type of preparation of the fish by the retailer, and the frequency and type of injury associated with handling of the fish by the consumer. A questionnaire was administered to 100 consecutive, consenting customers leaving a random sample of Toronto fish retailers that stocked live fish. Compared to non-Asians, Asians were more likely to purchase live or whole fish and to take it home whole or partially prepared rather than fully dressed. In addition, people of Asian ethnic origin were more likely to purchase tilapia (the last raw fish purchase was tilapia for 28% of Asians but none of the non-Asians). More than half (53%) of the people who prepared their own fish to some extent reported at least one prior injury, and 52% of the injuries occurred while they were preparing tilapia.

The Vancouver Experience

Following the report of *S. iniae* infections in Toronto in the winter of 1995 and 1996, Press et al. (27) carried out an epidemiologic and microbiologic investigation to determine whether fresh fish in Vancouver carried *S. iniae*. Eleven tilapia and six other fish species sharing circulated tank water and purchased live from five fish markets in the Greater Vancouver Regional District were swabbed, and the swabs were cultured for *S. iniae* on sheep blood agar and colistin-nalidixic acid medium. Seven of 11 tilapia and 4 of 6 other fish (rock cod, trout, and sculpin) were culture positive by standard microbiologic methods. PFGE with restriction endonucleases *Sma*I and *Apa*I revealed that the *S. iniae* strains from Vancouver had the same pattern as the isolates that caused an epidemic among humans and some, but not all, of the isolates from fish from Toronto. In 1997, surveillance in Vancouver identified two cases of cellulitis and bacteremia caused by *S. iniae* in patients who sustained inoculation injuries while preparing tilapia. In both patients the *S. iniae* strain had the same PFGE pattern as the strain responsible for the outbreak in Toronto. Whereas fish farms that supply Toronto markets were located in Tennessee, Arkansas, North Dakota, Delaware, and Illinois, the Vancouver tilapia were traced to a fish farm in North Dakota that did not supply fish to markets in Toronto.

EVIDENCE TO SUPPORT THE HYPOTHESIS THAT *S. INIAE* IS A NEW PATHOGEN

Whether *S. iniae* infections in humans are the result of the emergence of a new human pathogen or are a previously unrecognized disease cannot be known with certainty. *S. iniae* infections may not have been recognized in the past for several reasons. Cellulitis that occurs following a local injury or spontaneously is by far most frequently due to *Streptococcus pyogenes* or *Staphylococcus aureus*, and disease due to *S. iniae* cannot be clinically distinguished from disease caused by *S. pyogenes* and *S. aureus* (18). Cultures are not usually useful for the diagnosis of *S. iniae* infection in patients with cellulitis. Hook et al. (12) were able to isolate pathogens from only 26% of patients with cellulitis, even though they cultured punch biopsy specimens, aspirates, and blood (12). Since cultures are rarely performed, illness due to particular pathogens may be missed. Infections due to *S. iniae* may also not be recognized, because under certain growth conditions, the beta-hemolysis of *S. iniae* may not be evident. Isolates would then be misidentified as a viridans group streptococcus and may be considered contaminants. Even if identification to the species level was carried out with current commercial identification systems, *S. iniae* would not likely be correctly identified since it is not found in the databases of those systems.

Substantial evidence, however, does support the hypothesis that *S. iniae* is a new pathogen (16). Weinstein et al. (38) note that significant numbers of cases would not likely have been missed in retrospective surveillance studies because of failure of identification, since the majority of hospitals routinely refer viridans group streptococci isolated from sterile sites to a reference laboratory. In addition, *S. iniae* has only recently been identified as a pathogen in fish produced by the aquaculture industry. Overcrowding in farms and during transport may have contributed to the increasing importance of streptococcal infections in fish (8). Finally, although *S. iniae* commonly colonized the surfaces of tilapia and other species of fish, isolates are genetically diverse. Only two distinct, highly related clones (those with PFGE patterns A and A') have been identified to be associated with invasive disease in humans and fish. This situation is similar to that for other bacteria that cause disease in humans (22) and suggests the presence of one or more virulence factors, not present in all strains, that may be important for pathogenicity in both humans and fish.

The association of disease with tilapia may have occurred for a number of reasons. One possible explanation is that, although tilapia are no more likely than other cultured fish to be colonized with *S. iniae*, they are the most commonly purchased cultured fish, and they are more likely to be associated with injury than other fish. However, the data of Liu et al. (19) suggest that some clones of *S. iniae* may preferentially colonize different fish species and that the invasive clone is restricted primarily to tilapia. It may also be that conditions on farms or in ponds where tilapia are cultured are more conducive to growth of the invasive clone than conditions on other farms.

CONCLUSIONS

The demonstration of yet another new pathogen linked to the food industry is not surprising in view of the fact that rapid changes in patterns of food production, storage, distribution, and preparation provide increased opportunities for the exposure of humans to new organisms (3, 36). Although *S. iniae* is capable of causing invasive disease in humans, serious disease appears to be rare, and if people take the proper precautionary measures when handling whole, uncooked fish, infections caused by *S. iniae* can be prevented.

REFERENCES

1. **Ahmed, F. E.** 1991. *Seafood Safety.* National Academy Press, Washington, D.C.
2. **Anonymous.** 1996. Invasive infection due to *Streptococcus iniae*—Ontario, 1995–1996. *Morbid. Mortal. Weekly Rep.* **45:**650–653.
3. **Baird-Parker, A. C.** 1994. 1993 Fred Griffith Review Lecture. Foods and microbiological risks. *Microbiology* **140:**687–695.
4. **Berridge, B. R., J. D. Fuller, J. C. de Azavedo, D. E. Low, H. Bercovier, and P. F. Frelier.** 1998. Development of specific nested oligonucleotide PCR primers for the *Streptococcus iniae* 16S-23S ribosomal DNA intergenic spacer. *J. Clin. Microbiol.* **36:**2778–2781.
5. **Childs, J., R. E. Shope, D. Fish, F. X. Meslin, C. J. Peters, K. Johnson, E. Debess, D. Dennis, and S. Jenkins.** 1998. Emerging zoonoses. *Emerg. Infect. Dis* **4:**453–454.
6. **Durack, D. T., A. S. Lukes, and D. K. Bright.** 1994. New criteria for diagnosis of infective endocarditis: utilization of specific echocardiographic findings. *Am. J. Med.* **96:**200–209.
7. **Eldar, A., Y. Bejerano, and H. Bercovier.** 1994. *Streptococcus shiloi* and *Streptococcus difficile*: two new streptococcal species causing a meningoencephalitis in fish. *Curr. Microbiol.* **28:**139–143.
8. **Eldar, A., Y. Bejerano, A. Livoff, A. Horovitcz, and H. Bercovier.** 1995. Experimental streptococcal meningo-encephalitis in cultured fish. *Vet. Microbiol.* **43:**33–40.
9. **Eldar, A., P. F. Frelier, L. Assenta, P. W. Varner, S. Lawhon, and H. Bercovier.** 1995. *Streptococcus shiloi*, the name for an agent causing septicemic infection in fish, is a junior synonym of *Streptococcus iniae*. *Int. J. Syst. Bacteriol.* **45:**840–842.
10. **Goh, S. H., D. Driedger, S. Gillett, D. E. Low, S. M. Hemmingsen, M. Amos, D. Chan, M. Lovgren, B. M. Willey, C. Shaw, and J. A. Smith.** 1998. *Streptococcus iniae*, a human and animal pathogen: specific identification by the chaperonin 60 gene identification method. *J. Clin. Microbiol.* **36:**2164–2166.
11. **Hackney, C. R., and M. D. Pierson.** 1994. *Environmental Indicators and Shellfish Safety*, p. 523. Chapman & Hall, New York, N.Y.
12. **Hook, E. W., T. M. Hooton, C. A. Horton, M. B. Coyle, P. G. Ramsey, and M. Turck.** 1986. Microbiologic evaluation of cutaneous cellulitis in adults. *Arch. Intern. Med.* **146:**295–297.
13. **Huss, H. H.** 1994. *Assurance of Seafood Quality*. FAO Fisheries Technical Paper No. 334. Food and Agriculture Organization, Rome, Italy.
14. **Kaige, N., T. Miyazaki, and S. Kubota.** 1984. The pathogen and histopathology of vertebral deformity in cultured yellowtail *Seriola quinqueradiata*. *Fish Pathol.* **19:**173–180.
15. **Kitao, T., T. Aoki, and R. Sakoh.** 1981. Epizootic caused by β-haemolytic Streptococcus species in cultured freshwater fish. *Fish Pathol.* **15:**301–307.
16. **Kusuda, R.** 1992. Bacterial fish diseases in mariculture in Japan with special emphasis on streptococcosis. *Isr. J. Aquacult.* **44:**140.

17. **Kusuda, R., K. Kawai, F. Salati, C. R. Banner, and J. L. Fryer.** 1991. *Enterococcus seriolicida* sp. nov., a fish pathogen. *Int. J. Syst. Bacteriol.* **41:**406–409.
18. **Lee, P. C., J. Turnidge, and P. J. McDonald.** 1985. Fine-needle aspiration biopsy in diagnosis of soft tissue infections. *J. Clin. Microbiol.* **22:**80–83.
19. **Liu, E. T. H., C. D'Cunha, B. Yaffe, C. Ostach, J. Urquhuart, K. Gorman, W. Lee, J. Ying, L. Landry, M. Armstrong-Evans, The Fish Team, D. E. Low, and A. McGeer.** 1998. Understanding the epidemiology of S*treptococcus iniae* infections—results of a survey of fish buying and handling in the greater Toronto area. *In Abstracts of the 66th Conjoint Meeting on Infectious Diseases.*
20. **Morse, S. S.** 1995. Factors in the emergence of infectious diseases. *Emerg. Infect. Dis* **1:**7–15.
21. **Murphy, F. A.** 1998. Emerging zoonoses. *Emerg. Infect. Dis* **4:**429–435.
22. **Musser, J. M.** 1996. Molecular population genetic analysis of emerged bacterial pathogens: selected insights. *Emerg. Infect. Dis.* **2:**1–17.
23. **Perera, R. P., S. K. Johnson, M. D. Collins, and D. H. Lewis.** 1994. *Streptococcus iniae* associated with mortality of *Tilapia nilotica* × *T. aurea* hybrids. *J. Aquat. Anim. Health* **6:**335–340.
24. **Pier, G. B., and S. H. Madin.** 1976. *Streptococcus iniae* sp. nov., a beta-hemolytic streptococcus isolated from an Amazon freshwater dolphin, *Inia geoffrensis. Int. J. Syst. Bacteriol.* **26:**545–553.
25. **Pier, G. B., S. H. Madin, and S. Al-Nakeeb.** 1978. Isolation and characterization of a second isolate of *Streptococcus iniae. Int. J. Syst. Bacteriol.* **28:**311–314.
26. **Pillay, T. V. R.** 1993. *Aquaculture Principles and Practices*, p. 360–376. Fishing News Books, Oxford, United Kingdom.
27. **Press, N., E. Bryce, and G. Stiver.** 1998. Strain characteristics of S*treptococcus iniae* isolated from tilapia species in Vancouver, British Columbia. *Can. Commun. Dis Rep.* **24:**181–182.
28. **Rana, K., and A. Immink.** 1997. Trends in global aquaculture production: 1984–1996. Report FIRE/C886. *Anonymous Review of the State of World Aquaculture.* Food and Agriculture Organization, Rome, Italy.
29. **Rana, K. J.** 1997. Aquatic environment and use of species groups. Report FIRI/C886. *Anonymous Review of the State of World Aquaculture.* Food and Agriculture Organization, Rome, Italy.
30. **Reilly, P. J. A., P. Howgate, and F. Kaferstein.** 1997. Safety hazards and the application of the hazard analysis critical control point system (HACCP) in aquaculture, p. 353–373. *In* R. E. Martin, R. L. Collette, and J. W. Slavi (ed.), *Fish Inspection Quality Control and HACCP: A Global Focus.* Technomic Publishing Company, Lancaster, United Kingdom.
31. **Robinson, J. A., and F. P. Meyer.** 1966. Streptococcal fish pathogen. *J. Bacteriol.* **92:**512.
32. **Ruoff, K. L.** 1995. *Streptococcus*, p. 299–307. *In* P. R. Murray, E. J. Baron, M. A. Pfaller, F. C. Tenover, and R. H. Yolken (ed.), *Manual of Clinical Microbiology*, 6th ed. ASM Press, Washington, D.C.
33. **Stiassny, M. L., and A. Meyer.** 1999. Cichlids of the Rift Lakes. *Sci. Am.* **280:**64–69.
34. **Teixeira, L. M., V. L. C. Merquior, M. D. C. E. Vianni, M. D. G. S. Carvalho, S. E. L. Fracalanzza, A. G. Steigerwalt, D. J. Brenner, and R. R. Facklam.** 1996. Phenotypic and genotypic characterization of atypical *Lactococcus garvieae* strains isolated from water buffalos with subclinical mastitis and confirmation of *L. garvieae* as a senior subjective synonym of *Enterococcus seriolicida. Int. J. Syst. Bacteriol.* **46:**664–668.
35. **Vandamme, P., P. A. Vevriese, B. Pot, K. Kersters, and P. Melin.** 1997. *Streptococcus difficile* is a nonhemolytic group B, type Ib streptococcus. *Int. J. Syst. Bacteriol.* **47:**81–85.
36. **Vidaver, A.** 1996. Emerging and remerging infectious diseases: perspective on plants, animals and humans. *ASM News* **62:**583–585.
37. **Weinstein, M., D. Low, A. McGeer, B. Willey, D. Rose, M. Coulter, P. Wyper, A. Borczyk, M. Lovgren, and R. Facklam.** 1996. Invasive infection due to Streptococcus iniae: a new or previously unrecognized disease—Ontario, 1995–1996. *Can. Commun. Dis Rep.* **22:**129–131.
38. **Weinstein, M. R., M. Litt, D. A. Kertesz, P. Wyper, D. Rose, M. Coulter, A. McGeer, R. Facklam, C. Ostach, B. M. Willey, A. Borczyk, D. E. Low, and The Investigation Team.** 1997. Invasive infections due to a fish pathogen: *Streptococcus iniae. N. Engl. J. Med.* **337:**589–594.
39. **World Health Organization.** 1995. *Control of Food-Borne Trematode Infections.* Report of a WHO Study Group, Manila, Philippines. World Health Organization, Geneva, Switzerland.

Emerging Infections 3
Edited by W. M. Scheld, W. A. Craig, and J. M. Hughes
© 1999 ASM Press, Washington, D.C.

Chapter 5

Epidemic Typhus: a Forgotten but Lingering Threat

James G. Olson

HISTORY OF EPIDEMIC TYPHUS

The impact of louse-borne, or epidemic, typhus, which is caused by *Rickettsia prowazekii*, on populations is of historical significance but has passed from current concern. Whenever large numbers of people were crowded together under less than sanitary conditions, typhus appeared.

The association between typhus epidemics and war is one that can be traced from the earliest times. Typhus was responsible for the plague of Athens (430 to 428 B.C.). In 1489, Spanish soldiers who fought the Turks in Cyprus brought typhus to Spain. At the siege of Granada, 17,000 Spanish troops died of typhus, more than five times the number killed by the Moors (10). In 1528, the French army besieging Naples was stricken with typhus, causing 30,000 deaths and forcing the French to withdraw. In 1632, during the Thirty Years' War, the Swedish army was decimated by typhus, resulting in 16,000 deaths and causing the army to withdraw.

Typhus was responsible for the defeat of Napoleon's army of half a million men in Russia in 1812 and 1813. Before the French army reached Moscow, more than 80,000 soldiers had contracted typhus. When they began their retreat from Moscow, they left several thousand of the sickest soldiers and carried the strongest with them on wagons. Typhus spread rapidly through Napoleon's entire retreating army, reducing it to 20,000 sick and disheartened men. Nearly all of the 3,000 who survived were infected with typhus and were responsible for spreading the disease to the civilian populations (5).

In 1915, the Serbian epidemic resulted in 150,000 deaths and resulted in the cessation of military operations by the Serbian army for 6 months. In military hospitals alone, 2,500 patients were hospitalized each day (9). During the epidemic, the case-fatality ratio (CFR) varied between 30 and 60%. In the Polish epidemic

---

James G. Olson • Division of Viral and Rickettsial Diseases, National Center for Infectious Diseases, Centers for Disease Control and Prevention, Mailstop A-26, 1600 Clifton Rd. NE, Atlanta, GA 30333.

of 1916 to 1920, more than 422,000 cases of typhus occurred in a population of 2.5 million. Between 1917 and 1923, the typhus epidemic in European Russia resulted in 30 million cases of typhus with 3 million deaths (10).

During the Second World War, there were severe epidemics of typhus in the areas that had experienced regular but small outbreaks each winter. Morocco, Algeria, Tunisia, Egypt, Iran, Turkey, Yugoslavia, Rumania, Bulgaria, Hungary, Germany, and Poland each reported thousands of civilian cases annually (8). In 1942, there were 23,000 cases with 5,000 deaths in the civilian population of Egypt, and 77,000 cases were reported in French North Africa (3). During the years 1939 to 1945, typhus spread from Russia and Central Europe to German concentration camps and then to Italy, where it affected British and U.S. troops. The hospital admission rate due to typhus among the British forces serving in the Middle East was greater than 5 per 10,000 population during the entire war (3).

CURRENT STATUS OF EPIDEMIC TYPHUS

Louse-borne typhus remains endemic in the mountainous regions of the Americas, the Himalayas, Afghanistan, and Africa. The disease is maintained in an endemic cycle of transmission that remains barely detectable. Key ingredients common to each area where typhus remains active include poverty and the absence of a reliable water supply. These factors result in crowding and infrequent bathing and laundering of clothing and bedding, which lead to the infestation of the populations with the human body louse, *Pediculus humanus corporis*, the arthropod vector. The incidence rates and CFRs remain very low. Figure 1 shows the reported incidence of epidemic typhus in Ethiopia for the years 1985 to 1991. Occasionally, conditions that favor epidemic transmission occur. Epidemics have recently occurred in Addis Ababa, Ethiopia (1990); Nigeria (1990); Cuzco, Peru (1995); and Ngozi, Burundi (1995).

Following a civil war that began in 1993, thousands of refugees were relocated throughout Burundi in large camps with poor hygiene and marginal nutrition. The

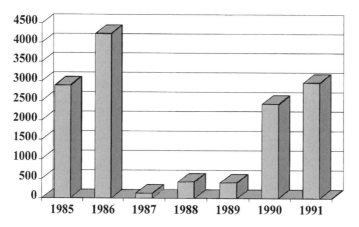

Figure 1. Epidemic typhus cases, Ethiopia, 1985 to 1991. Data from the Ethiopian Health and Nutrition Research Institute.

cholera and typhoid fever epidemics that occurred were well publicized, but the more than 45,000 cases of typhus were almost unnoticed. The epidemic spread from an outbreak among prisoners in Ngozi in 1995 to the local civilian population. Epidemic typhus then spread into populations at higher elevations, where colder conditions prevailed and infestations with lice were prevalent. Figure 2 shows the number of clinically diagnosed typhus cases by month from January to September of 1997. At its peak in February, more than 11,000 cases per month occurred in 28 Burundian refugee camps that accommodated over 760,000 displaced persons. The incidence rate of epidemic typhus in Burundi for the entire period of the epidemic was 5,960 per 100,000 population. Table 1 shows the incidence rate of epidemic typhus cases for the same period in the refugee camps located in the three provinces in the central highlands above elevations of 2,000 m. The incidence rates per 100,000 population were 31,680 in Muramvya, 15,709 in Gitega, and 14,979 in Kayanza. With the exception of camps located in Ngozi Province (incidence rate, 18,508/100,000), provinces at lower elevations had lower incidences. Camps located in Bujumbura, Makamba, Karuzi, Muyinga, and Cibitoke Provinces at elevations of between 1,000 and 2,000 m had incidence rates of between 300 and 4,000 per 100,000 population. Epidemic typhus was absent from camps located in the remaining six provinces, which were situated at elevations below 1,000 m (6).

The CFR was in excess of 15% in the initial outbreaks that occurred in prisons. Once typhus was suspected and treatment with appropriate antimicrobial agents was initiated, the CFR fell to <0.5%. A nationwide program of treatment was begun in March 1997. A single oral dose of doxycycline (200 mg) was administered to each patient with suspected typhus. In July, inhabitants of refugee camps were treated with permethrin (1%) dusting powder to eliminate body lice (6).

CONTINUING THREAT

The threat of louse-borne typhus remains wherever there is or has been endemic transmission. Brill-Zinsser disease, or recrudescent typhus, may occur years fol-

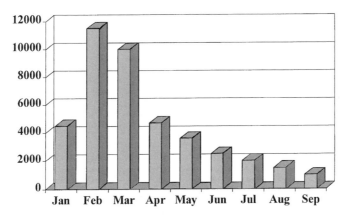

Figure 2. Epidemic typhus cases by month, refugee camps, Burundi, 1997.

Table 1. Typhus surveillance in refugee camps, Burundi, 1997

Province	Refugee population	No. of cases	Incidence/100,000 population
Muramvya	47,885	15,170	31,680
Ngozi	2,869	531	18,508
Gitega	66,224	10,441	15,709
Kayanza	99,244	14,886	14,979
All provinces	764,334	43,971	5,763

lowing a typhus infection. Patients who recover from louse-borne typhus remain chronically infected for life. Between 10 and 20% of patients have recrudescences of their illnesses in response to stress, severe malnutrition, other infectious diseases, or diminished immune function. When Brill-Zinsser disease occurs in a population infested with body lice, an epidemic of louse-borne typhus can be initiated (7).

Epidemic typhus is characterized clinically by sudden onset, sustained high fever of about 2 weeks' duration, a maculopapular rash, and altered mental state (1). The incubation period usually is from 8 to 12 days. The disease may be divided into the prodromal, early, and late phases. Prodromes of vague malaise and headache are common. The early phase is usually ushered in by the abrupt onset of fever, severe headache, myalgia of the back and legs, and chills or chilly sensations. The headache is intense and intractable and persists day and night. Over the first 2 or 3 days, the temperature reaches about 39 to 41°C and continues at that level until death or recovery. The skin is usually hot and dry. The face is flushed or dusky; the conjunctivas are suffused; photophobia is frequent. The mental state is dull. Weakness and prostration may be mild early after onset, but it may become profound after 2 or 3 days. Unproductive cough with sparse physical findings occurs in about two-thirds of the patients. Nausea, vomiting, and diarrhea occur but are uncommon. Constipation is usually present.

The characteristic rash appears between the 4th and 7th days and is the hallmark of the late phase of disease. In some instances, it is preceded by a diffuse, transient erythema. The lesions first appear on the trunk and axillary folds and spread to the extremities, sparing the face, palms, and soles except in severely ill patients. At first, the lesions are pinkish red macules that blanch on pressure. The evolution of the rash depends on the severity of the illness. In mild cases, it may fade completely in 1 or 2 days; in cases of moderate severity, it may become maculopapular, petechial (4), or possibly hemorrhagic, changing to a reddish brown color and lasting for 1 to 2 weeks before fading. In severe cases, the lesions may be exceedingly numerous, almost confluent, quickly becoming hemorrhagic or purpuric. The rash may be absent in 5 to 10% of patients. Cardiopulmonary findings include undulating and irregular pulse, low blood pressure with brief episodes of hypotension below 80 mm Hg, and occasionally cyanosis. The mental state progresses from dullness to stupor or, occasionally, coma. The stupor may be interrupted by periods of delirium, excitement, or vigorous activity, during which the patient may exhibit self-destructive action or wander off. Cranial nerves are selectively and variably involved (e.g., tinnitus, deafness, dysphagia, and dysphonia may occur). Coarse tremors may appear. Urinary and fecal incontinence is encountered in moderately or severely ill patients.

Common findings include oliguria, proteinuria, and azotemia. Jaundice is rare, but elevations in serum aminotransferase levels may appear early. The leukocyte count may be decreased early in the course of illness; in the 2nd and 3rd weeks of the disease, the leukocyte count is normal or only slightly elevated unless complications ensue. Eosinophils are absent or rare in the early stages of typhus. Anemia may develop in the 2nd or 3rd week.

Complications are common in untreated patients and include secondary bacterial bronchopneumonia, otitis media, and parotitis. Thrombosis may affect the large arteries, with serious results, e.g., hemiplegia. Thrombosis of small vessels in the skin may lead to gangrene, particularly of the toes, fingers, or ear lobes. Necrosis of the skin over the bony prominences may occur, especially over the sacrum or greater trochanter. The severity of disease and the CFR increase with age, being less severe and often uncharacteristic in younger children but increasing rapidly in those over the age of 40 years.

Recrudescent typhus is similar to primary typhus except that it is milder. On the average, the fever is lower and of shorter duration, the rash is less intense and often absent, and the CFR ratio is less than 1%.

Epidemic typhus may be difficult to diagnose. The early clinical signs and symptoms are remarkably nonspecific and may mimic those of other infectious diseases including measles, meningococcemia, leptospirosis, toxic shock syndrome, and thrombotic thrombocytopenic purpura, as well as noninfectious causes. Successful patient outcomes are guided more by the clinical acumen of the evaluating health care provider than by the sensitivities and specificities of laboratory tests, since results of testing are not available in time to benefit the patient. Therapeutic decisions must be based on a presumptive diagnosis developed from clinical suspicion and the epidemiologic setting. Confirmatiory laboratory tests are available at only a few reference center laboratories but are serologic in nature and serve to confirm the etiology retrospectively.

There is effective antimicrobial therapy for the typhus fevers (4). The response to tetracyclines or chloramphenicol is rapid and efficacious. Most patients become afebrile within 48 h of treatment, and single-dose doxycycline therapy is effective in epidemic situations (2). It is important for the medical personnel that make up disaster relief teams and refugee health programs to become aware of the continuing threat of typhus. Despite evidence that vaccines that contain killed typhus rickettsiae have been effective in the control of epidemics, conventional typhus vaccines composed of killed rickettsiae are no longer available in the United States. Strategies for control of epidemics of louse-borne typhus in refugee camps must include two elements of intervention: (i) antimicrobial treatment of patients with suspected cases and (ii) delousing of the entire population at risk.

Infected lice and louse feces on a patient with typhus present a special threat to all nonimmune contacts, including physicians and attendants, among whom infection is a common occupational hazard. Decontamination and delousing of the patient with typhus, including the patient's clothing and blankets, are performed immediately on hospitalization. Clothing and bedding are best decontaminated by heat, because this will kill the lice as well as the rickettsiae. After the patient is decontaminated and deloused, isolation and quarantine are not necessary. Depending on the circumstances, it may be necessary to apply insecticides at appropriate intervals to prevent reinfestation with lice.

Control of louse-borne typhus currently depends heavily on control of the louse vector. When simple hygienic measures, e.g., bathing and laundering of clothes in hot water with detergent, cannot be followed, the application of insecticide dusts (10% dichlorodiphenyltrichloroethane, 1% malathion, 1% lindane, or 1% permethrin) to fully clothed persons is effective at reducing louse populations and controlling disease in acute outbreaks. Insecticide resistance among body lice is a widespread and growing problem. Kits for the testing of insecticide susceptibility are available from the World Health Organization. The older methods of subjecting clothes and bedding to heat or fumigants, e.g., methyl bromide, are effective but cumbersome. Insecticides alone are less effective for long-term louse control in areas where conditions conducive to louse infestation persist and where louse strains resistant to insecticides can be and are selected. Long-term louse control or eradication depends on correction of the complex environmental, economic, cultural, educational, and political factors that contribute to louse infestations.

CONCLUSIONS

The war-ravaged countries of the former Yugoslavia are at risk if the poverty, war, and discontinuance of social services continue. Similarly, the countries of the former Soviet Union are at risk for epidemic typhus outbreaks. To date only anecdotal evidence of louse-borne typhus has been reported. However, as the magnitudes of the outbreaks increase, the likelihood that they will be etiologically confirmed and investigated increases.

REFERENCES

1. **Kamal, A. M., and G. A. Messih.** 1943. Typhus fever (review of 11,410 cases) symptomatology, laboratory investigations and treatment. *J. Egypt. Public Health Assoc.* **1:**126–213.
2. **Krause, D. W., P. L. Perine, J. E. McDade, and S. A. Awoke.** 1975. Treatment of louse-borne typhus fever with chloramphenicol, tetracycline or doxycycline. *East Afr. Med. J.* **52:**421–427.
3. **Moe, J. B., and C. E. Pederson.** 1980. The impact of rickettsial diseases on military operations. *Mil. Med.* **145:**780–785.
4. **Perine, P. L., B. P. Chandler, D. K Krause, P. McCardle, S. Awoke, E. Habte-Gabr, C. L. Wisseman, Jr., and J. E. McDade.** 1992. A clinico-epidemiological study of epidemic typhus in Africa. *Clin. Infect. Dis.* **14:**1149–1158.
5. **Prinzing, F.** 1916. *Epidemics Resulting from Wars.* The Clarendon Press, Oxford, United Kingdom.
6. **Raoult, D., J. B. Ndihokubwayo, H. Tissot-Dupont, V. Roux, B. Faugere, R. Abegbinni, and R. J. Birtles.** 1998. Outbreak of epidemic typhus associated with trench fever in Burundi. *Lancet* **352:**353–358.
7. **Reilly, P. J., and R. W. Kalinske.** 1980. Brill-Zinsser disease in North America. *West. J. Med.* **133:** 338–340.
8. **Snyder, J. C.** 1947. Typhus fever in the Second World War. *Calif. Med.* **66:**3–10.
9. **Strong, R. P., G. C. Shattuck, A. W. Sellards, H. Zinsser, and J. G. Hopkins.** 1920. *Typhus Fever with Particular Reference to the Serbian Epidemic.* American Red Cross, Cambridge, Mass.
10. **Zinsser, H.** 1944. *Rats, Lice and History.* The Atlantic Monthly Press (Little, Brown & Co.), Boston, Mass.

Emerging Infections 3
Edited by W. M. Scheld, W. A. Craig, and J. M. Hughes
© 1999 ASM Press, Washington, D.C.

Chapter 6

The Microsporidial Infections: Progress in Epidemiology and Prevention

David A. Schwartz and Ralph T. Bryan

Microsporidia have risen from obscure and anecdotal causes of keratitis and systemic disease in humans to become one of the most medically significant groups of emerging infectious agents. Their belated recognition as important causes of gastrointestinal, respiratory, renal, ocular and disseminated disease has come about largely as a result of the human immunodeficiency virus (HIV) pandemic. The initial recognition of ocular microsporidial disease in HIV-infected persons was believed to be due to a common microsporidial pathogen of mammals, *Encephalitozoon cuniculi*. However, directly as a result of increased interest in these organisms by physicians and scientists, at least 12 microsporidial agents which infect humans have been characterized, and several others are under investigation. The velocity with which knowledge of the human microsporidial infections has progressed is evident by the fact that 7 of these 12 species are newly described organisms since the recognition of AIDS. It is increasingly recognized that the microsporidia not only parasitize HIV-infected persons but parasitize immunosuppressed, non-HIV-infected organ transplant recipients and immunocompetent persons as well (14–16, 47, 70, 79, 88, 100).

The first decade of the investigation of human microsporidiosis was characterized by tremendous advances in the clinical recognition of the spectrum of disease caused by these protozoal agents, antigenic and molecular characterization of the microsporidia with production of an array of diagnostic reagents, descriptive pathology of the effects of microsporidia on human tissues, and the search for effective modes of therapy. The second decade of microsporidial research with humans will almost certainly focus on the search for mechanisms of acquisition and transmission of the microsporidia to humans. The past 2 years have already been witness to significant advances in the understanding of the epidemiology of microsporidiosis, including identification of animal reservoirs and potential environmental

David A. Schwartz • Department of Pathology, Emory University School of Medicine, Atlanta, GA 30335. *Ralph T. Bryan* • National Center for Infectious Diseases, Centers for Disease Control and Prevention, Albuquerque, NM 87110.

sources of infection. This chapter focuses on what is known regarding the epidemiology of human microsporidiosis and what we may be poised to better understand in the very near future. Topics to be covered include prevalence and geographic distribution, case demographics and populations at risk, and potential modes of transmission.

THE MICROSPORIDIA

The microsporidia are a unique group of obligately intracellular, spore-forming protozoa. They are true eukaryotes because they have a membrane-bound nucleus, an intracytoplasmic membrane system, and chromosome separation on mitotic spindles, but they are unusual among the eukaryotes in that they have 70S ribosomes, no mitochondria, and simple vesicular Golgi membranes. Microsporidia are diverse organisms that are capable of infecting a wide variety of both vertebrate and invertebrate hosts. These unusual protozoa are truly ubiquitous in our environment and infect familiar insects such as mosquitoes, fleas, grasshoppers, and honeybees; common food fish such as salmon, flounder, and monkfish; and freshwater snails. They can also be found in common environmental sources such as ditch water, and in the western United States, certain species are intentionally released into the environment for the biological control of destructive grasshoppers and locusts.

The microsporidial spore is a highly specialized, environmentally resistant structure that varies in size and shape according to species. Those species that infect mammals, including humans, tend to be smaller, ranging in size from 1.0 to 3.0 μm by 1.5 to 4.0 μm, and are usually ovoid in shape. The ultrastructural characteristics of microsporidial spores are distinctive.

Although different microsporidial genera can display significant variations in their methods of cell division, their life cycles share several general features that can be described in three phases. Phase I, the infective phase, begins with the ingestion, or possibly inhalation, of spores by a susceptible host. Thereafter, the spore is stimulated by conditions such as shifting pH or ionic concentrations to evert its coiled polar filament, which is actually a tubular structure analogous to a telescoping fishing rod or radio antenna. Upon eversion, this filament becomes a tubule through which the infective sporoplasm is injected into a host cell. During phase II, the injected sporoplasm develops into proliferative stages, or meronts, which multiply, depending on the species, either by repeated binary fission or by multiple fission with the formation of multinucleate plasmodial forms. This process, also known as merogony, is followed by phase III, or sporogony, which begins as meront cell membranes thicken to form sporonts. After subsequent divisions, sporonts give rise to sporoblasts, which develop into mature spores without undergoing further multiplication. As mature spores accumulate in an infected cell, that cell eventually expands to the point of rupture, thereby releasing infectious spores and completing the life cycle. This combination of merogonous and sporogonous multiplication gives the microsporidia enormous reproductive potential with resultant heavy host infestations and environmental contamination. Released spores may infect nearby host cells or escape into the environment via stool, urine, or respiratory secretions (12, 14–16, 20).

Among the numerous microsporidial species, at least 12 have been implicated in human disease (Table 1). There are also other human-infecting microsporidia for which appropriate genera and species have not been determined, such as those termed "*Nosema*-like" or assigned to the "collective group" *Microsporidium*. *Nosema* and *Pleistophora* are generally considered to be pathogens of insects and fish, respectively, whereas *E. cuniculi* usually infects nonhuman mammals and, occasionally, birds. *Enterocytozoon bieneusi*, *Encephalitozoon hellem*, *Encephalitozoon intestinalis*, *Trachipleistophora hominis*, *Trachipleistophora anthropophthera*, *Vittaforma corneae*, and *Brachiola vesicularum* were all originally described in humans, but animal hosts have recently been identified for *E. bieneusi*, *E. hellem*, and *E. intestinalis* (9, 10, 14–16, 21, 33, 57, 66, 74, 79, 100).

MICROSPORIDIA INFECTING HUMANS

E. bieneusi

E. bieneusi was initially described by Desportes and colleagues (35) as a new species of microsporidian that occurs in the intestines and stools of AIDS patients with chronic diarrhea. It shares the family Enterocytozoonidae with one other organism, *Enterocytozoon salmonis*, an intranuclear parasite of salmonid fish.

Enterocytozoon is one of the most prevalent intestinal pathogens identified in patients with AIDS, and in addition, the organisms can spread into the hepatobiliary tree to infect biliary and pancreatic duct epithelial cells. The most common anatomic location of *E. bieneusi* is within the cytoplasm of superficial lining epithelial cells of the small intestine (73, 75, 79, 82). *Enterocytozoon* infection is associated with chronic diarrhea and wasting syndrome. In patients with hepatobiliary infection, it can cause papillary stenosis, sclerosing cholangitis of both intra- and extrahepatic bile ducts, and acalculous cholecystitis. Unlike infections due to other microsporidial species in HIV-infected patients, *E. bieneusi* rarely produces systemic infections (14–16, 62, 99).

Enterocytozoon is the smallest microsporidian reported to infect humans. All developmental stages are formed in direct contact with the host cell cytoplasm, and no sporophorous vesicles or pansporoblastic membranes are present. Early in development it produces elongated nuclei, which are unique to this genus. The proliferative and sporogonial stages are rounded, multinucleated plasmodia measuring up to 6 μm in diameter. Also unique to this genus is the presence of electron-dense discs, which are precursors to the polar tubule and anchoring discs. The mature spores are oval, measure approximately 1 to 1.6 μm in length and 0.7 to 1 μm in width, and contain five to seven turns of the coiled polar tubule which appear in two rows by electron microscopy (75, 79, 82, 99).

E. (Formerly Septata) intestinalis

E. intestinalis was first identified by Cali and colleagues (18) in clinical samples from AIDS patients with diarrhea in 1993. The agent was initially named *Septata intestinalis* because of the ultrastructural observation of unique septations between spores in the cytoplasm of infected cells. It is the second most prevalent micro-

Table 1. Microsporidial species pathogenic for humans, their clinical manifestations, and recognized animal hosts or reservoirs

Microsporidial agent	Clinical manifestations (humans)	Reservoir or other hosts
Enterocytozoon bieneusi	Chronic or acute diarrhea, wasting syndrome, biliary tract disease	Pig, rhesus macaque
Encephalitozoon cuniculi	Disseminated infection, keratoconjunctivitis, sinusitis, pneumonitis, urinary tract infection, nephritis, hepatitis, peritonitis, encephalitis	Rabbit, mouse, rat, muskrat, hamster, guinea pig, ground shrew, cat, fox, leopard, puma, squirrel and rhesus monkeys, baboon, goat, sheep, dog, pig, horse
Encephalitozoon hellem	Disseminated infection, keratoconjunctivitis, sinusitis, nasal polyps, bronchiolitis, pneumonitis, nephritis, ureteritis, cystitis, prostatitis	Parakeet, parrot
Encephalitozoon intestinalis (formerly *Septata intestinalis*)	Disseminated infection, chronic diarrhea, weight loss, sinusitis, urinary tract infection, nephritis	Donkey, pig, cow, dog, goat
Pleistophora spp.	Myositis	None
Trachipleistophora hominis	Myositis, sinusitis, keratoconjunctivitis	None
Trachipleistophora anthropophthera	Disseminated infection (brain, heart, kidneys)	None
Brachiola vesicularum	Myositis	None
Vittaforma corneae (formerly *Nosema corneum*)	Keratitis, corneal ulcer	None
Nosema algerae	Corneal infection	Mosquito
Nosema connori	Disseminated infection	None
Nosema ocularum	Keratitis, corneal ulcer	None

sporidial infection reported in AIDS patients. In a study from the United States, intestinal infection with *E. intestinalis* occurred in a 1:10 ratio compared with the rate of *E. bieneusi* infection (53). A recent German investigation of 20 HIV-positive patients with intestinal microsporidiosis, including both persons with and persons without diarrhea, also found that *E. intestinalis* occurs with approximately 10% of the frequency of *Enterocytozoon* (89). *E. intestinalis* is present throughout the small intestine, where developing stages and spores are found in the cytoplasm of enterocytes and in the cytoplasm of fibroblasts, macrophages, and endothelial cells of the lamina propria. It can also infect the colon and hepatobiliary tree. The most common clinical presentation of *E. intestinalis* infection, similar to that of *E. bieneusi* infection, is severe chronic diarrhea, which often progresses to malabsorption and wasting syndrome. Unlike *Enterocytozoon*, however, *E. intestinalis* frequently disseminates to involve other organs including the bronchi, renal tubules, nasal epithelium, and the eye (14–16, 18, 40, 59, 63, 64).

E. intestinalis has developmental stages which are somewhat similar to those of the other two species of *Encephalitozoon* (*E. cuniculi* and *E. hellem*) which infect humans. Meronts of *Encephalitozoon* spp. proliferate by cellular elongation and development of cytoplasmic invaginations between nuclei. Sporonts also divide by fission. Similar to *E. hellem* and *E. cuniculi*, sporogony of *E. intestinalis* occurs in the cytoplasm within a parasitophorous vacuole of host origin. The proliferative cells of *E. intestinalis* are uni-, bi-, or tetranucleated. Sporogony is tetrasporous. The most obvious diagnostic ultrastructural feature which characterizes *E. intestinalis* is the formation of a parasite-secreted fibrillar matrix surrounding the developing organisms. This gives the parasitophorous vacuole a septated or honeycombed appearance. Another unique finding is the presence of tubular appendages that are up to 1.2 μm in length and 50 nm in diameter and that originate from the sporont surface and end in a bulbar structure. The mature spores of *E. intestinalis* measure 2.0 by 1.2 μm and contain a single row of polar tubule coils with four to seven turns (79, 82, 99–101).

Recommendations were made to change the taxonomic status of this agent from *S. intestinalis* to *E. intestinalis* on the basis of the results of genetic and immunological analysis (48); most investigators now designate this agent *E. intestinalis* in the medical literature.

E. cuniculi

E. cuniculi, the first microsporidian to be recognized as a parasite of mammals, was first described as an infection in rabbits in 1922. It has a broad host range, infecting birds, carnivores, rodents, and mammals including primates. In nonhuman hosts, *E. cuniculi* has a predilection for the brain and kidneys, but it also infects macrophages, vascular endothelium, and epithelial cells in a variety of organs (20, 45).

Encephalitozoon infections of humans were rarely reported prior to the AIDS pandemic (14–16). Before the identification of *E. hellem* as a separate species in 1991, all *Encephalitozoon* infections in patients with AIDS were believed to be due to *E. cuniculi*. Most of these patients had microsporidial keratoconjunctivitis, but extraocular infections due to *E. cuniculi* were described from one patient with hepatitis and another with peritonitis. Since 1991, most human infections with *Encephalitozoon* have been found to be due to *E. hellem*. Patients with widely disseminated *E. cuniculi* infections have been reported, including infections that involve the central nervous system, heart, kidneys, spleen, lymph nodes, adrenal glands, and trachea (14–16, 31, 75, 77, 79, 82, 101).

E. cuniculi develops in an intracytoplasmic parasitophorous vacuole bounded by a membrane presumably of host cell origin. The nuclei of all stages of both *E. cuniculi* and *E. hellem* are unpaired. Meronts divide by binary fission, are round to ovoid structures measuring 2 to 6 by 1 to 3 μm, and lie in close proximity to the vacuolar membrane. Sporonts lie free in the center of the vacuole and divide into two sporoblasts, which then mature into spores. The spores of both *E. hellem* and *E. cuniculi* measure 2 to 2.5 by 1 to 1.5 μm and have five to seven turns of the coiled polar tubule in a single row (75, 79).

E. hellem

E. hellem is a newly described microsporidian which is morphologically indistinguishable from *E. cuniculi* (79). Before 1991, it was assumed that all *Encephalitozoon* infections in humans were due to *E. cuniculi*. However, in that year Didier and colleagues (36) used biochemical and antigenic methods to describe a new species of *Encephalitozoon*, which they named *E. hellem*, from the eyes of three patients with AIDS and keratoconjunctivitis (Color Plate 1). This new microsporidian was morphologically indistinguishable from *E. cuniculi* by light and electron microscopy. Shortly thereafter, the first patient with disseminated infection and renal failure due to *E. hellem* was described by Schwartz and colleagues (76), and following this, a second patient with systemic *E. hellem* infection and bronchiolitis was reported, also by Schwartz et al. (80). The potential of *E. hellem* to cause disseminated disease in patients with AIDS has now been clearly demon-

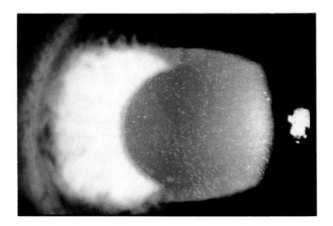

Color Plate 1. Keratoconjunctivitis due to *E. hellem* showing the characteristic finding of punctate epithelial keratopathy by slit-lamp examination.

strated. Infections of trachea, bronchus, lungs, kidneys, ureters, bladder, prostate, nose and paranasal sinuses, cornea, conjunctiva, liver, and peritoneum have been described (14–16, 55, 77, 79, 81, 100, 101). An autopsy of one untreated patient with disseminated *E. hellem* infection demonstrated numerous organisms within the lining epithelium of almost the entire length of the tracheobronchial tree, suggesting a respiratory tract portal of entry and dissemination (76). The developmental stages and ultrastructural features of *E. hellem* are similar to those of *E. cuniculi* (79).

Pleistophora spp.

Pleistophora spp. are microsporidial parasites of insects and fish, including neon tetras, a common aquarium fish. A *Pleistophora* sp. has been reported from the skeletal muscles of two persons (22a, 54a), one of whom was confirmed to have AIDS.

Pleistophora spp. develop within the cytoplasm of host skeletal muscle cells. The parasite secretes a thick, amorphous vesicle that surrounds and isolates the parasite from the host cell cytoplasm. It is termed a sporophorous vesicle. The nuclei of all developmental stages are unpaired, and merogonic proliferation results in multinucleated plasmodia. Sporogony is multisporous and produces large numbers of spores within the sporophorous vesicle. Mature spores measure 2.8 by 3.2 to 3.4 μm and have 9 to 12 coils of the polar tubule (100).

T. hominis and *T. anthropophthera*

Two newly identified microsporidian species, *T. hominis* and *T. anthropophthera*, have been described as agents of myositis and disseminated disease in patients with AIDS, adding to the growing list of microsporidial pathogens of humans (43a, 94, 107). The initial recognition of this new genus of microsporidian occurred in 1996 from the skeletal muscle of a patient with AIDS and myositis (43a). Since then, it has also been identified as causing ring-enhancing lesions of the cerebrum and hippocampus; such lesions are associated with seizures and other symptoms referable to the central nervous system. Autopsy of these patients has revealed disseminated disease also involving the heart, thyroid, pancreas, parathyroids, liver, spleen, bone marrow, and lymph nodes. In culture, meronts of this microsporidian have two to four nuclei and divide by binary fission. A sporophorous vesicle is present, and in this vesicle sporoblasts are formed by repeated binary fission. The number of sporoblasts and later spores within the sporophorous vesicle varies from 2 to greater than 32. Mature spores measure 4.0 by 2.4 μm and have a prominent posterior vacuole. This parasite differs from *Pleistophora* in that it does not form multinucleated sporogonial plasmodia and in that the sporophorous vesicle enlarges during sporogony and its wall is not multilayered (16, 100, 101).

B. vesicularum

B. vesicularum is a newly described microsporidian agent that was first identified in 1998 as a cause of myositis in a patient with AIDS. Because it has only been described from a single patient, little is currently known of its pathogenic potential or biological features (19).

V. corneae (Formerly Nosema corneum)

Nosema spp. are well-described parasites of a variety of invertebrates. Human infections with *Nosema corneum* that cause ocular disease have been reported. *N. corneum* has recently been reassigned to the genus *Vittaforma* (85). *V. corneae* infections have been described in persons with AIDS (34). Rare infections of humans with other *Nosema* spp. have also been described (see below).

The ultrastructural features of *V. corneae* are sufficient for this parasite to be distinguished from the other microsporidian pathogens of humans. Development of the parasite takes place in direct contact with the host cell cytoplasm. Nuclei are diplokaryotic, sporogony is polysporoblastic, and sporonts are ribbon shaped, constricting to give rise to linear arrays of sporoblasts. Each parasite is enveloped by a complete cisterna of host endoplasmic reticulum. The spores of *Vittaforma* measure 3.8 by 1 μm and have five to seven turns of the coiled polar tubule (101).

Nosema algerae and Other Nosema spp.

Nosema connori infection was first described in 1973. It was associated with disseminated infection in an athymic child which involved almost all of the tissues examined at autopsy. Not all stages of the parasite were seen, and only sporoblasts with immature and mature spores could be identified in these tissues. The mature spores of *N. connori* are diplokaryotic, measure 4 to 4.5 by 2 to 2.5 μm, and have approximately 11 turns of the coiled polar tubule. This microsporidian develops in direct contact with the host cell cytoplasm. Another *Nosema* sp., termed *Nosema ocularum*, was identified from biopsy samples from a person with a corneal ulcer. The spores measured 3 by 5 μm and contained polar tubules with 11 to 12 turns (99, 101).

Recently *N. algerae*, a ubiquitous microsporidian parasite of mosquitoes, was isolated from the cornea of an immunocompetent Mexican man with ocular symptoms. Spores had a typical *Nosema* configuration by ultrastructure, and the identity of the agent was confirmed by PCR analysis (95).

Uncharacterized Microsporidia

Microsporidian pathogens of humans which are not sufficiently characterized to be confidently assigned to a known genus are designated by the collective term *Microsporidium*. These include *Microsporidium africanum*, a parasite found in the stroma of a perforated corneal ulcer from a woman from Botswana, and *Microsporidium ceylonensis*, which was isolated from a corneal ulcer in a young boy from Sri Lanka (14, 99–101).

PREVALENCE AND GEOGRAPHIC DISTRIBUTION

There have been no systematic, routine state-sponsored or federally sponsored surveillance programs for microsporidial infections anywhere in the world, and it is not a reportable disease in the United States. As a result, and because studies based on truly random samples have rarely, if ever, been conducted for microsporidiosis, reliable estimates of its prevalence are not available. Those reports of prevalence in the literature generally refer to highly selected population groups such as AIDS patients with chronic diarrhea and have relied upon studies with noncontrolled, nonrandom designs, including prospective cohort studies, retrospective specimen and chart reviews, and limited surveys with primarily convenience samples. Also problematic has been the lack of consistency in terms of diagnostic approaches and case selection criteria. These factors, in conjunction with the multiple species and diverse clinical manifestations of human microsporidian infections, make it very difficult to understand the true burden of disease attributable to microsporidiosis.

Despite these drawbacks, investigations conducted worldwide reveal reasonably consistent results for some patient populations. Most of what is now known about human microsporidiosis can be attributed to experience with patients with HIV infection or AIDS. Since 1985 and the first recognition of *E. bieneusi* as an AIDS-associated opportunistic infection (35), several hundred patients with chronic diarrhea attributed to this organism have been reported. Worldwide, between 1989 and 1998, at least 25 published studies of AIDS patients with chronic diarrhea have reported prevalences of *E. bieneusi* infections ranging from 4 to 50%. Combined, these studies have evaluated over 2,400 patients and have confirmed some 375 cases of *E. bieneusi* infection, for an overall prevalence of approximately 15% (15). These observations suggest that we can reasonably expect that *E. bieneusi* accounts for a significant proportion of the chronic diarrheal disease observed in patients with AIDS. Although closer scrutiny is needed, there appears to be no consistent trends or variations in prevalence on the basis of country of origin or other demographic characteristics (11–14, 30, 41, 54, 89, 93, 96, 99).

Although human disease associated with microsporidia has been reported predominantly from developed nations in North America, Western Europe, and Australia, the recognition of human microsporidiosis is on the rise worldwide. Persons suffering from a variety of microsporidian disease manifestations have been identified from all continents except Antarctica. With new interest in the organisms and improved diagnostic approaches, recognition of microsporidian disease in the Third World is increasingly common. Human infections are now well documented in several African nations (5, 22, 41, 49, 56, 93), southeast Asia (60), and Central and South America (11, 43, 106).

SEROLOGIC STUDIES

Surveys for antibodies to microsporidia in human sera have focused exclusively on human exposure to *Encephalitozoon* species. The frequency of positive specimens ranged from 0 to 38% for the various population groups evaluated prior to 1991 (7, 12, 50, 87). Those studies, however, lacked clinical or pathologic correlations and failed to produce any definitive epidemiologic conclusions. Since that time, only a few serologic investigations have been performed. Earlier studies targeted (presumably) *E. cuniculi*, but recent publications have reported results based on human immunoreactivity to *E. intestinalis* and *E. hellem* as well. In three studies published in 1997, human sera from France, The Netherlands, Slovakia, and the Czech Republic were variably screened for antibodies to *Encephalitozoon* species by such techniques as enzyme-linked immunosorbent assay (ELISA), the indirect fluorescent-antibody test, counterimmunoelectrophoresis, and the complement fixation test. Van Gool and colleagues (92) found antibodies to *E. intestinalis* among pregnant French women (5%) and Dutch blood donors (8%). HIV-infected Czech patients were screened by Pospisilova and colleagues (65), who found that 5.3% were seropositive for *E. cuniculi*, while 1.3% were seropositive for *E. hellem*; all (presumably HIV-negative) blood donors who were screened were seronegative for both species. In Slovakia, Cislakova and colleagues (23) found that 5.1% of slaughterhouse workers were seropositive for *Encephalitozoon* species (not specified) but that 92 forestry workers, 22 dog breeders, and 150 blood donors were all seronegative. These more recent studies suffer from many of the same limitations as those of earlier years, including the use of convenience rather than random sampling techniques, but they do suggest that human infections with *Encephalitozoon* species may be more common than was previously recognized.

CASE DEMOGRAPHICS AND POPULATIONS AT RISK

The overwhelming majority of serious illnesses which have been reported to result from infections with the various human-infecting microsporidia appears to occur predominantly in adults suffering from HIV-associated immunosuppression (100). Human microsporidiosis, however, is increasingly being recognized in persons with other forms of immunosuppression. Infections with *E. bieneusi*, for example, have been confirmed in (one patient each) HIV-negative liver and heart-lung transplant recipients (67, 71). Cotte and colleagues (28) also noted a number of *E. bieneusi* infections in bone marrow, heart-lung, liver, and kidney transplant recipients during a possible outbreak of intestinal microsporidiosis in France in 1995. *E. cuniculi* was recently identified in a kidney-pancreas transplant recipient (47) (Fig. 1), and a case of pulmonary microsporidial infection (presumably infection with an *Encephalitozoon* species) was confirmed at autopsy in a patient with chronic myeloid leukemia who had undergone bone marrow transplantation (52). Transplant recipients, however, do not appear to be the only HIV-negative, immunosuppressed populations at risk for microsporidiosis. Silverstein and colleagues (86) described a patient who developed chronic bilateral microsporidial keratoconjunctivitis while taking systemic prednisone (20 mg per day) for severe asthma. Although the infecting species was not reported, the organisms pictured were consistent with *Encephalitozoon*, and the patient responded successfully to therapy with albendazole. In yet another case of non-HIV-associated immunosuppression, Wanke and colleagues (98) observed a patient with *E. bieneusi*-associated diarrhea who had an unexplained decreased CD4-cell count and a history of cryptococcal meningitis. Interestingly, this patient also responded successfully to therapy with albendazole. With these various reports in mind, it is reasonable to anticipate that the recognition of microsporidiosis in association with other, non-HIV-associated forms of immunosuppression will continue to increase.

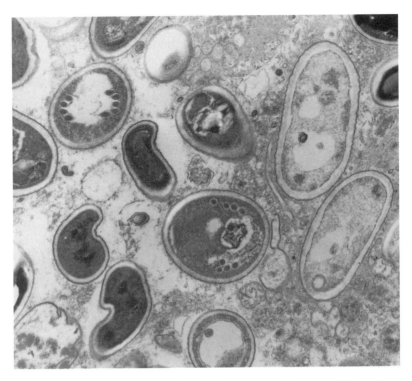

Figure 1. Sample from a transplanted kidney removed from an HIV-negative kidney-pancreas transplant recipient following development of renal failure. Microsporidiosis due to *E. cuniculi* was identified as the cause of renal failure. This electron micrograph shows mature spores of *E. cuniculi* within necrotic renal tubules. Magnification, ×20,000.

Although most recognized cases of human microsporidiosis are associated with some form of immunosuppression, reports describing microsporidial infections in HIV-negative, immunocompetent patients are also increasing. These reports have included instances of *E. bieneusi* infections in travelers as well as in adults and children who reside in various countries in tropical regions (2, 17, 22, 28, 49, 56, 70, 88, 98). Also, Raynaud and colleagues (68) have reported on the first association of *E. intestinalis* with chronic diarrhea in immunocompetent travelers. It is interesting to speculate, therefore, that intestinal microsporidiosis may be an underappreciated cause of traveler's diarrhea that warrants further investigation. Heightened awareness of this disease by clinicians who care for travelers returning from tropical destinations should help to increase our recognition and, ultimately, our understanding of the epidemiology of this disease.

POTENTIAL MODES OF TRANSMISSION

Zoonotic Infections

E. cuniculi

Microsporidian infections in a wide variety of invertebrates and vertebrates were well recognized prior to the initial report of human infection in 1959. *E. cuniculi* was first described in a rabbit with motor paralysis by Wright and Craighead in 1922 (105). Because it is the first mammalian microsporidian which was grown in culture, it is the most extensively studied microsporidian that infects mammals. It has a broad host range, and a partial listing of potential hosts include the rabbit, mouse, rat, muskrat, guinea pig, hamster, ground shrew, fox, cat, leopard, puma, squirrel monkey, rhesus monkey, baboon, goat, sheep, dog, swine, and horse (20). *E. cuniculi* was for many years the sole member of its genus. Many of the initially described microsporidian infections of humans, both prior to and during the AIDS pandemic, have been due to *Encephalitozoon*-like organisms. These isolates microscopically resembled *E. cuniculi*, and thus, they were believed to be due to this microsporidian. However, the isolation from three AIDS patients in 1991 of a morphologically identical but antigenically and biochemically distinct species of *Encephalitozoon, E. hellem*, raised the possibility that some previously reported human infections had resulted from this newly discovered agent and not from *E. cuniculi*. Additional confirmation of the importance of *E. hellem* as a human pathogen was obtained in 1993, when Schwartz and colleagues (77), using antibody-based methods, identified *E. hellem* but not *E. cuniculi* from the eyes of seven patients with AIDS and keratoconjunctivitis. The existence of *E. cuniculi* infections in humans was in doubt until 1995, when disseminated *E. cuniculi* was confirmed in an AIDS patient by both nucleic acid-based and tissue culture methods (31). Since then, additional molecular typing method- and antibody-confirmed cases of *E. cuniculi* infection in patients with AIDS have been reported (33, 37, 58).

Because of differences in the parasite distribution and lesions seen in animals with natural *E. cuniculi* infections, Weiser (102, 103) believed that strain differences might exist. In 1995 Didier and colleagues (38) found that *E. cuniculi* isolates obtained from rabbits, dogs, and mice could be differentiated on the basis of subtle differences in protein profiles in the 54- to 59-kDa range using sodium dodecyl sulfate-polyacrylamide gel electrophoresis and antigenic analysis and differences in the 5′-GTTT-3′ repeats present in the internal transcribed spacer region of the ribosomal DNA identified by PCR. They designated these isolates strain I (rabbits and one mouse), strain II (murine only), and strain III (domestic dogs only). Using similar methods, Didier and colleagues (37) examined an isolate of *E. cuniculi* obtained from a patient with AIDS and disseminated microsporidiosis. They found that the ribosomal DNA internal transcribed spacer region of this isolate was identical to that of *E. cuniculi* III, which had been isolated only from domestic dogs. Although the patient owned a dog, no microsporidia were detected in the pet's urine (37).

Additional evidence is accumulating that human *E. cuniculi* infections may result from animal sources. Deplazes and colleagues (32) reported that *E. cuniculi* I, originally described from rabbits, has been identified as infecting humans in Switzerland. Four *E. cuniculi* isolates from HIV-infected patients living in Switzerland were indistinguishable by immunological and molecular methods from isolates obtained from Swiss rabbits (58). None of these patients either owned a rabbit or remembered having been exposed to a rabbit as an adult. However, one patient grew up on a farm where rabbits and other animals were raised, and another two patients kept a variety of pets.

Natural infections of nonhuman primates with an *Encephalitozoon* species have been described. In a primate colony housing 250 squirrel monkeys (*Saimiri sciureus*), immunofluorescence and dot-ELISA techniques revealed serum antibodies to *E. cuniculi* at least once in 179 monkeys and three or more times in 56 monkeys (84). The animals had organisms and granulomatous infections in a variety of organs including brains, kidneys, lungs, adrenal glands, and livers (108). Nonhuman primates are also susceptible to experimental infection with several microsporidian agents which also infect humans, including *E. cuniculi* (39), *E. hellem* (39), and *E. bieneusi* (see below).

The source of human *E. cuniculi* infections and the mechanism(s) of transmission are still not clear. Although too few *E. cuniculi* infections of humans have been analyzed to provide firm evidence of zoonotic transmission, it appears likely that at least some cases of human infection are acquired from animals.

E. hellem

Several reports based upon light and electron microscopy have described *Encephalitozoon* infection of psittacine birds, and considerable interest regarding the possible role of these animals as potential reservoirs of human infection has been raised. Following the discovery of *E. hellem* in 1991 by Didier and colleagues (36), efforts to isolate this agent from nonhuman sources proved to be unsuccessful, and for several years it was believed that the organism was confined to human hosts. However, in 1997 an *Encephalitozoon* species was reported to cause fatal microsporidian disease in young birds from a budgerigar, or parakeet (*Melopsittacus undulatus*), aviary in Mississippi. The birds, chicks from 1 to 2 weeks of age, had heavy microsporidian infection of the intestines and multifocal microsporidian hepatic necrosis. Southern blotting and PCR confirmed that the etiologic agent was *E. hellem* (9). This was followed by a report in 1998 of *E. hellem* infection in a different avian host, *Eclectus roratus* (the eclectus parrot). Microsporidia were identified in this bird from liver and kidney sections submitted following autopsy and were confirmed to be *E. hellem* by PCR (66). *E. hellem* has not been identified thus far from nonhuman mammals, but it is possible that mammalian isolates which were previously believed to be *E. cuniculi* by morphological methods are, in fact, *E. hellem*. Although some patients with AIDS who have developed *E. hellem* infection keep companion animals and birds (76), there has been no documentation of concurrent infection of both humans and their companion animals with this microsporidian.

E. (Formerly *Septata*) *intestinalis*

E. intestinalis is the most recent addition to the genus *Encephalitozoon*. Humans remained the only recognized host of this agent until 1998, when Bornay-Llinares (10) and colleagues described *E. intestinalis* in stools from a variety of mammals in Mexico. Spores of *E. intestinalis* were identified in stool specimens from five different animals (donkey, pig, dog, cow, and goat) collected during an epidemiologic survey in two rural villages in Pueblo State. Light microscopic examination of stools showed within the cytoplasms of shed epithelial cells clusters of microsporidian spores morphologically consistent with an *Encephalitozoon* spp. In those stool samples with a high parasite burden, there was ultrastructural evidence of an *Encephalitozoon*-type infection (Fig. 2). The identity of the microsporidia as *E. intestinalis* was confirmed with an anti-*E. intestinalis* antiserum and by PCR.

Prior to the AIDS pandemic, an intestinal microsporidian was identified in 1973 at necropsy from a female *Callicebus moloch* monkey which had been housed in a primate colony (83). Although the morphologic features of this agent were somewhat unclear, it was believed to resemble an *Encephalitozoon* spp. on the basis of light and electron microscopy. In retrospect, it is possible that this agent might have represented the then-undiscovered microsporidian *E. intestinalis*.

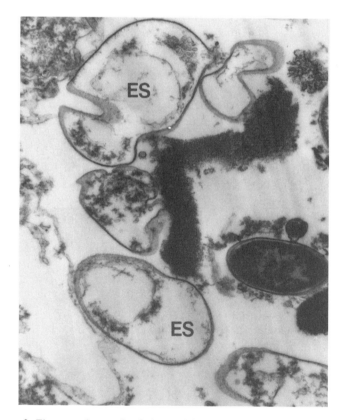

Figure 2. Electron micrograph of pig stool from Mexico showing empty microsporidian spores (ES). These microsporidia were identified as *E. intestinalis* by species-specific fluorescent-antibody examination and PCR. Magnification, ca. ×31,500.

E. bieneusi

Following the initial description of *E. bieneusi* as a cause of diarrhea and wasting syndrome in patients with AIDS in 1985, this agent has been found to be the most prevalent cause of microsporidian infection of humans. However, its potential environmental source(s) continues to elude the scientific community. *E. bieneusi* was first identified in a nonhuman host in 1996, when Deplazes and colleagues (33) described spores from immature and adult pigs in Switzerland. The identity of these spores was confirmed to be *E. bieneusi* by DNA analysis. Following that report, there were independent reports on two geographically disparate primate colonies describing naturally acquired *E. bieneusi* infections in captive macaques (4, 21, 57, 74). All of the animals had been experimentally infected with the simian immunodeficiency virus (SIV) prior to the diagnosis of microsporidiosis at the time of necropsy. Although most infected macaques were *Macaca mulatta*, a few *Macaca cyclopis* and *Macaca nemestrina* macaques also had *E. bieneusi* infections. An interesting feature of the pathology of these primates was that the majority of the parasite burden resided in the gallbladder and not, as has been described for human infections, in the small intestine (57, 74). More recently, Mansfield and colleagues (21) have found *E. bieneusi* infections in immunocompetent, non-SIV-infected macaques from the same primate colony. The environmental source for both human and nonhuman primate infections remains unknown.

In addition to the occurrence of natural infections of macaques with *Enterocytozoon*, this agent has been experimentally transmitted from a human with AIDS and intestinal microsporidiosis to SIV-infected macaques via oral inoculation with concentrated spores (91). Infected animals began to shed spores within 1 week after inoculation and continued to shed spores until they were killed 7 to 8 months later. Microscopic examination of the intestine and hepatobiliary tract revealed that the parasite burden was so sparse that *E. bieneusi* could be detected only by in situ hybridization techniques.

Waterborne Transmission

Some intestinal protozoa, such as *Giardia*, *Cyclospora*, and *Cryptosporidium*, are commonly acquired by ingestion of contaminated water (or food), suggesting that the same may be true for *E. bieneusi* and *E. intestinalis* (27). Unfortunately, the potential environmental sources of the microsporidia that infect humans have been poorly researched. Recent observations, however, are beginning to provide a stronger scientific foundation for the theory of waterborne transmission of some forms of human microsporidiosis.

Microsporidia have been isolated from ditch water in a mosquito larval habitat in Florida (6). Several genera, including two which were potentially infective to humans, *Pleistophora* and *Nosema*, were identified. The first identification of a pathogenic human microsporidian from a natural water source was reported in 1997 (90). Spores of *E. bieneusi*, the most prevalent microsporidian that infects humans, were identified by a novel filtration-PCR method in samples of environmental surface water from the River Seine in France. Other microsporidian species potentially infective for humans, including *Pleistophora* sp. and *V. corneae*, were identified in water from the Rivers Loire and Seine by this technique.

Several groups of investigators working separately in different parts of the world have found that water contact may be an independent risk factor for intestinal microsporidiosis. A case-control study was conducted in clinics serving HIV-infected persons in Massachusetts and Texas to identify environmental risk factors for acquiring intestinal infection (98a). Twelve patients with intestinal microsporidiosis and 54 uninfected controls were enrolled. Risk factors for the acquisition of microsporidiosis in HIV-infected persons included swimming in rivers, ponds, and lakes and drinking unfiltered tap water. In 1997, another prospective unmatched case-control study of risk factors for the acquisition of intestinal microsporidiosis was conducted among HIV-infected patients ($<$200 CD4 cells/mm^3) in France (51). The only two factors which were associated with microsporidian infection were swimming in a pool and male homosexuality. These investigators suggested that the mode of transmission of intestinal microsporidiosis is fecal-oral, including water-borne and person-to-person transmission.

In 1998 Cotte and colleagues (28) reported on an outbreak of intestinal microsporidiosis in HIV-infected persons which occurred in mid-1995 in France. In a retrospective study of 1,453 patients (978 HIV-infected and 395 HIV-uninfected patients) who underwent stool examinations for microsporidia in Lyon, France, between April 1993 and December 1996, a cluster of microsporidiosis cases was noted to occur from May to November 1995. Two hundred infected patients were identified during this outbreak, whereas 138 "endemic" cases of infection were found outside the outbreak period. Both HIV-infected and HIV-uninfected persons were found to have intestinal microsporidiosis in each period. Variations in the geographic distribution of the affected patients during the outbreak were suggestive of an association between the municipal water distribution system and the occurrence of the outbreak. However, none of the typical markers for fecal contamination of water were identified during or outside the outbreak period.

In the most recent study to address the potential for waterborne transmission, Enriquez and colleagues (43) assessed the prevalence of *E. intestinalis* in two rural, agricultural communities in central Mexico. This cross-sectional survey revealed that 15 (21.4%) of 70 households had at least one member who was infected with this organism. They also found that the use of untreated water from an indoor faucet and the use of community wells as a primary water source were significantly more common in those households with an *E. intestinalis*-infected resident. Furthermore, the use of a private well as the primary household water source appeared to be protective.

Two studies have failed to show an association of water with intestinal microsporidiosis. In Brazil, Wuhib and colleagues (106) examined stool specimens from 166 HIV-infected persons to determine the prevalence of intestinal parasites. In addition to their finding that cryptosporidiosis and microsporidiosis were the most common intestinal parasites, cryptosporidial but not microsporidial infection was found to be associated with the rainy season. That study, however, did not examine the specific forms of water contact (swimming, drinking, and humidifier use) which were observed as risk factors in the previously discussed investigations. Conteas and colleagues (24) examined 8,439 stool specimens from HIV-infected persons in southern California from 1993 to 1996 and found no seasonal association with either recreational water use or seasonal contamination of the water supply.

In summary, although data in support of waterborne transmission are accumulating, some uncertainty remains. It is likely, however, that waterborne transmission of human microsporidiosis does indeed occur. Further studies are needed to confirm a definitive link between human infections and contaminated water sources before appropriate public health initiatives are considered.

Airborne Transmission and Respiratory Tract Acquisition

The occurrence of upper and lower respiratory tract infections suggests that microsporidiosis can be acquired by inhalation or can be transmitted via aerosolized infected materials. In the mouse model of microsporidiosis, oral, intranasal, and intratracheal applications of *E. cuniculi* lead to disseminated infections (29, 104). Transmission via the aerosol route has especially been implicated as a likely route of infection in some of the reported cases of *E. hellem* infection. The initial evidence for respiratory acquisition was based upon the unexpected autopsy findings of prominent respiratory epithelial *E. hellem* infection that extended confluently from the proximal trachea down to the terminal bronchioles in the first patient with AIDS and disseminated microsporidiosis to be described (76). This superficial pattern of respiratory epithelial infection was similar to that seen in other infections which have a respiratory route of acquisition. Since then many additional cases of microsporidial respiratory infection have been reported (55, 80). Several cases of *E. hellem* infection limited to the paranasal sinuses but in which intestinal infection was notably absent have been described (1, 42, 72), providing indirect evidence for primary respiratory tract infection. Many patients with *Encephalitozoon* infections present with initial symptoms of sinonasal disease, suggesting an upper respiratory portal of entry in these cases.

The presence of *Encephalitozoon* spores in respiratory secretions as well as urine has led to the suggestion that ocular infections with these agents may be acquired by external autoinoculation, perhaps by contaminated fingers (77). Ingestion or inhalation of spore-laden urine contaminating animal cages is an established means of *E. cuniculi* transmission in rabbits and other laboratory animals, suggesting that comparable forms of environmental exposure could lead to human infection. Because *E. hellem* has recently been isolated from bird feces, it is conceivable that this agent is acquired through inhalation of aerosolized fecal material containing infective spores, a route of transmission that is well documented for *Cryptococcus neoformans*.

Transmission via Insects

Microsporidia are parasitic in a broad range of insects. There had been no evidence for transmission of these agents to humans until recently, when a 61-year-old immunocompetent non-HIV-infected man from Mexico developed ocular symptoms due to a *Nosema*-like microsporidian. The agent was ultimately isolated and was identified by ultrastructure, immunofluorescence, and Western blot and

PCR analyses as *N. algerae* (95). This microsporidian is a common parasite of anopheline mosquitoes and represents the first insect microsporidian to be reported as a human pathogen. The mechanism by which this infection occurred remains unknown. Although a parasite of mosquitoes, *N. algerae* has been cultivated in continuous culture of mammalian cells at 37°C, indicating that this microsporidian can survive and replicate at human body temperature (61). These observations may have important consequences in identification of future *Nosema* isolates from humans.

Direct Person-to-Person Transmission

Diffuse involvement of the urinary tract is typical of disseminated infections due to all *Encephalitozoon* species. The identification of a prostatic abscess (81) and urethral infection (8, 26, 76) in some male patients raises the possibility that person-to-person transmission by sexual means may be at least anatomically feasible.

The recent identification of concurrent microsporidial infection in homosexual male sexual partners has drawn attention to the potential of person-to-person transmission. In one set of infections involving a cohabitating pair of male partners who were both infected with microsporidia, the sexual partner of a patient with intestinal microsporidiosis was diagnosed with microsporidial urethritis, which did not resolve until he abstained from unprotected sexual intercourse and treatment with albendazole was initiated (8). The patient's good response to albendazole therapy and the organ systems affected together seem to indicate infection with an *Encephalitozoon* spp., but the etiologic agent was not further characterized by the investigators. They concluded that sexual transmission of microsporidia was the most probable explanation for the patient's urethritis.

Four additional cohabitating homosexual male partner pairs have been found to have concurrent microsporidiosis (78). Three of these four sets of men were concurrently infected with HIV. In the fourth partner pair, one partner was HIV infected and the other was not. In all four pairs the partners were alive and infected with microsporidia concurrently with one another, were infected with the same microsporidian species, and were shedding spores in either feces or body fluids. Two partner pairs were infected with *E. hellem*, one pair was infected with *E. bieneusi*, and the HIV-discordant pair was infected with *E. intestinalis*.

Other investigators have reported that microsporidiosis is more prevalent among their homosexual patients than among other risk groups (96). Two prospective case-control studies have shown that male homosexuality (51) and having an HIV-infected cohabitant (98a) are risk factors for the acquisition of intestinal microsporidiosis. Interestingly, in the mouse, rectal installation of *E. cuniculi* has been shown to cause disseminated infections (45).

Although the circumstantial evidence seems strong, the documentation of infections of sexual partners does not prove the sexual transmissibility of microsporidia. It is conceivable that infections of sexual partners are the result of fecal-oral, urinary-oral, or common-source transmission. The well-documented presence of viable, infective spores in multiple body fluids and excreta is consistent with all of these potential modes of transmission.

PREVENTION

Microsporidian spores can survive and can remain infective in the environment for extended periods of time. In vitro data evaluating the potential efficacy of preventive measures have been published only for *E. cuniculi* (97). These experiments indicate that spores can survive in the environment for months to years, depending on humidity and temperature. Even in a typical dry hospital environment (22°C) spores can survive for at least a month. Exposure to recommended working concentrations of most disinfectants for 30 min, boiling for 5 min, and autoclaving at 120°C were reported to kill the spores. Freezing may not be an effective means of disinfection, as it has been possible to grow *E. hellem* successfully after storing it at −70°C for months. Because *E. intestinalis* has only recently been sustained in culture and *E. bieneusi* has been grown successfully only in short-term cultures, the potential infectivities of both parasites as well as the efficacies of preventive measures have not been evaluated.

For these reasons, data in support of effective preventive strategies are limited. However, the presence of infective spores in body fluids and feces suggests that standard precautions in health care and other institutional settings, general attention to hand washing, and other personal hygiene measures may be helpful in preventing primary infections. Meticulous hand washing may be of particular importance in preventing ocular infection, which may occur as a result of inoculation of conjunctival surfaces by fingers contaminated with respiratory fluids or urine. Whether respiratory precautions might be efficacious for persons documented to have spores in sputum or other respiratory secretions is unknown. Similarly, precautions pertinent to environmental or zoonotic exposure to microsporidia are as yet undefined (13).

Whether primary prophylaxis with antimicrobial agents is possible remains to be determined. Co-trimoxazole and atovaquone (for *Pneumocystis carinii* and *Toxoplasma gondii* infections) and azithromycin (for mycobacterial infections) are effective or are under investigation for prophylactic treatment of other opportunistic infections in patients with AIDS. It is possible that the use of these agents could also reduce the incidence of microsporidiosis. *E. bieneusi* infection, however, has been detected in patients receiving clindamycin, trimethoprim-sulfamethoxazole (TMP-SMX), dapsone, pyrimethamine, and itraconazole. In a prospective evaluation of a series of 76 patients in Hamburg, Germany, 3 of 22 patients (14%) who were on TMP-SMX for *P. carinii* prophylaxis developed *E. bieneusi* infection, whereas 11 of 54 patients (20%) who were on inhalational pentamidine prophylaxis or who did not receive any prophylaxis developed *E. bieneusi* infection ($P > 0.2$) (3). Even though these numbers are small, it seems that the currently used prophylactic dosage of 960 mg per day will offer no or, at best, minimal protection from *E. bieneusi* infection. Four of five patients with disseminated *E. intestinalis* infection reported by Molina and associates (59) also received TMP-SMX prior to the diagnosis of infection, indicating that TMP-SMX is also ineffective in preventing *E. intestinalis* infection. Future trials that evaluate prophylactic strategies that use drugs with potential antimicrosporidial activities should attempt to address this question. Finally, although its efficacy as a therapeutic agent for *Encephalito-*

zoon infections is well confirmed (26, 31, 40, 59), rigorous clinical trials with albendazole for primary or secondary prophylaxis have yet to be performed.

One of the most exciting observations in the prevention of microsporidiosis in persons with AIDS has been the role of highly active antiretroviral therapy (HAART) in raising CD4 lymphocyte counts and heightening immunity. Several small studies have now shown that administration of a protease inhibitor together with one or two nucleoside analogues has resulted in remission of the diarrheal symptoms of most patients with microsporidian-associated diarrhea (25, 44, 46). In some patients, the stool was persistently negative for microsporidian-spores for up to 10 months after treatment. Although HAART is a promising treatment regimen for the prevention of microsporidiosis in patients with AIDS, long-term follow-up is needed to assess whether these patients are actually free of the intracellular stages of microsporidia or are temporarily in remission with an inactive infection.

A high standard of personal hygiene seems mandatory for patients infected with microsporidia. HIV-positive persons are already advised to avoid raw eggs and undercooked meat in order to avoid exposure to *Salmonella* spp. and *Toxoplasma gondii*. Because *E. cuniculi* can infect eggs and consumable animals such as rabbits, this general recommendation should be reinforced (69). In addition, infected patients should be warned that sexual transmission of microsporidiosis cannot be excluded. Cohabitating sexual partners of infected patients should be offered screening for microsporidiosis regardless of their HIV status.

REFERENCES

1. **Albrecht, H., and D. A. Schwartz.** 1998. Unpublished data.
2. **Albrecht, H., and I. Sobottka.** 1997. *Enterocytozoon bieneusi* infection in patients who are not infected with human immunodeficiency virus. *Clin. Infect. Dis.* **25:**344.
3. **Albrecht, H., I. Sobottka, H. J. Stellbrink, and H. Greten.** 1995. Does the choice of *Pneumocystis carinii* prophylaxis influence the prevalence of *Enterocytozoon bieneusi* microsporidiosis in AIDS-patients? *AIDS* **9:**302–303.
4. **Anderson, D. C., S. A. Klumpp, A. J. Da Silva, N. J. Pieniazek, H. M. McClure, and D. A. Schwartz.** 1997. Naturally-acquired *Enterocytozoon bieneusi* (Microsporida) hepatobiliary infection in rhesus monkeys with simian immunodeficiency virus (SIV): a possible animal model of disease, abstr. K-120b, p. 349. *In Abstracts of the 37th Interscience Conference on Antimicrobial Agents and Chemotherapy.* American Society for Microbiology, Washington, D.C.
5. **Aoun, K., A. Bouratbine, A. Datry, S. Biligui, and R. Ben Ismail.** 1997. Presence of intestinal microsporidia in Tunisia: apropos of 1 case. *Bull. Soc. Pathol. Exot.* **90:**176. (In French.)
6. **Avery, S. W., and A. H. Undeen.** 1987. The isolation of microsporidia and other pathogens from concentrated ditch water. *J. Am. Mosq. Control Assoc.* **3:**54–58.
7. **Bergquist, R., L. Morfeldt-Mansson, P. O. Pherson, B. Petrini, and J. Wasserman.** 1984. Antibody against *Encephalitozoon cuniculi* in Swedish homosexual men. *Scand. J. Infect. Dis.* **16:**389–391.
8. **Birthistle, K., P. Moore, and P. Hay.** 1996. Microsporidia: a new sexually transmissible cause of urethritis. *Genitourin. Med.* **72:**445.
9. **Black, S. S., L. A. Steinohrt, D. C. Bertucci, L. B. Rogers, and E. S. Didier.** 1997. *Encephalitozoon hellem* in budgerigars (*Melopsittacus undulatus*). *Vet. Pathol.* **34:**189–198.
10. **Bornay-Llinares, F. J., A. J. da Silva, H. Moura, D. A. Schwartz, G. S. Visvesvara, N. J. Pieniazek, A. Cruz-Lopez, P. Hernandez-Jauregui, and J. Enriquez.** 1998. Immunological, mi-

croscopic and molecular evidence of *Encephalitozoon* (*Septata*) *intestinalis* infection in mammals other than man. *J. Infect. Dis.* **178:**820–826.

11. **Brasil, P., F. C. Sodre, T. Cuzzi-Maya, M. C. Gutierrez, H. Mattos, and H. Moura.** 1996. Intestinal microsporidiosis in HIV-positive patients with chronic unexplained diarrhea in Rio de Janeiro, Brazil: diagnosis, clinical presentation, and follow-up. *Rev. Inst. Med. Trop. Sao Paulo* **38:**97–102.

12. **Bryan, R. T., A. Cali, R. L. Owen, and H. C. Spencer.** 1991. Microsporidia: opportunistic pathogens in patients with AIDS, p. 1–26. *In* T. Sun (ed.), *Progress in Clinical Parasitology*, vol. 2. Field & Wood, Philadelphia, Pa.

13. **Bryan, R. T.** 1995. Microsporidiosis as an AIDS-related opportunistic infection. *Clin. Infect. Dis.* **21**(Suppl.):S62–S65.

14. **Bryan, R. T.** 1995. Microsporidia, p. 2513–2524. *In* G. L. Mandell, J. E. Bennett, and R. Dolin (ed.), *Principles and Practice of Infectious Diseases*, 4th ed. Churchill Livingstone, New York, N.Y.

15. **Bryan, R. T., and D. A. Schwartz.** 1999. Epidemiology of microsporidiosis, p. 502–516. *In* M. Wittner and L. M. Weiss (ed.), *The Microsporidia and Microsporidiosis*. ASM Press, Washington, D.C.

16. **Bryan, R. T., R. Weber, and D. A. Schwartz.** Microsporidiosis. *In* R. L. Guerrant, D. J. Krogstad, J. H. Maguire, D. H. Walker, and P. F. Weller (ed.), *Tropical Infectious Diseases: Principles, Pathogens, and Practice,* in press. Churchill Livingstone, Edinburgh, United Kingdom.

17. **Bryan, R. T., R. Weber, and D. A. Schwartz.** 1997. Microsporidiosis in persons without HIV. *Clin. Infect. Dis.* **24:**534–535. (Letter.)

18. **Cali, A., D. P. Kotler, and J. M. Orenstein.** 1993. *Septata intestinalis* n.g., n.sp., an intestinal microsporidian associated with chronic diarrhea and dissemination in AIDS patients. *J. Eukaryot. Microbiol.* **40:**101–112.

19. **Cali, A., P. M. Takvorian, S. Lewin, et al.** 1998. *Brachiola vesicularum*, n.g., n.sp., a new microsporidium associated with AIDS and myositis. *J. Eukaryot. Microbiol.* **45:**240–251.

20. **Canning, E. U., and W. S. Hollister.** 1987. Microsporidia of mammals—widespread pathogens or opportunistic curiosities? *Parasitol. Today* **3:**267–273.

21. **Carville, A., K. Mansfield, K. C. Lin, J. McKay, L. Chalifoux, and A. Lackner.** 1997. Genetic and ultrastructural characterization of *Enterocytozoon bieneusi* in simian immunodeficiency virus infected and immunocompetent rhesus macaques. *Vet. Pathol.* **34:**515.

22. **Cegielski, J. P., Y. R. Ortega, S. McKee, J. F. Madden, L. Gaido, D. A. Schwartz, K. Manji, A. F. Jorgensen, S. E. Miller, U. P. Pulipaka, A. E. Msengi, D. H. Mwakyusa, C. R. Sterling, and L. B. Reller.** 1999. *Cryptosporidium, Enterocytozoon,* and *Cyclospora* infections in pediatric and adult patients with diarrhea in Tanzania. *Clin. Infect. Dis.* **28:**314–321.

22a.**Chupp, G. L., J. Alroy, L. S. Adelman, J. C. Breen, and P. R. Skolnik.** 1993. Myositis due to *Pleistophora* (microsporidia) in a patient with AIDS. *Clin. Infect. Dis.* **16:**15–21.

23. **Cislakova, L., H. Prokopcakova, M. Stefkovic, and M. Halanova.** 1997. *Encephalitozoon cuniculi*—clinical and epidemiologic significance. Results of a preliminary serologic study in humans. *Epidemiol. Mikrobiol. Imunol.* **46:**30–33.

24. **Conteas, C. N., O. G. W. Berlin, M. J. Lariviere, S. S. Pandhumas, C. E. Speck, R. Porschen, and T. Nakaya.** 1998. Examination of the prevalence and seasonal variation of intestinal microsporidiosis in the stools of persons with chronic diarrhea and human immunodeficiency virus infection. *Am. J. Trop. Med. Hyg.* **58:**559–561.

25. **Conteas, C. N., O. G. W. Berlin, C. E. Speck, S. S. Pandhumas, M. J. Lariviere, and C. Fu.** 1998. Modification of the clinical course of intestinal microsporidiosis in acquired immunodeficiency syndrome patients by immune status and anti-human immunodeficiency virus therapy. *Am. J. Trop. Med. Hyg.* **58:**555–558.

26. **Corcoran, G. D., J. R. Isaacson, C. Daniels, and P. L. Chiodini.** 1996. Urethritis associated with disseminated microsporidiosis: clinical response to albendazole. *Clin. Infect. Dis.* **22:**592–593.

27. **Cornet, M., S. Romand, J. Warszawski, and P. Bouree.** 1996. Factors associated with microsporidial and cryptosporidial diarrhea in HIV infected patients. *Parasite* **3:**397–401.

28. **Cotte, L., M. Rabodonirina, C. Raynal, F. Chapuis, M. A. Piens, and C. Trepo.** 1998. Outbreak of intestinal microsporidiosis in HIV-infected and non-infected patients, abstr. 483. *In Abstracts of the 5th Conference on Retroviruses and Opportunistic Infections*.

29. **Cox, J. C., R. C. Hamilton, and H. D. Attwood.** 1979. An investigation of the route and progression of *Encephalitozoon cuniculi* in adult rabbits. *J. Protozool.* **26:**260–265.

30. **Coyle, C. M., M. Wittner, D. P. Kotler, C. Noyer, J. M. Orenstein, H. B. Tanowitz, and L. M. Weiss.** 1996. Prevalence of microsporidiosis due to *Enterocytozoon bieneusi* and *Encephalitozoon intestinalis* among patients with AIDS-related diarrhea: determination by polymerase chain reaction to the microsporidian small-subunit rRNA gene. *Clin. Infect. Dis.* **23:**1002–1006.

31. **De Groote, M. A., G. S. Visvesvara, M. L. Wilson, N. J. Pieniazek, S. B. Slemenda, A. J. da Silva, G. J. Leitch, R. T. Bryan, and R. Reves.** 1995. Polymerase chain reaction and culture confirmation of disseminated *Encephalitozoon cuniculi* in a patient with AIDS: successful therapy with albendazole. *J. Infect. Dis.* **171:**1375–1378.

32. **Deplazes, P., A. Mathis, R. Baumgartner, I. Tanner, and R. Weber.** 1996. Immunologic and molecular characteristics of *Encephalitozoon*-like microsporidia isolated from humans and rabbits indicate that *Encephalitozoon cuniculi* is a zoonotic parasite. *Clin. Infect. Dis.* **22:**557–559.

33. **Deplazes, P., A. Mathis, C. Muller, and R. Weber.** 1996. Molecular epidemiology of *Encephalitozoon cuniculi* and first detection of *Enterocytozoon bieneusi* in faecal samples of pigs. *J. Eukaryot. Microbiol.* **43:**93S.

34. **Deplazes, P., A. Mathis, and M. van Saanen.** Dual microsporidial infection due to *Vittaforma corneae* and *Encephalitozoon hellem* in an AIDS patient. *Clin. Infect. Dis.*, in press.

35. **Desportes, I., Y. Le Charpentier, A. Galian, F. Bernard, B. Cochand-Priollet, A. Lavergne, P. Ravisse, and R. Modigliani.** 1985. Occurrence of a new microsporidian: *Enterocytozoon bieneusi* n.g., n.sp., in the enterocytes of a human patient with AIDS. *J. Protozool.* **32:**250–254.

36. **Didier, E. S., P. J. Didier, D. N. Friedberg, S. M. Stenson, J. M. Orenstein, R. W. Yee, F. W. Tio, R. M. Davis, C. Vossbrinck, N. Millichamp, and J. A. Shadduck.** 1991. Isolation and characterization of a new human microsporidian, *Encephalitozoon hellem* (n. sp.), from three AIDS patients with keratoconjunctivitis. *J. Infect. Dis.* **163:**617–621.

37. **Didier, E. S., G. S. Visvesvara, M. D. Baker, L. B. Rogers, D. C. Bertucci, M. A. DeGroote, and C. R. Vossbrinck.** 1996. A microsporidian isolated from an AIDS patient corresponds to *Encephalitozoon cuniculi* III, originally isolated from domestic dogs. *J. Clin. Microbiol.* **34:**2835–2837.

38. **Didier, E. S., C. R. Vossbrinck, M. D. Baker, L. B. Rogers, D. C. Bertucci, and J. A. Shadduck.** 1995. Identification and characterization of three *Encephalitozoon cuniculi* strains. *Parasitology* **111:**411–421.

39. **Didier, P. J., E. S. Didier, and M. Murphey-Corb.** 1995. Experimental microsporidiosis in immunodeficient monkeys, abstr. 5614. *FASEB J.* **9:**A967.

40. **Dore, G. J., D. J. Marriott, M. C. Hing, J. L. Harkness, and A. S. Field.** 1995. Disseminated microsporidiosis due to *Septata intestinalis* in nine patients infected with the human immunodeficiency virus: response to therapy with albendazole. *Clin. Infect. Dis.* **21:**70–76.

41. **Drobniewski, F., P. Kelly, A. Carew, B. Ngwenya, N. Luo, C. Pankhurst, and M. Farthing.** 1995. Human microsporidiosis in African AIDS patients with chronic diarrhea. *J. Infect. Dis.* **171:**515–516.

42. **Dunand, V. A., S. M. Hammer, R. Rossi, M. Poulin, M. A. Albrecht, J. P. Doweiko, P. C. DeGirolami, E. Coakley, E. Piessens, and C. A. Wanke.** 1997. Parasitic sinusitis and otitis in patients infected with human immunodeficiency virus: report of five cases and review. *Clin. Infect. Dis.* **25:**267–272.

43. **Enriquez, F. J., D. Taren, A. Cruz-López, M. Muramoto, J. D. Palting, and P. Cruz.** 1998. Prevalence of intestinal encephalitozoonosis in Mexico. *Clin. Infect. Dis.* **26:**1227–1229.

43a. **Field, A. S., D. J. Marriott, S. T. Milliken, B. J. Brew, E. U. Canning, J. G. Kench, P. Darveniza, and J. L. Harkness.** 1996. Myositis associated with a newly described microsporidian, *Trachipleistophora hominis*, in a patient with AIDS. *J. Clin. Microbiol.* **34:**2803–2811.

44. **Foudraine, N. A., G. J. Weverling, T. van Gool, M. T. L. Roos, F. de Wolf, P. P. Koopmans, P. J. van den Broek, P. L. Meenhorst, R. van Leeuwen, J. M. A. Lange, and P. Reiss.** 1998. Improvement of chronic diarrhoea in patients with advanced HIV-1 infection during potent antiretroviral therapy. *AIDS* **12:**35–41.

45. **Fuentealba, I. C., N. T. Mahoney, J. A. Shadduck, J. Harvill, V. Wicher, and K. Wicher.** 1992. Hepatic lesions in rabbits infected with *Encephalitozoon cuniculi* administered per rectum. *Vet. Pathol.* **29:**536–540.

46. **Goguel, J., C. Katlama, C. Sarfati, C. Maslo, C. Leport, and J. M. Molina.** 1997. Remission of AIDS-associated intestinal microsporidiosis with highly active antiretroviral therapy. *AIDS* **11:** 1658–1659.

47. **Goodman, H., R. T. Bryan, and D. A. Schwartz.** 1998. Unpublished data.

48. **Hartskeerl, R. A., T. Van Gool, A. R. J. Schuitema, E. S. Didier, and W. J. Terpstra.** 1995. Genetic and immunological characterization of the microsporidian *Septata intestinalis* Cali, Kotler and Orenstein, 1993: reclassification to *Encephalitozoon intestinalis*. *Parasitology* **110:**277–285.

49. **Hautvast, J. L. A., J. J. M. Tolboom, T. J. M. M. Derks, P. Beckers, and R. W. Sauerwein.** 1997. Asymptomatic intestinal microsporidiosis in a human immunodeficiency virus-seronegative, immunocompetent Zambian child. *Pediatr. Infect. Dis. J.* **16:**415–416.

50. **Hollister, W. S., and E. U. Canning.** 1987. An enzyme-linked immunosorbent assay (ELISA) for detection of antibodies to *E. cuniculi* and its use in determination of infections in man. *Parasitology* **94:**209–219.

51. **Hutin, Y., M. N. Sombardier, C. Sarfati, J. M. Decazes, J. Modai, and J. M. Molina.** 1997. Risk factors for intestinal microsporidiosis in patients infected with human immunodeficiency virus (HIV), abstr. I-150, p. 271. *In Abstracts of the 37th Interscience Conference on Antimicrobial Agents and Chemotherapy.* American Society for Microbiology, Washington, D.C.

52. **Kelkar, R., P. S. Sastry, S. S. Kulkarni, T. K. Saikia, P. M. Parikh, and S. H. Advani.** 1997. Pulmonary microsporidial infection in a patient with CML undergoing allogeneic marrow transplant. *Bone Marrow Transplant.* **19:**179–182.

53. **Kotler, D. P., and J. M. Orenstein.** 1994. Prevalence of intestinal microsporidiosis in HIV-infected individuals referred for gastroenterological evaluation. *Am. J. Gastroenterol.* **89:**1998–2002.

54. **Kyaw, T., A. Curry, V. Edwards-Jones, J. Craske, and B. K. Mandal.** 1997. The prevalence of *Enterocytozoon bieneusi* in acquired immunodeficiency syndrome (AIDS) patients from the north west of England: 1992–1995. *Br. J. Biomed. Sci.* **54:**186–191.

54a. **Ledford, D. K., M. D. Overman, A. Gonzalvo, A. Cali, S. W. Mester, and R. F. Lockey.** 1985. Microsporidiosis myositis in a patient with acquired immunodeficiency syndrome. *Ann. Intern. Med.* **102:**628–630.

55. **Lucas, S. B., D. A. Schwartz, and P. A. Hasleton.** 1996. Pulmonary parasitic diseases, p. 316–319. *In* P. S. Hasleton (ed.), *Spencer's Pathology of the Lung,* 5th ed. McGraw-Hill, Inc., New York, N.Y.

56. **Maiga, I., O. Doumba, M. Dembele, H. Traore, I. Desportes-Livage, I. Hilmarsdottir, E. Giboyau, L. Maiga, L. Kassambara, Y. el Fakhry, A. Datry, M. Gentilini, and E. Pichard.** 1997. Human intestinal microsporidiosis in Bamako (Mali): the presence of *Enterocytozoon bieneusi* in HIV seropositive patients. *Sante* **7:**257–262. (In French.)

57. **Mansfield, K. G., A. Carville, D. Shvetz, J. MacKey, S. Tzipori, and A. A. Lackner.** 1997. Identification of an *Enterocytozoon bieneusi*-like microsporidian parasite in simian-immunodeficiency-virus-inoculated macaques with hepatobiliary disease. *Am. J. Pathol.* **150:**1395–1405.

58. **Mathis, A., M. Michel, H. Kuster, C. Muller, R. Weber, and P. Deplazes.** 1997. Two *Encephalitozoon cuniculi* strains of human origin are infectious to rabbits. *Parasitology* **114:**29–35.

59. **Molina, J. M., E. Oksenhendler, B. Beauvais, C. Sarfati, A. Jaccard, F. Derouin, and J. Modai.** 1995. Disseminated microsporidiosis due to *Septata intestinalis* in patients with AIDS: clinical features and response to albendazole therapy. *J. Infect. Dis.* **171:**245–249.

60. **Morakote, N., P. Siriprasert, S. Piangjai, P. Vitayasai, B. Tookyan, and P. Uparanukraw.** 1995. Microsporidium and Cyclospora in human stools in Chiang Mai, Thailand. *Southeast Asian J. Trop. Med. Hyg. Public Health* **26:**799–800.

61. **Moura, H., A. J. Da Silva, I. N. Moura, D. A. Schwartz, S. Wallace, G. J. Leitch, R. A. Wirtz, and G. S. Visvesvara.** Characterization of *Nosema algerae* isolates after continuous cultivation in mammalian cells at 37°C. *J. Eukaryot. Microbiol.,* in press.

62. **Orenstein, J., J. Chiang, W. Steinberg, P. Smith, H. Rotterdam, and D. Kotler.** 1990. Intestinal microsporidiosis as a cause of diarrhea in human immunodeficiency virus-infected patients, a report of 20 cases. *Hum. Pathol.* **21:**475–481.

63. **Orenstein, J. M., D. T. Dieterich, and D. P. Kotler.** 1992. Systemic dissemination by a newly recognized intestinal microsporidia species in AIDS. *AIDS* **6:**1143–1150.

64. **Orenstein, J. M., M. Tenner, A. Cali, and D. P. Kotler.** 1992. A microsporidian previously undescribed in humans, infecting enterocytes and macrophages, and associated with diarrhea in an acquired immunodeficiency syndrome patient. *Hum. Pathol.* **23:**722–728.
65. **Pospisilova, Z., O. Ditrich, M. Stankova, and P. Kodym.** 1997. Parasitic opportunistic infections in Czech HIV-infected patients—a prospective study. *Cent. Eur. J. Public Health* **5:**208–213.
66. **Pulparampil, N., D. Graham, D. Phalen, and K. Snowden.** 1998. *Encephalitozoon hellem* infection in an Eclectus parrot—zoonotic potential?, p. 64. *In Proceedings of the International Conference on Emerging Infectious Diseases.*
67. **Rabodonirina, M., M. Bertocchi, I. Desportes-Livage, L. Cotte, H. Levrey, M. A. Piens, G. Monneret, M. Celard, J. F. Mornex, and M. Mojon.** 1996. *Enterocytozoon bieneusi* as a cause of chronic diarrhea in a heart-lung transplant recipient who was seronegative for human immunodeficiency virus. *Clin. Infect. Dis.* **23:**114–117.
68. **Raynaud, L., F. Delbac, V. Broussolle, M. Rabodonirina, V. Girault, M. Wallon, G. Cozon, C. P. Vivares, and F. Peyron.** 1998. Identification of *Encephalitozoon intestinalis* in travelers with chronic diarrhea by specific PCR amplification. *J. Clin. Microbiol.* **36:**37–40.
69. **Reetz, J.** 1994. Natürliche Übertragung von Mikrosporidien (*Encephalitozoon cuniculi*) über das Hühnerei. *Tieraerztl Praxis* **22:**147–150.
70. **Sandfort, J., A. Hannerman, H. Gelderblom, K. Stark, R. L. Owen, and B. Ruf.** 1994. *Enterocytozoon bieneusi* infection in an immunocompetent patient who had acute diarrhea and who was not infected with the human immunodeficiency virus. *Clin. Infect. Dis.* **19:**514–516.
71. **Sax, P. E., J. D. Rich, W. S. Pieciak, and Y. M. Trnka.** 1995. Intestinal microsporidiosis occurring in a liver transplant recipient. *Transplantation* **60:**617–618.
72. **Scaglia, M., S. Gatti, L. Sacchi, S. Corona, G. Chichino, A.M. Bernuzzi, G. Barbarini, G. P. Croppo, A. J. Da Silva, N. J. Pieniazek, and G. S. Visvesvara.** 1998. Asymptomatic respiratory tract microsporidiosis due to *Encephalitozoon hellem* in three patients with AIDS. *Clin. Infect. Dis.* **26:**174–176.
73. **Schmidt, W., T. Schneider, W. Heise, J.-D. Schulzke, T. Weinke, R. Ignatius, R. L. Owen, M. Zeitz, E.-O. Riecken, and R. Ullrich.** 1997. Mucosal abnormalities in microsporidiosis. *AIDS* **11:**1589–1594.
74. **Schwartz, D. A., D. C. Anderson, S. A. Klumpp, and H. M. McClure.** 1998. Ultrastructure of atypical (teratoid) sporogonial stages of *Enterocytozoon bieneusi* (Microsporidia) in naturally infected rhesus monkeys (*Macacca mulatta*). *Arch. Pathol. Lab. Med.* **122:**423–429.
75. **Schwartz, D. A., and R. T. Bryan.** 1997. Microsporidia, p. 61–93. *In* C. R. Horsburgh, Jr., and A. M. Nelson (ed.), *Pathology of Emerging Infections.* ASM Press, Washington, D.C.
76. **Schwartz, D. A., R. T. Bryan, K. O. Hewan-Lowe, G. S. Visvesvara, R. Weber, A. Cali, and P. Angritt.** 1992. Disseminated microsporidiosis (*Encephalitozoon hellem*) and acquired immunodeficiency syndrome: autopsy evidence for respiratory acquisition. *Arch. Pathol. Lab. Med.* **116:**660–668.
77. **Schwartz, D. A., G. S. Visvesvara, M. C. Diesenhouse, R. Weber, R. L. Font, L. A. Wilson, G. Corrent, D. F. Rosberger, P. C. Keenen, H. E. Grossniklaus, K. O. Hewan-Lowe, and R. T. Bryan.** 1993. Ocular pathology of microsporidiosis: role of immunofluorescent antibody for diagnosis of *Encephalitozoon hellem* in biopsies, smears, and intact globes from seven AIDS patients. *Am. J. Ophthalmol.* **115:**285–292.
78. **Schwartz, D. A., M. Flepp, G. S. Visvesvara, R. T. Bryan, and R. Weber.** Unpublished data.
79. **Schwartz, D. A., I. Sobottka, G. J. Leitch, A. Cali, and G. S. Visvesvara.** 1996. Pathology of microsporidiosis. Emerging parasitic infections in patients with the acquired immunodeficiency syndrome. *Arch. Pathol. Lab. Med.* **120:**173–188.
80. **Schwartz, D. A., G. S. Visvesvara, G. J. Leitch, L. S. Tashjian, M. Pollack, and R. T. Bryan.** 1993. Pathology of symptomatic microsporidial (*Encephalitozoon hellem*) bronchiolitis in AIDS: a new respiratory pathogen diagnosed by biopsy, bronchoalveolar lavage, sputum cytology, and tissue culture. *Hum. Pathol.* **24:**937–943.
81. **Schwartz, D. A., G. S. Visvesvara, R. Weber, and R. T. Bryan.** 1994. Male genital tract microsporidiosis and AIDS: prostatic abscess due to *Encephalitozoon hellem. J. Eukaryot. Microbiol.* **41:**61S.

82. **Schwartz, D. A., G. S. Visvesvara, R. Weber, C. M. Wilcox, and R. T. Bryan.** 1994. Microsporidiosis in HIV positive patients: current methods for diagnosis using biopsy, cytologic, ultrastructural, immunological and tissue culture techniques. *Folia Parasitol.* **41**:91–99.

83. **Seibold, H. R., and E. N. Fussell.** 1973. Intestinal microsporidiosis in *Callicebus moloch. Lab. Anim. Sci.* **23**:115–118.

84. **Shadduck, J. A., and G. Baskin.** 1989. Serologic evidence of *Encephalitozoon cuniculi* infection in a colony of squirrel monkeys (*Saimiri sciureus*). *Lab. Anim. Sci.* **39**:328–330.

85. **Silveira, H., and E. U. Canning.** 1995. *Vittaforma corneae* n. comb. for the human microsporidium *Nosema corneum* Shadduck, Meccoli, Davis, & Font, 1990, based on its ultrastructure in the liver of experimentally infected athymic mice. *J. Eukaryot. Microbiol.* **42**:158–165.

86. **Silverstein, B. E., E. T. Cunningham, T. P. Margolis, V. Cevallos, and I. G. Wong.** 1997. Microsporidial keratoconjunctivitis in a patient without human immunodeficiency virus infection. *Am. J. Ophthalmol.* **124**:395–396.

87. **Singh, M., G. J. Kane, L. MacKinlay, I. Quaki, E. H. Yap, B. C. Ho, L. C. Ho, and L. C. Kim.** 1982. Detection of antibodies to *Nosema cuniculi* (protozoa: microsporidia) in human and animal sera by the indirect fluorescent antibody technique. *Southeast Asia J. Trop. Med. Public Health* **13**:110–113.

88. **Sobottka, I., H. Albrecht, J. Schottelius, C. Schmetz, M. Bentfield, R. Laufs, and D. A. Schwartz.** 1995. Self-limited traveller's diarrhea due to a dual infection with *Enterocytozoon bieneusi* and *Cryptosporidium parvum* in an immunocompetent HIV-negative child. *Eur. J. Clin. Microbiol. Infect. Dis.* **14**:919–920.

89. **Sobottka, I., D. A. Schwartz, J. Schottelius, G. S. Visvesvara, N. J. Pieniazek, C. Schmetz, N. P. Kock, R. Laufs, and H. Albrecht.** 1998. Prevalence and clinical significance of intestinal microsporidiosis in German HIV-infected patients. *Clin. Infect. Dis.* **26**:475–480.

90. **Sparfel, J. M., C. Sarfati, O. Ligoury, B. Caroff, N. Dumoutier, B. Gueglio, E. Billaud, F. Raffi, J. M. Molina, M. Miegeville, and F. Derouin.** 1997. Detection of microsporidia and identification of *Enterocytozoon bieneusi* in surface water by filtration followed by specific PCR. *J. Eukaryot. Microbiol.* **44**:78S.

91. **Tzipori, S., A. Carville, G. Widmer, D. Kotler, K. Mansfield, and A. Lackner.** 1997. Transmission and establishment of a persistent infection of *Enterocytozoon bieneusi*, derived from a human with AIDS, in simian immunodeficiency virus-infected rhesus monkeys. *J. Infect. Dis.* **175**:1016–1020.

92. **Van Gool, T., J. C. M. Vetter, B. Weinmayr, A. Van Dam, F. Derouin, and J. Dankert.** 1997. High seroprevalence of *Encephalitozoon* species in immunocompetent subjects. *J. Infect. Dis.* **175**: 1020–1024.

93. **Van Gool, T., E. Luderhoff, K. J. Nathoo, C. F. Kiire, J. Dankert, and P. R. Mason.** 1995. High prevalence of *Enterocytozoon bieneusi* infections among HIV-positive individuals with persistent diarrhea in Harare, Zimbabwe. *Trans. R. Soc. Trop. Med. Hyg.* **89**:478–480.

94. **Vávra, J., A. T. Yachnis, J. A. Shadduck, and J. M. Orenstein.** Microsporidia of the genus *Trachipleistophora*—causative agents of human microsporidiosis: description of *Trachipleistophora anthropophthera* n.sp. (Protozoa: Microsporidia). *J. Eukaryot. Microbiol.*, in press.

95. **Visvesvara, G. S., M. Belloso, H. Moura, A. J. Da Silva, I. N. Moura, G. J. Leitch, D. A. Schwartz, P. Chevez-Barrios, S. Wallace, and J. D. Goosey.** Isolation of *Nosema algerae* from the cornea of an immunocompetent patient. *J. Eukaryot. Microbiol.*, in press.

96. **Voglino, M. C., G. Donelli, P. Rossi, A. Ludovisi, V. Rinaldi, F. Goffredo, R. Paloscia, and E. Pozio.** 1996. Intestinal microsporidiosis in Italian individuals with AIDS. *Ital. J. Gastroenterol.* **28**:381–386.

97. **Waller, T.** 1980. Sensitivity of *Encephalitozoon cuniculi* to various temperatures, disinfectants and drugs. *Lab. Anim. Sci.* **13**:277–280.

98. **Wanke, C. A., P. DeGirolami, and M. Federman.** 1996. *Enterocytozoon bieneusi* infection and diarrheal disease in patients who were not infected with human immunodeficiency virus: case report and review. *Clin. Infect. Dis.* **23**:816–818.

98a.**Watson, D. A. R., D. Asmuth, and C. A. Wanke.** 1996. Environmental risk factors for acquisition of microsporidia in HIV-infected persons. *Clin. Infect. Dis.* **23**:816–818.

99. **Weber, R., R. T. Bryan, D. A. Schwartz, and R. L. Owen.** 1994. Human microsporidial infections. *Clin. Microbiol. Rev.* **7**:426–461.

100. **Weber, R., D. A. Schwartz, and R. T. Bryan.** Microsporidiosis. *In* G. L. Mandell, J. E. Bennett, and R. Dolin (ed.), *Principles and Practice of Infectious Diseases*, 5th ed., in press. Churchill Livingstone, Edinburgh, United Kingdom.

101. **Weber, R., D. A. Schwartz, and P. Deplazes.** 1999. Laboratory diagnosis of microsporidiosis, p. 315–362. *In* M. Wittner and L. M. Weiss (ed.), *The Microsporidia and Microsporidiosis.* ASM Press, Washington, D.C.

102. **Weiser, J.** 1965. Microsporidian infections of mammals and the genus *Encephalitozoon. Int. Congr. Parasitol.* **1:**445–446.

103. **Weiser, J.** 1964. On the taxonomic position of the genus *Encephalitozoon* Levaditi, Nicolau & Schoen, 1923 (Protozoa:*Microsporidia*). *Parasitology* **54:**749–751.

104. **Wicher, V., R. E. Baughn, C. Fuentealba, J. A. Shadduck, F. Abbruscato, and K. Wicher.** 1991. Enteric infection with an obligate intracellular parasite, *Encephalitozoon cuniculi*, in an experimental model. *Infect. Immun.* **59:**2225–2231.

105. **Wright, J. H., and E. M. Craighead.** 1922. Infectious motor paralysis in young rabbits. *J. Exp. Med.* **36:**135–140.

106. **Wuhib, T., T. M. J. Silva, R. D. Newman, L. S. Garcia, M. L. D. Pereira, C. S. Chaves, S. P. Wahlquist, R. T. Bryan, R. L. Guerrant, A. Q. de Sousa, T. R. B. S. de Queiroz, and C. L. Sears.** 1994. Cryptosporidial and microsporidial infections in human immunodeficiency virus-infected patients in northeastern Brazil. *J. Infect. Dis.* **170:**494–497.

107. **Yachnis, A. T., J. Berg, A. Martinez-Salazar, B. S. Bender, L. Diaz, A. M. Rojiani, T. A. Eskin, and J. M. Oremstein.** 1996. Disseminated microsporidiosis especially infecting the brain, heart, and kidneys—report of a newly recognized pansporoblastic species in two symptomatic AIDS patients. *Am. J. Clin. Pathol.* **106:**535–543.

108. **Zemen, D. H., and G. B. Baskin.** 1985. Encephalitozoonosis in squirrel monkeys (*Saimiri sciureus*). *Vet. Pathol.* **22:**24–31.

Emerging Infections 3
Edited by W. M. Scheld, W. A. Craig, and J. M. Hughes
© 1999 ASM Press, Washington, D.C.

Chapter 7

Leishmania: a Parasite on the Move

James H. Maguire

The first cases of human leishmaniasis date back perhaps as far as to the first century A.D., when pre-Incan pottery from the Andes portrayed skin lesions and facial deformities (10, 13, 48). While therefore not a new disease, leishmaniasis does represent a major health problem. Currently 12 million persons in 88 countries are affected, 350 million persons are exposed to the risk of infection, and 1.5 million to 2 million new cases occur each year (48).

During the past decade, there has been an explosive increase in numbers of new cases, spread of the disease into new regions, and even appearance of new clinical syndromes (13, 48). This resurgence of leishmaniasis reflects the remarkable adaptability of the *Leishmania* parasite to changing conditions, such as those resulting from economic development, human modification of the environment, and population movements.

LEISHMANIASIS: BACKGROUND

Transmission and Ecology

Leishmaniae, like the trypanosomes, are flagellate protozoa of the order Kinetoplastida (10). They are transmitted between phlebotomine sand flies and a variety of vertebrate hosts. Infected sand flies inoculate the 10- to 20-μm-long, motile promastigote forms while taking a blood meal from the host (22). Promastigotes invade macrophages and transform into the round, aflagellate amastigote form, which measures 3 to 6 μm in diameter. Amastigotes replicate intracellularly by binary fission, rupture the host cell, and invade other mononuclear phagocytic cells locally or at a distance. Feeding sand flies ingest amastigotes from the blood or skin of the host. Amastigotes transform into promastigotes, replicate by binary fission in the insect's gut, and become infective in roughly a week's time.

James H. Maguire • Division of Infectious Disease, Brigham and Women's Hospital, and Department of Immunology and Infectious Diseases, Harvard School of Public Health, Boston, MA 02115.

There are over 30 species of *Leishmania*, of which at least one dozen infect human beings (10, 28). In general, leishmaniasis is a zoonotic infection of rodents, edentates, or other wild mammals, or of wild and domestic canids (10). Human beings usually are accidental hosts and not important for maintaining the cycle of transmission except in the case of *Leishmania donovani* in south Asia and *Leishmania tropica* in the Middle East, central Asia, and the Mediterranean littoral.

Transmission of leishmaniasis occurs in diverse ecological settings and on all continents except Australia and Antarctica. Requirements of the vector and reservoir hosts determine the distribution of infection. Approximately 30 of the 500 known species of sand flies have been identified as vectors of leishmaniasis (10, 28, 48), and each has specific habitats. Breeding sites must meet specific requirements of temperature, humidity, and abundance of organic material in order for emerging larvae to develop. Female sand flies, measuring 2 to 3 mm in length, require mammalian blood to produce eggs and a suitable environment in which to deposit them. Because they are weak fliers, their search for a blood meal takes place within a radius seldom greater than several hundred meters. Different species of sand flies have different preferences for the source of blood meals, but are capable of taking blood from a wide variety of vertebrates when necessary. Feeding usually takes place after dark, and types of daytime resting places vary among the species. Male sand flies and female sand flies between blood meals feed on sugars of certain plants.

Human infection occurs when persons intrude upon the natural transmission cycle between vector and reservoir or enter sand fly resting and breeding sites (3, 10, 13, 18, 19, 23–26). Hence, transmission may take place in the vicinity of an animal burrow where flies encounter a source of blood and organic debris in which to deposit eggs. Animal pens near houses or organic debris in the floors or in cracks in the walls of houses may support dense populations of flies. In forests, sand flies breed in holes in trees or leaf litter on the ground and rest on tree trunks, branches, and leaves. Because of the diversity of sand fly behavior and requirements, appropriate conditions for transmission are found in a variety of different settings including temperate zones, tropical areas, mountains, deserts, plains, and even cities (10).

Clinical Features

Leishmania infection produces a spectrum of clinical manifestations. With most species of parasite, the majority of persons experience subclinical infections that are only detectable in retrospect by skin testing or serological tests (5, 8, 16). When disease does develop, it falls into one of three major categories: visceral, cutaneous, or mucocutaneous. In the past, it was believed that each species of parasite produced a single category of disease. Hence, *Leishmania tropica*, *L. major*, *L. aethiopica*, *L. mexicana*, *L. amazonensis*, and *L. peruviana* were considered causes of only cutaneous leishmaniasis; *L. braziliensis*, *L. guyanensis*, and *L. panamensis* caused mucocutaneous leishmaniasis; and *L. donovani*, *L. infantum*, and *L. chagasi* caused visceral leishmaniasis. It is now known that certain species can produce different syndromes, especially in persons with impaired cell-mediated immunity.

For example, infection with *L. chagasi* and *L. donovani* can result in isolated skin lesions (37), while visceral infection is well documented for *L. amazonensis* and *L. tropica* (6).

The reasons that persons exposed to the same species or strain of parasite develop different types of syndrome are not well understood. There is strong evidence for genetic susceptibility to infection and types of disease in inbred mice, but similar data for human beings are limited (27). Impaired cell-mediated immunity, as in persons with AIDS or recipients of organ transplants, increases the incidence of disease among infected persons and may result in more severe or unusual manifestations (1, 7, 8, 36). Previous infection offers partial protection against reinfection with organisms of the same species and may modify the clinical manifestations of infection should reinfection occur (42).

Visceral Leishmaniasis

In visceral leishmaniasis, or kala-azar, there is infection of reticuloendothelial cells throughout the body and particularly in the liver, spleen, bone marrow, and lymphoid tissue. Disease is characterized by fever, weight loss, hepatosplenomegaly, hyperglobulinemia, and pancytopenia. Without treatment, mortality from secondary infection, bleeding, anemia, or heart failure approaches 100% (29, 36). Young age, malnutrition, human immunodeficiency virus (HIV) infection, and immunosuppressive therapy are all known to be risk factors for the development of full-blown visceral leishmaniasis after infection with the parasite (3, 5, 16).

In the Indian subcontinent, persons who recover from infection with *L. donovani* frequently develop the syndrome of post-kala-azar dermal leishmaniasis, in which huge numbers of parasites infect the skin and produce a variety of lesions (10). These persons are highly infective to sand flies, as are persons with classic Indian kala-azar, who have high numbers of parasites circulating in the peripheral blood. Indeed, infected humans are the only known reservoir of infection in this region. Elsewhere in Asia, Europe, the Americas, and parts of Africa, domestic and wild canids are the major reservoir of visceral leishmaniasis. In East Africa, rodents and perhaps human beings and canids are believed to be the reservoir.

More than 90% of the world's cases of visceral leishmaniasis are reported from Bangladesh, Brazil, India, and the Sudan (48). Other endemic regions include parts of Burma, China, central Asia, the Mediterranean littoral, sub-Saharan Africa, Mexico, and Central and South America. In 1990, when there were an estimated 400,000 new cases of visceral leishmaniasis and 50,000 deaths worldwide, the global burden of this form of the disease was calculated to exceed 2 million disability-adjusted life years (DALYs), or more than the DALYs estimated for other tropical infectious diseases such as schistosomiasis, trypanosomiasis, dengue, and leprosy.

Cutaneous Leishmaniasis

In cutaneous leishmaniasis, parasite replication is confined primarily to the skin. Infected macrophages, cells damaged by parasites, and the host's cell-mediated immune response are responsible for the lesions, which typically ulcerate, but also may be papular, nodular, or verrucous (8, 10, 29, 36). Depending on the species of parasite, lesions may be slow to heal or not heal at all without treatment, and lesions on the face or genitalia may damage mucous membranes. Certain persons infected with *L. amazonensis* or *L. aethiopica* appear to be unable to mount a specific immune response against the parasite and develop diffuse cutaneous leishmaniasis in which nonhealing lesions loaded with parasites cover the body and resemble the lesions of lepromatous leprosy.

More than 90% of cases of cutaneous leishmaniasis emanate from Brazil and Peru in the New World and four Middle Eastern countries in the Old World (48). There is a human reservoir of *L. tropica* infection in the Middle East, Mediterranean basin, and central Asia, but lower mammals are the reservoir for other species that cause cutaneous lesions (10). Gerbils and other rodents are the reservoir hosts for *L. major* in Africa, the Middle East, Central Asia, and the Indian subcontinent, and hyraxes are the reservoir for *L. aethiopica* in Kenya and Ethiopia. In the Americas, rodents, marsupials, edentates, and canids are the reservoirs of the different species of *Leishmania* that produce cutaneous disease.

Mucocutaneous Leishmaniasis

In a small proportion of infected persons, parasites of *L. braziliensis* and, to a lesser extent, *L. panamensis* and *L. guyanensis* spread from the skin to the mucous membranes of the nose and oropharynx, where they produce hideously deforming, destructive lesions (10). Mucosal involvement may precede, occur simultaneously, or occur even decades after the appearance and resolution of the cutaneous lesions. The lesions do not heal without treatment and often relapse after treatment. The incidence of mucosal involvement varies from less than 1 to about 5% in areas of Central and South America where leishmaniasis is endemic.

Treatment

Treatment is required for persons with clinically apparent visceral leishmaniasis, mucocutaneous leishmaniasis, and cases of cutaneous leishmaniasis in which spontaneous healing is slow, lesions involve the face, or infection is due to species that can cause mucocutaneous leishmaniasis or diffuse cutaneous leishmaniasis. The gold standard treatment is pentavalent antimony (either sodium stibogluconate [Pentostam] or meglumine antimoniate [Glucantime]) given intravenously or intramuscularly at a dose of 20 mg/kg/day for a minimum of 20 days (10, 17, 43). There are numerous problems with antimony therapy: the drug is expensive and available only in parenteral form, and it causes frequent side effects and is not 100% effective. Alternative therapies with drugs such as pentamidine, amphotericin B, liposomal amphotericin, and aminosidine each share several of the disadvantages of antimony. Oral antifungal drugs such as ketoconazole, fluconazole, and itraconazole are active in cases of infections with *L. major* and *L. mexicana*, species in which the rate of spontaneous healing is high and for which treatment is often not necessary.

GROWING INCIDENCE AND SPREAD OF LEISHMANIASIS

The World Health Organization (WHO) has noted a marked increase in almost all forms of leishmaniasis during the past two decades (48). Some of the increase is due to increased reporting. Official figures are thought to represent a gross underestimate. There have been, however, an unequivocal increase in the number of cases worldwide, a widening of the distribution of infection within areas of endemicity, and reports of leishmaniasis from areas where the disease was not previously endemic. WHO cites as examples official data in which there were increases of 460, 730, and 160% in the number of cases of cutaneous leishmaniasis in Tunisia, Turkey, and Syria, respectively, over periods of 4 to 8 years (48). The number of cases of visceral leishmaniasis in Bangladesh rose from 2,300 in 1988 to 15,000 in 1995. In Brazil, the number of reported cases of visceral leishmaniasis doubled in the period from 1993 to 1997 compared with the period from 1988 to 1992, and in northeast Brazil alone there has been a fivefold increase in the number of cases of cutaneous leishmaniasis since 1980 (17, 48).

In many cases, such increases are linked to human activities and behavior (9, 18, 19, 28, 33, 34, 46, 47). Economic development leads to environmental modifications that expose populations to cycles of transmission. Migration and travel bring nonimmune persons into areas of transmission. Other population movements result in introduction of parasites, infected reservoirs, and perhaps sand flies into areas where the disease was not previously endemic. Rapid urbanization may create conditions that facilitate the rapid spread among crowded populations. Cessation of vector control activities for malaria and other vector-borne diseases allows sand fly populations to prosper. In the following section, specific illustrations of factors underlying increases and spread of leishmaniasis are presented.

Resurgence and Reemergence of Leishmaniasis: Examples

Visceral Leishmaniasis in the Sudan: a "Killing Disease"

An epidemic of visceral leishmaniasis began in southern Sudan following the civil war in 1983 (4, 12, 39, 40). Initially, there were reports of numerous deaths of unknown cause in the area. Later, this so-called "killing disease" was shown to be visceral leishmaniasis. The area of the epidemic was outside previously known areas of endemicity. Of approximately 280,000 persons living in the region of endemicity, over 100,000 are estimated to have died from the disease. Treatment became available in 1989, but access to treatment was not available in some areas, and fighting interrupted treatment in other areas. By 1996, some 17,000 persons had been treated, but in some areas, the case-fatality rate was as high as 70%.

Several explanations were considered for the epidemic. Flooding of the area in the early 1960s followed construction of the Owen Falls Dam, which controlled the flow of water from Lake Victoria to the Nile River. The floods initially eliminated most of the existing forest, but by the beginning of the epidemic in 1984, a closed-canopy acacia forest had returned and become populated with *Phlebotomus orientalis*, a known vector of visceral leishmaniasis. Because of the armed conflict, infected persons, including soldiers, were forced to travel through the forests, and perhaps some of them introduced the parasite into the region. Inhabitants of the area had no prior exposure to infection or immunity, nor did the tens of thousands of persons who later crossed through the area in search of food during the dry or "hunger" season or to escape fighting. Attack rates and high rates of clinical disease during the epidemic were attributable to malnutrition that resulted from the drought and disruption of agriculture and cattle raising by the war. Because of the civil war and lack of health services, neither good epidemiological data nor treatment were initially available. Subsequently, treatment by expatriate health workers, primarily Médecins sans Frontières, has been successful in treating persons under extremely difficult conditions, but there has been a sharp rise in number of cases from the end of 1997 to 1998 (31).

Visceral Leishmaniasis in Southern Croatia

Human and canine visceral leishmaniasis has been reported in southern coastal Croatia since 1931 (38). Probably because of mass antimalarial insecticide use (38, 44, 45), there had been only sporadic human cases since 1950 until recently. At the University Hospital in Split, there had been no cases between 1986 and 1991, but between 1992 and 1997, there were 11 cases (38). The increase in numbers of cases was attributed to the war from 1992 to 1995, in which many persons became malnourished, numbers of stray dogs increased, and spraying of insecticides for vector control was disrupted.

Visceral Leishmaniasis in Eastern India

Bihar State in eastern India has been the site of a series of huge epidemics of visceral leishmaniasis for several decades. In 1994, as many as 250,000 persons were estimated to have contracted the disease, and 38 of the 42 districts experienced the worst epidemic since the late 1970s (48). In several villages, onset of the epidemic was traced to a single person with post-kala-azar dermal leishmaniasis. Because visceral leishmaniasis in this region is an anthroponosis, interventions to interrupt transmission rely on application of insecticides and detection and treatment of cases. The rapid increase in numbers of cases may reflect resistance of local strains of *L. donovani* to antimony and of the local vector *Phlebotomus argentipes* to DDT under the pressure of intense control efforts (43).

Leishmania and HIV Coinfection

There have been over 1,000 cases of leishmaniasis in persons coinfected with HIV, the majority in southern Europe where *L. infantum* is endemic (1, 8, 28). Currently in southern Europe, 25 to 75% or more of adult cases of visceral leishmaniasis occur in HIV-infected persons, 1.5 to 9.5% of persons with AIDS suffer from newly acquired or reactivated visceral leishmaniasis, and 7 to 17% of HIV-infected persons with fever have leishmaniasis (1, 47). Needle sharing among intravenous drug users appears to be an important route of transmission (2).

Because of unusual characteristics of leishmaniasis in HIV-infected persons, *Leishmania* and HIV coinfection has been considered by some to be a true "new or emerging" disease. Visceral disease occurs in HIV-positive persons infected with not only visceralizing strains of *L. donovani*, but also dermotropic strains of *L. donovani*, zoonotic strains of *Leishmania* that previously had not been recognized as human pathogens, and even insect trypanosomatids. Visceral leishmaniasis in HIV-infected persons is associated with higher levels of parasitemia than is seen in non-HIV-infected persons, and sand flies readily acquire parasites from coinfected persons (1).

The clinical manifestations of visceral leishmaniasis in HIV-infected persons are often atypical (1). Compared to persons without HIV infection, organomegaly is less common, serological tests for leishmaniasis are more likely to be negative, and infections of the skin, gastrointestinal tract, and respiratory tract occur more frequently among HIV-infected persons. Relapses following treatment occur nearly always unless prophylactic treatment is given.

There are reports of *Leishmania* and HIV coinfection from other parts of the world, including India and Brazil (1, 48). There have also been cases of infection with dermotropic *Leishmania* species such as *L. braziliensis* in which the presentation resembled that of diffuse cutaneous leishmaniasis or visceral leishmaniasis.

Leishmaniasis in the United States

Most cases of leishmaniasis seen in the United States are cutaneous cases imported by civilian and military travelers returning from areas where the disease is endemic (20, 30). Increased tourism to tropical areas has increased the numbers of civilians at risk for infection. In a review of cases of American cutaneous leishmaniasis for which sodium stibogluconate had been released by the Centers for Disease Control and Prevention between 1985 and 1990, almost 40% occurred among tourists, tour guides, and visitors (20).

U.S. military personnel have acquired cutaneous infections in a number of settings such as jungle training classes in Panama or military operations in the Middle East. A "new" clinical form of *L. tropica* infection, "viscerotropic leishmaniasis," was recently described among veterans of Operation Desert Storm (28). There were nine parasitologically documented cases out of a total of 500,000 soldiers who had been deployed to eastern Saudi Arabia. None of the nine persons had skin lesions or classic symptoms of visceral leishmaniasis. The onset of illness was delayed for months to several years. Common complaints included chronic fatigue, cough, abdominal pain, and intermittent diarrhea. Because of a concern for transfusion-induced transmission, all veterans of the operation were prohibited from donating blood for several years after return to the United States.

During the past 25 years, over two dozen cases of cutaneous or disseminated cutaneous leishmaniasis due to *L. mexicana* have been reported from Texas (32). The enzootic cycle in Texas involves the southern plains wood rat and a sand fly that is associated with wood rat burrows. The emergence of human cases was attributed to the location of dwellings near the typical mesquite-cactus habitat of the wood rat. Competent human-biting sand fly vectors can be found in other parts of the United States, and cases of locally acquired *L. donovani* infections in dogs and *L. mexicana* infections in cats have been identified.

Emergence and Resurgence of Leishmaniasis: Case Histories from Brazil

Cutaneous Leishmaniasis on the Outskirts of Manaus, Amazonas

In the Brazilian Amazon basin, most cases of cutaneous leishmaniasis are caused by *L. guyanensis* (3, 23–26). In the natural transmission cycle, the mammalian reservoirs of the parasite are sloths and anteaters that live in the canopy of the forest. The sand fly vector, *Lutzomyia umbratilis*, feeds on these animals at night in the tree tops. During the day, female sand flies descend to the floor to deposit their eggs and can be found in great numbers resting on tree trunks. *Lutzomyia umbratilis* prefers not to feed on human beings but will do so when disturbed. Hence, most human infections traditionally occurred among forest workers who were attacked by sand flies during the day while felling a tree or leaning against a tree trunk.

In the early 1980s, cutaneous leishmaniasis due to *L. guyanensis* began to emerge as a periurban disease when forest on the outskirts of the city of Manaus was cleared for construction of a large housing settlement called Cidade Nova. As settlers moved into the houses, as many as 10% or more of the inhabitants of certain neighborhoods developed cutaneous leishmaniasis. Destruction of the natural habitat appeared to have resulted in high rates of exposure to infected sand flies, even among children and other persons who did not enter the forest (3). It was hypothesized that the sloths and anteaters disappeared after their habitat had been destroyed, and at the same time, opossums began to scavenge in the residential area. A high rate of infection among opossums was detected, suggesting that a new reservoir host had emerged to replace the former hosts; indeed, infection in opossums is rare in areas of undisturbed forest.

Cutaneous Leishmaniasis in Baturité, Ceará

The *municipio* or county of Baturité is thought to be the oldest focus of cutaneous and mucocutaneous leishmaniasis due to *L. braziliensis* in Brazil and is the largest focus of cutaneous disease in the state of Ceará (42). The disease is endemic in the rural zone of Baturité, which extends up the sides of a small mountain approximately 800 m in altitude. In addition to a steady incidence of new cases among 1 to 2% of the population each year, there are periodic epidemics with rates 10 times or higher than the yearly average. Transmission occurs primarily in and around the house, and the domestic dog is the presumed primary reservoir for human infection. A sylvatic reservoir that maintains the cycle in the forest has not yet been identified.

The reason for periodic epidemics is not well understood. There may be some association with climate, since transmission seems to increase following droughts. However, prior exposure and immunity to reinfection may be important as well (42). During the first year or two after new families move into the area from regions where the disease is less common, the household attack rate is high. Immunity to reinfection is strong (although not 100%) and long-lasting, even among persons who experience sublinical infections, which are twice as common as clinically apparent infections. It may be that exposure rates in the population do not vary greatly from year to year, and epidemics become apparent only when there are a large number of susceptible children or newcomers to the area.

In Baturité, a new clinical syndrome was reported among persons with *L. braziliensis* infections (42). Approximately 70% of persons who presented with cutaneous lesions had massively enlarged regional lymph nodes that appeared about the same time as their cutaneous ulcers. Aspirates of the nodes revealed large numbers of parasites, and some persons were febrile and had hepatosplenomegaly, suggesting that systemic dissemination of infection occurred early in the course of disease. Because of the size of the nodes, the illness was called "bubonic leishmaniasis." Baturité in fact is an important focus of plague, and during a large plague epidemic over a decade ago, there were cases of buboes in which the diagnosis of plague was not confirmed; in retrospect, these may have been cases of leishmaniasis.

Urban Leishmaniasis in Teresina, Piauí

Visceral leishmaniasis has long been a major health problem in northeast Brazil. Traditionally it was a disease of rural areas and the periphery of small towns in the countryside. Since 1980, however, at least six major Brazilian cities have reported cases or even epidemics of visceral leishmaniasis (11, 21). The first reports of urban visceral leishmaniasis in Brazil came from Teresina, a city of approximately 600,000 inhabitants and the capital of Piauí, Brazil's poorest state. Locally acquired cases of visceral leishmaniasis were virtually unknown in Teresina before 1980 (11), but cases acquired within the city limits have been reported every year since then, including two major outbreaks in 1983 to 1985 and 1993 to 1994, with approximately 1,000 cases of full-blown visceral leishmaniasis and at least seven cases of coinfection with HIV and *Leishmania chagasi* on the latter occasion (29, 35). Over 90% of cases required hospitalization, and 5% were fatal despite treatment. In 1996, a survey showed that 49% of 200 residents of Teresina had a reactive leishmanin skin test, indicating prior infection, and the ratio of asymptomatic to symptomatic infections was as high as 175:1 in some areas.

The emergence of visceral leishmaniasis in Teresina is believed to have resulted from massive drought-driven movements of people and their domestic animals from rural areas to crowded and precarious housing settlements on the periphery of the city (11). It is believed that sand flies had infested the city decades before the first cases occurred, and the new and impoverished housing settlements favored increases in their abundance. It is believed that domestic dogs or even people who had been infected in the rural environment were responsible for the introduction of the parasite when they migrated to the city.

Recurrent epidemics of visceral leishmaniasis appear to occur every 5 to 10 years in urban areas such as Teresina (as well as in rural zones). The reasons for the cycles are not clear, but climate or patterns of immunity among reservoirs or human hosts are likely to be important (14, 15, 41, 44). In the absence of effective interventions, a third epidemic can be anticipated in Teresina during the next 5 years. There is justifiable concern that HIV infection in the population will have increased considerably by that time and will amplify both the size of the epidemic and the severity of illness.

Measures to control the spread of visceral leishmaniasis in Teresina have focused on identifying and killing infected dogs, and application of insecticide in the neighborhoods surrounding new cases of frank kala-azar. These measures have not interrupted transmission, and the impression of health workers in Teresina is that the epidemics of 1983 to 1985 and 1993 to 1994 resolved spontaneously, since the number of cases already had decreased substantially before widespread implementation of control measures began (11, 15, 29, 44). The effectiveness of current control efforts is limited by financial constraints, a lack of surveillance tools to distinguish areas that require intervention from those that do not, and an imperfect understanding of the epidemiology of urban kala-azar. In the latter regard, there is evidence that perpetuation of transmission may be maintained by reservoir hosts in addition to dogs, such as foxes, marsupials, or human beings. Recently, a high rate of infection of laboratory-reared sand flies after feeding on patients with kala-azar was documented in a hospital in Teresina.

CONCLUSIONS

The impressive adaptability of *Leishmania* species to changing environments indicates that leishmaniasis will continue to be an unwelcome consequence of human behavior and economic development. At present, tools for interrupting transmission are limited: currently available drugs are less than satisfactory, an effective vaccine to prevent infection does not exist, and better techniques for diagnosis and surveillance are needed. High among the priorities for research on leishmaniasis is the development of new methods for predicting the occurrence of outbreaks and establishment of new foci of transmission. This will require a better understanding of the epidemiology and ecology of the infection and the reasons for its continued emergence and reemergence.

REFERENCES

1. **Alvar, J., C. Canavate, B. Gutierrez-Solar, M. Jimenez, F. Laguna, R. Lopez-Velez, R. Molina, and J. Moreno.** 1997. *Leishmania* and human immunodeficiency virus coinfection: the first 10 years. *Clin. Microbiol. Rev.* **10**:298–319.
2. **Alvar, J., and M. Jimenez.** 1994. Could infected drug-users be potential *Leishmania infantum* reservoirs? *AIDS* **8**:854. (Letter.)
3. **Arias, J. R., and R. D. Naiff.** 1981. The principal reservoir host of cutaneous leishmaniasis in the urban areas of Manaus, Central Amazon of Brazil. *Mem. Inst. Oswaldo Cruz* **76**:279–286.
4. **Ashford, R. W., and M. C. Thomson.** 1991. Visceral leishmaniasis in Sudan. A delayed development disaster? *Ann. Trop. Med. Parasitol.* **85**:571–572.
5. **Badaró, R., T. C. Jones, C. R. Lorenço, B. J. Cerf, D. Sampaio, E. M. Carvalho, H. Rocha, R. Teixeira, and W. D. Johnson, Jr.** 1986. A prospective study of visceral leishmaniasis in an endemic area of Brazil. *J. Infect. Dis.* **154**:639–649.
6. **Barral, A., R. Badaró, M. Barral-Netto, G. Grimaldi, Jr., H. Momem, and E. M. Carvalho.** 1986. Isolation of *Leishmania mexicana amazonensis* from the bone marrow in a case of American visceral leishmaniasis. *Am. J. Trop. Med. Hyg.* **35**:732–734.
7. **Berenguer, J., F. Gomez-Campdera, B. Padilla, M. Rodriguez-Ferrero, F. Anaya, S. Moreno, and F. Valderrabano.** 1998. Visceral leishmaniasis (Kala-Azar) in transplant recipients: case report and review. *Transplantation* **65**:1401–1404.
8. **Berman, J. D.** 1997. Human leishmaniasis: clinical, diagnostic, and chemotherapeutic developments in the last 10 years. *Clin. Infect. Dis.* **24**:684–703.
9. **Brandão-Filho, S., and J. Shaw.** 1994. Leishmaniasis in Brazil. *Parasitol. Today* **10**:329–330.
10. **Bryceson, A. D.** 1996. Leishmaniasis, p. 1213–1245. *In* G. C. Cook (ed.), *Manson's Tropical Diseases*, 20th ed. The W. B. Saunders Co., Philadelphia, Pa.
11. **Costa, C. H., H. F. Pereira, and M. V. Araújo.** 1990. Epidemia de leishmaniose visceral no estado do Piauí, Brasil, 1980–1986. *Rev. Saúde Pública* **24**:361–372.
12. **de Beer, P., A. el Harith, M. van Grootheest, and A. Winkler.** 1990. Outbreak of kala-azar in the Sudan. *Lancet* **335**:224. (Letter.)
13. **Desjeux, P.** 1992. Human leishmaniases: epidemiology and public health aspects. *World Health Stat. Q.* **45**:267–275.

14. **Dye, C.** 1992. Leishmaniasis epidemiology: the theory catches up. *Parasitology* **104**(Suppl.):S7–S18.

15. **Dye, C.** 1996. The logic of visceral leishmaniasis control. *Am. J. Trop. Med. Hyg.* **55**:125–130.

16. **Evans, T. G., M. J. Teixeira, I. T. McAuliffe, I. Vasconcelos, A. Vasconcelos, A. Sousa, J. Lima, and R. A. Pearson.** 1992. Epidemiology of visceral leishmaniasis in Northeast Brazil. *J. Infect. Dis.* **166**:1124–1132.

17. **Fundação Nacional de Saúde.** 1998. Statistics on leishmaniasis. Fundação Nacional de Saúde, Brasilia, Brazil.

18. **Giladi, M., C. Block, Y. L. Danon, E. Schinder, and C. L. Greenblatt.** 1988. Local environmental risk factors in the acquisition of cutaneous leishmaniasis. *Isr. J. Med. Sci.* **24**:185–187.

19. **Gratz, N. G.** 1999. Emerging and resurging vector-borne diseases. *Annu. Rev. Entomol.* **44**:51–75.

20. **Herwaldt, B. L., S. L. Stokes, and D. D. Juranek.** 1993. American cutaneous leishmaniasis in U.S. travelers. *Ann. Intern. Med.* **118**:779–784.

21. **Jeronimo, S. M., R. M. Oliveira, S. Mackay, R. M. Costa, J. Sweet, E. T. Nascimento, K. G. Luz, M. Z. Fernandes, J. Jernigan, and R. D. Pearson.** 1994. An urban outbreak of visceral leishmaniasis in Natal, Brazil. *Trans. R. Soc. Trop. Med. Hyg.* **88**:386–388.

22. **Killick-Kendrick, R.** 1990. The life-cycle of *Leishmania* in the sandfly with special reference to the form infective to the vertebrate host. *Ann. Parasitol. Hum. Comp.* **65**(Suppl. 1):37–42.

23. **Lainson, R.** 1988. Ecological interactions in the transmission of the leishmaniases. *Philos. Trans. R. Soc. Lond.* **321**:389–404.

24. **Lainson, R., and J. J. Shaw.** 1978. Epidemiology and ecology of leishmaniasis in Latin-America. *Nature* **273**:595–600.

25. **Lainson, R., L. Ryan, and J. J. Shaw.** 1987. Infective stages of *Leishmania* in the sandfly vector and some observations on the mechanism of transmission. *Mem. Inst. Oswaldo Cruz* **82**:421–424.

26. **Lainson, R.** 1985. Our present knowledge of the ecology and control of leishmaniasis in the Amazon region of Brazil. *Rev. Soc. Bras. Med. Trop.* **18**:47–56.

27. **Lara, M. L., Z. Layrisse, J. V. Scorza, E. Garcia, Z. Stoikow, J. Granados, and W. Bias.** 1991. Immunogenetics of human American cutaneous leishmaniasis. Study of HLA haplotypes in 24 families from Venezuela. *Hum. Immunol.* **30**:129–135.

28. **Magill, A. J.** 1995. Epidemiology of the leishmaniases. *Dermatol. Clin.* **13**:505–523.

29. **Maguire, J. H., C. H. Costa, D. Lamounier, L. Beck, B. Lobitz, S. Dister, and B. Wood.** 1999. Application for remote sensing and geographical information systems (GIS) technology to study transmission of *Leishmania chagasi* in Teresina, Piauí, Brazil. http://geo.arc.nasa.gov/sge/health/projects/leishb/leishb.

30. **Maguire, J. H., N. M. Gantz, S. Moschella, and S. C. Pan.** 1983. Leishmanial infections: a consideration in travellers returning from abroad. *Am. J. Med. Sci.* **285**:32–40.

31. **McGregor, A.** 1998. WHO warns of epidemic leishmania. *Lancet* **351**:575.

32. **McHugh, C. P., P. C. Melby, and S. G. Lafon.** 1996. Leishmaniasis in Texas: epidemiology and clinical aspects of human cases. *Am. J. Trop. Med. Hyg.* **55**:547–555.

33. **Molyneux, D. H.** 1997. Patterns of change in vector-borne diseases. *Ann. Trop. Med. Parasitol.* **91**:827–839.

34. **Molyneux, D. H.** 1998. Vector-borne parasitic diseases—an overview of recent changes. *Int. J. Parasitol.* **28**:927–934.

35. **National Aeronautics and Space Administration.** 1998. NASA: CHAART Satellite and Sensor Evaluation for Public Health. http://geo.arc.nasa.gov/sge/health/sensor/sensor.htm.

36. **Pearson, R. D., and A. Q. Sousa.** 1996. Clinical spectrum of leishmaniasis. *Clin. Infect. Dis.* **22**:1–13.

37. **Ponce, C., E. Ponce, A. Morrison, A. Cruz, R. Kreutzer, D. McMahon-Pratt, and F. Neva.** 1991. *Leishmania donovani chagasi*: new clinical variant of cutaneous leishmaniasis in Honduras. *Lancet* **337**:67–70.

38. **Punda-Polic, V., S. Sardelic, and N. Bradaric.** 1998. Visceral leishmaniasis in southern Croatia. *Lancet* **351**:188. (Letter.)

39. **Seaman, J., A. J. Mercer, and E. Sondorp.** 1996. The epidemic of visceral leishmaniasis in western Upper Nile, southern Sudan: course and impact from 1984 to 1994. *Int. J. Epidemiol.* **25**:862–871.

40. **Seaman, J., R. W. Ashford, J. Schorscher, and J. Dereure.** 1992. Visceral leishmaniasis in southern Sudan: status of healthy villagers in epidemic conditions. *Ann. Trop. Med. Parasitol.* **86:**481–486.

41. **Sherlock, I. A.** 1996. Ecological interactions of visceral leishmaniasis in the State of Bahia, Brazil. *Mem. Inst. Oswaldo Cruz* **91:**671–683.

42. **Sousa, A. Q., M. E. Parise, M. M. Pompeu, J. M. Coelho Filho, I. A. Vasconcelos, J. W. Lima, E. G. Oliveira, A. W. Vasconcelos, J. R. David, and J. H. Maguire.** 1995. Bubonic leishmaniasis: a common manifestation of *Leishmania* (*Viannia*) *braziliensis* infection in Ceara, Brazil. *Am. J. Trop. Med. Hyg.* **53:**380–385.

43. **Sundar, S., N. K. Agrawal, P. R. Sinha, G. S. Horwith, and H. W. Murray.** 1997. Short-course, low-dose amphotericin B lipid complex therapy for visceral leishmaniasis unresponsive to antimony. *Ann. Intern. Med.* **127:**133–137.

44. **Tesh, R. B.** 1995. Control of leishmaniasis: is it time to change strategies? *Am. J. Trop. Med. Hyg.* **52:**287–292.

45. **Tesh, R. B., and G. Papaevangelou.** 1977. Effect of insecticide spraying for malaria control on the incidence of sandfly fever in Athens, Greece. *Am. J. Trop. Med. Hyg.* **26:**163–166.

46. **Walton, B. C.** 1989. Leishmaniasis. A worldwide problem. *Int. J. Dermatol.* **28:**305–307.

47. **Wijeyaratne, P. M., L. K. Arsenault, and C. J. Murphy.** 1994. Endemic disease and development: the leishmaniases. *Acta Trop.* **56:**349–364.

48. **World Health Organization Division of Control of Tropical Diseases.** 1998. *Disease Sheet: Leishmaniasis.* http://www.who.ch.programmes/ctd/diseases/leis/.

Emerging Infections 3
Edited by W. M. Scheld, W. A. Craig, and J. M. Hughes
© 1999 ASM Press, Washington, D.C.

Chapter 8

Chagas' Disease (American Trypanosomiasis): a Tropical Disease Now Emerging in the United States

Louis V. Kirchhoff

Chagas' disease (American trypanosomiasis) is a zoonosis caused by *Trypanosoma cruzi*, a flagellated protozoan parasite that is found only in the Americas. The geographic distribution of *T. cruzi* infection in humans and its other mammalian hosts is determined primarily by the range of the various species of hematophagous triatomine insects that act as vectors. This range extends from central Argentina to the southern United States. Even though large portions of the range of *T. cruzi* endemicity lie in temperate regions, Chagas' disease is generally considered a tropical disease because the majority of persons with the illness live in the tropics.

THE ORGANISM AND MECHANISMS OF TRANSMISSION

The genus *Trypanosoma* contains about 20 species, but only *T. cruzi* and two African trypanosome subspecies, *Trypanosoma brucei rhodesiense* and *T. brucei gambiense*, are pathogenic in humans (77). *T. cruzi* was first described in 1909 by a Brazilian physician, Carlos Chagas, who observed the motile parasites while doing microscopic examinations of dissected intestines of triatomine insects (23). He named the organism after his mentor, Oswaldo Cruz. The complex life cycle of *T. cruzi* involves both mammalian hosts and insect vectors (Fig. 1) Various species of triatomines, or kissing bugs, transmit *T. cruzi* (Fig. 2). These vectors are found in great numbers in the wild, where the organism is transmitted among many mammalian species that make up the natural reservoir. In areas of endemicity the triatomines live in the nooks and crannies of the substandard dwellings that are so common in Latin America. The insects become infected with *T. cruzi* by taking blood meals from humans or other mammals that have circulating trypomastigotes

Louis V. Kirchhoff • Department of Internal Medicine, University of Iowa, and Department of Veterans Affairs Medical Center, Iowa City, IA 52242.

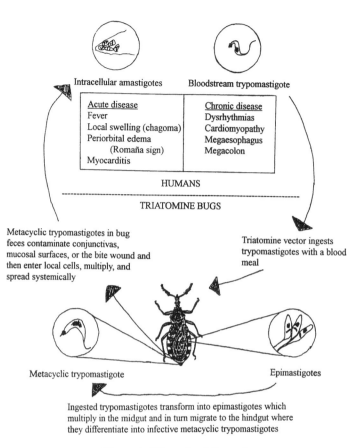

Figure 1. Life cycle of *T. cruzi.*

(Fig. 3). Ingested parasites multiply in the midgut of the insects after transformation into epimastigotes, which are flagellates of a distinct morphologic type. In the hindgut epimastigotes become infective metacyclic trypomastigotes that are discharged with the feces at the time of subsequent blood meals. Transmission to a second mammalian host occurs when conjunctivas, mucous membranes, or breaks in the skin are contaminated with bug feces containing infective trypomastigotes. The organisms then enter a variety of host cell types and multiply in the cytoplasm after differentiation into amastigotes. After multiplication amastigotes fill a host cell, they transform into trypomastigotes, and the cell ruptures. The released parasites invade local cells or spread via blood and lymph to distant tissues such as muscles, where they initiate further cycles of multiplication and maintain a parasitemia infective for insect vectors.

T. cruzi can also be transmitted by transfusion of blood donated by persons who harbor the parasite, and this mode of transmission constitutes a public health problem in some areas of endemicity (110). This usually takes place in cities when infected asymptomatic migrants from rural areas of endemicity donate blood. Con-

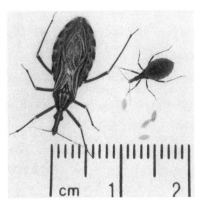

Figure 2. Eggs, second instar nymph, and adult of *Rhodnius prolixus*, a triatomine vector of *T. cruzi*.

genital transmission has also been reported and can be associated with spontaneous abortions as well as a high fatality rate and severe impairment in infants coming to term (9, 38). Finally, dozens of laboratory accidents that have resulted in the transmission of *T. cruzi* have occurred as a consequence of the ease with which infective forms can be produced in the laboratory (51, 53)

THE DISEASE

Acute and Indeterminate Phases of Chagas' Disease

The first sign of acute *T. cruzi* infection can be a chagoma, which is an erythematous and indurated inflammatory lesion at the site of parasite entry that ap-

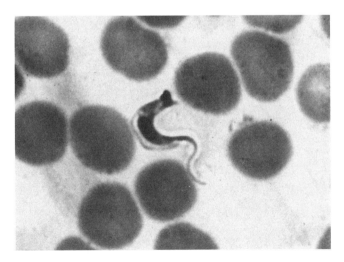

Figure 3. *T. cruzi* trypomastigote in human blood. Giemsa stain was used. Magnification, ×625. Courtesy of Maria A. Shikanai Yasuda, São Paulo, Brazil.

pears a week or two after transmission has taken place (97). When the parasite has entered through a conjunctiva, the patient may develop Romaña's sign, which consists of unilateral and painless periorbital edema (Fig. 4). Romaña's sign is found in only a small percentage of patients with acute Chagas' disease, however, and similar findings can result from several other processes. Spread of the parasites from the site of initial multiplication may be accompanied by fever, malaise, edema of the face and lower extremities, as well as generalized lymphadenopathy and hepatosplenomegaly. Some patients develop morbilliform rashes called schizotrypanides. Lymphocytosis may accompany the high parasitemias of acute *T. cruzi* infection, and mild elevation of transaminase levels may also be present. Cardiac and skeletal muscles can be heavily parasitized, and severe myocarditis develops in a small proportion of patients, occasionally causing death (72, 91) (Fig. 5). Nonspecific electrocardiographic abnormalities can occur, but the life-threatening conduction disturbances common in chronic cardiac Chagas' disease usually are not present. *T. cruzi* also can invade the central nervous system (52), but neurologic findings are uncommon. Meningoencephalitis, a rare complication of acute *T. cruzi* infection, is associated with a poor prognosis (120). Acute Chagas' disease resolves spontaneously in 4 to 8 weeks in the vast majority of patients, who then enter the *indeterminate phase* of the infection, which is characterized by a lack of symptoms, lifelong subpatent parasitemias, and easily detectable antibodies to *T. cruzi* antigens.

Chronic Chagas' Heart Disease

Although most patients with chronic *T. cruzi* infections remain in the indeterminate phase for life, roughly 10 to 30% develop symptomatic chronic Chagas'

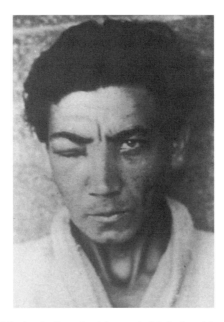

Figure 4. Romaña's sign (unilateral painless periorbital edema) in a Brazilian patient with acute Chagas' disease. Courtesy of Mário Shiroma, São Paulo, Brazil.

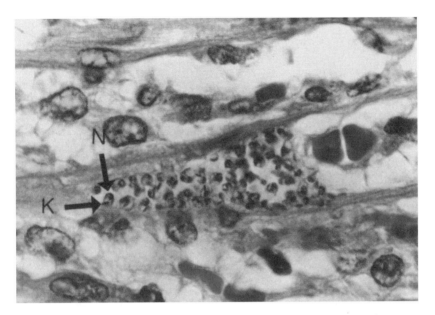

Figure 5. *T. cruzi* in the heart muscle of a child who died of acute Chagas' disease. The infected cardiomyocyte shown contains several dozen amastigotes. Arrows point to the kinetoplast (k) and nucleus (N) of one amastigote. The kinetoplast is characteristic of the order Kinetoplastida, to which *T. cruzi* belongs.

disease, typically years or even decades after the infection was acquired. Cardiac problems are the most frequent consequence of chronic *T. cruzi* infection. Hearts obtained at autopsy from patients who died of Chagas' cardiomyopathy usually have a global appearance due to chamber enlargement, and thrombi are frequently present. Apical aneurysms of the left ventricle are typical in patients with advanced cardiac Chagas' disease. The process underlying these gross pathologic lesions is chronic inflammation with mononuclear cell infiltration and diffuse fibrosis, which affect the conduction system as well as the cardiac muscle (4, 5). Parasites are rarely seen by light microscopy but can be detected by PCR. The inflammatory process results in a variety of dysrhythmias, including premature ventricular contractions, atrial bradyarrhythmias, and fibrillation; bundle branch blocks, typically of the right bundle; and complete atrioventricular block. Most instances of sudden death in patients with chronic Chagas' disease probably result from the latter or ventricular arrhythmias. The symptoms associated with chronic cardiac Chagas' disease reflect the rhythm disturbances, congestive failure, and thromboembolism that result from the fibrosing cardiopathy (66). The dysrhythmias can cause dizziness and syncope, and sudden death is a common occurrence (1, 96). Symptoms of right-sided failure are often present, as the cardiomyopathy frequently affects the right side of the heart more than the left side.

Chronic Gastrointestinal Chagas' Disease (Megadisease)

Dysfunction of the gastrointestinal tract is the second most common result of chronic Chagas' disease (62). As with Chagas' cardiopathy, chagasic gastrointestinal disease usually occurs years or decades after *T. cruzi* infection is acquired. Symptoms resulting from megaesophagus (Fig. 6) are the most typical clinical manifestations, but symptoms related to megacolon (Fig. 7) are also common. The process underlying megadisease is a loss of neurons in the gastrointestinal tract (69, 70). Quantitative evaluations of this degenerative process have shown that in severely affected patients up to 85% of the neurons in the esophagus and 50% of those in the colon may be lost (69). The factors that underlie the variable rate and pattern of neuronal destruction are not known.

Pathologic examination of esophageal specimens obtained surgically or at autopsy from patients with megaesophagus have shown various degrees of thickening of the muscular wall and dilatation. As in the case of cardiac tissue, microscopic examination shows fibrosis and mononuclear cell infiltration, but the finding of parasites is unusual. The symptom most commonly associated with chagasic megaesophagus is dysphagia. Many patients with megaesophagus sense substernal accumulation of swallowed food and take in water or more food or even eat in a

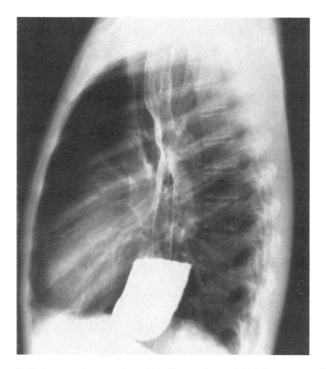

Figure 6. Barium esophagram in a Brazilian patient with dolicomegaesophagus caused by chronic Chagas' disease. Contrast material is pooled in the distal esophagus, which is markedly enlarged. Courtesy of Franklin A. Neva. Reprinted from reference 89a with permission from The McGraw-Hill Companies.

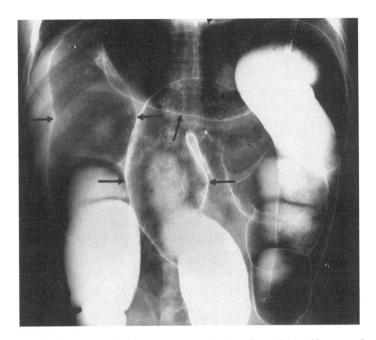

Figure 7. Air contrast barium enema examination of a patient with megacolon associated with chronic *T. cruzi* infection. Increased diameters of the ascending, transverse, and sigmoid segments of the colon are marked with opposing arrows.

standing position to facilitate its passage into the stomach. Pain, which often begins in the lower substernal region and which spreads upward, also is a frequent symptom in patients with megaesophagus. In patients with severe megaesophagus, regurgitation can be a problem, and if the underlying abnormality is not treated, it can lead to intermittent aspiration with associated bronchitis, chronic cough, and pneumonia.

As with chagasic megaesophagus, colonic disease is manifested by thickening of the wall and dilatation. The sigmoid colon is the most frequently affected segment. As the disease progresses, the colon can become markedly enlarged in both diameter and length, and with time the thickening of the wall can become less pronounced. The pathologic changes apparent on microscopic examination of affected colonic tissue are similar to those found in the esophagus. Constipation is the most common symptom associated with Chagas' disease of the colon. As the size of the colon gradually increases over time, the frequency of bowel movements decreases, and some patients have periods of constipation that last weeks. Pain resulting from ineffective and recurrent colonic contractions, as well as accumulation of feces and flatus, is also a common symptom.

Other organs can be affected by chronic gastrointestinal Chagas' disease. A common finding is hypertrophy of the parotid glands, which is present in as many as 25% of patients with chagasic megaesophagus. The stomach may also be involved, although much less commonly than the esophagus and colon, and affected patients usually have either megacolon or megaesophagus (28). Hypotonia, hypo-peristalsis, decreased acid secretion, and delayed emptying of the stomach have been described in patients with megaesophagus, but dilatation of the stomach is not found frequently (117).

The pathogenesis of the gastrointestinal and cardiac lesions associated with chronic *T. cruzi* infection has been debated for many years. Some investigators have held that autoimmune mechanisms cause the chronic pathology (27, 116). Studies showing that mammalian nerve and cardiac cells have epitopes that cross-react with antibodies to *T. cruzi* epitopes support this concept (31, 119, 125). Others have thought that injury resulting from the presence of parasites in tissues constitutes the fundamental pathogenic insult that leads to the lesions of the chronic phase (69). Considerable experimental work has been done in attempts to resolve this issue. Recently, a small number of studies with experimental animals and humans have provided evidence supporting the concept that a low-level presence of parasites in chronically affected cardiac tissue, detectable by PCR-based assays, stimulates a chronic inflammatory response that over time causes the pathology (18, 56). These findings and those of a limited number of treatment trials with experimental animals and humans suggest that elimination of the parasites may truncate the pathogenic process and have stimulated experts in the field to recommend an approach to specific treatment more aggressive than that used in the past.

Immunosuppression and *T. cruzi* Infection

Immunosuppression of patients chronically infected with *T. cruzi* can lead to a recrudescence of the infection, often with an intensity that is atypical of acute Chagas' disease in immunocompetent patients. The incidence of reactivation of *T. cruzi* in patients who are immunosuppressed is not known, and both its absence (10, 32, 80, 81) and its occurrence (71, 102, 106) have been described. Several reports of reactivations of chronic *T. cruzi* infections after renal transplantation have appeared, and in two of these cases there was involvement of the central nervous system (75, 86, 95). In my view chronic *T. cruzi* infection should not be considered a contraindication for kidney transplantation. *T. cruzi*-infected patients who have undergone the procedure, however, should be monitored periodically for signs and symptoms of reactivation.

Persons coinfected with the human immunodeficiency virus (HIV) and *T. cruzi* are also at risk for reactivation of the latter. Several dozen such cases have been described (103, 108), and it is noteworthy that a large proportion of these patients developed *T. cruzi* brain abscesses, which do not occur in immunocompetent persons with acute or chronic Chagas' disease. Calculations based on the epidemiologies of HIV and *T. cruzi* in Latin America suggest that the incidence of *T. cruzi* brain abscesses in persons infected with both organisms is extremely low. The diagnosis of *T. cruzi* brain abscesses in HIV-infected persons is complicated by the difficulty in distinguishing these lesions radiographically from those of cerebral toxoplasmosis.

DIAGNOSIS

Acute Chagas' Disease

The first item to look for when one considers the diagnosis of acute *T. cruzi* infection is a history of exposure to the parasite. This could take the form of residence in an environment in which vector-borne transmission occurs, a recent blood transfusion in an area of endemicity, birth to a mother who is chronically infected, or a laboratory accident involving *T. cruzi*. In the United States it is important to keep in mind that imported cases among tourists returning from countries where the disease is endemic have not been reported and that autochthonous *T. cruzi* infections are extremely rare.

The diagnosis of acute *T. cruzi* infection is made by detecting parasites, and serologic tests play a limited role. Circulating organisms are highly motile, and they often can be seen in wet preparations of anticoagulated blood or buffy coat. In many cases, the parasites can also be seen in Giemsa-stained smears of these specimens. In acutely infected immunocompetent patients examination of blood preparations is the cornerstone of *T. cruzi* detection. In immunocompromised patients suspected of having acute Chagas' disease, however, microscopic examination of other specimens such as lymph node and bone marrow aspirates and cerebrospinal fluid and pericardial fluid specimens may give positive results. When these approaches fail to detect *T. cruzi* in a patient whose epidemiologic and clinical histories suggest the presence of the parasite, as is often the case (112), attempts to grow the organism can be made. This can be done by culturing blood or other specimens in liquid media (24) or by xenodiagnosis (84), which involves allowing laboratory-reared insect vectors to feed on a patient suspected of being infected with *T. cruzi*. A major disadvantage of these two methods is the fact that they take at least a month to complete, and this is beyond the time at which decisions regarding treatment must be made. Moreover, although xenodiagnosis and hemoculture are 100% specific, their sensitivities may be no greater than 50 to 70%. In view of this, it is clear that improved methods for the diagnosis of acute Chagas' disease are needed, and PCR-based assays may fulfill this role (see below).

Chronic Chagas' Disease

Chronic Chagas' disease is usually diagnosed by detecting immunoglobulin G antibodies that react specifically with parasite antigens, and finding the parasite is not of primary importance. A number of sensitive serologic tests are used in Latin America, such as the indirect immunofluorescence, indirect hemagglutination, complement fixation, and enzyme-linked immunosorbent assays (22, 92). A persistent shortcoming of these serodiagnostic assays has been the occurrence of false-positive results. This occurs typically with specimens from patients having illnesses such as toxoplasmosis, malaria, leishmaniasis, syphilis, and other parasitic and nonparasitic diseases. Because of this problem, most authorities recommend that sera be tested by two or three serologic tests. The latter approach carries with it enormous logistical and economic burdens, both in clinical settings and in blood banks. For example, in the largest blood donor center in São Paulo, Brazil, 3.4%

of donated units are thrown out because of reactivity in one or more of the three assays used. As many as two-thirds of these may in fact come from donors not infected with *T. cruzi* but must be discarded because of inconsistent test results (22). Thus, as is the case with acute Chagas' disease, improved tests for the detection of chronic *T. cruzi* infection are needed.

A variety of test kits for the detection of antibodies to *T. cruzi* are available commercially in Latin America. These kits are used in many areas to screen donated blood and for clinical testing, but in some regions of endemicity screening of the blood supply is limited by a lack of appreciation of the problem of transfusion-associated transmission of *T. cruzi* and financial constraints (21). In the United States there are several options for serologic testing for *T. cruzi* infection. Abbott Laboratories has received Food and Drug Administration (FDA) clearance for marketing of an assay for clinical testing but not blood bank screening (Chagas EIA, Abbott Laboratories, Abbott Park, Ill.) (92). Clearance for clinical use has also been obtained for tests manufactured by Gull Laboratories (Chagas' IgG ELISA, Gull Laboratories, Salt Lake City, Utah) and Hemagen Diagnostics (Chagas' Kit [EIA method], Hemagen Diagnostics, Waltham, Mass.). Limited comparative studies of the Abbott and Gull assays suggest that the former may have a slight advantage in terms of sensitivity and specificity (12, 22). Finally, in my laboratory we perform a confirmatory radioimmune precipitation assay that was shown to be highly sensitive and specific when used to test geographically diverse groups of positive and negative specimens (65).

Considerable effort has been invested in developing new assays for the detection of both acute and chronic *T. cruzi* infections. Several laboratories have focused on the development of tests in which synthetic peptides or recombinant *T. cruzi* proteins are used as target antigens. Most of these efforts have been directed toward the detection of antibodies to *T. cruzi* in chronically infected persons (20, 22, 37, 54, 82). When taken together, these studies suggest that tests with recombinant proteins that have higher specificities than the conventional assays but that still maintain high levels of sensitivity will be developed. The tests described to date have not been evaluated in large field trials, however, and none are available commercially.

The possibility of using PCR-based assays for direct detection of *T. cruzi* has also been studied (61, 63). Although the number of parasites in the blood of patients with chronic *T. cruzi* infection is extremely low, PCR-based assays have the potential to detect such low numbers because the organisms have highly repetitive kinetoplast DNA and nuclear sequences that can be amplified by PCR. Moser et al. (88) described a PCR-based test in which a 188-bp repetitive nuclear DNA sequence, of which there are ~100,000 copies per parasite, is amplified. In contrived experiments as little as 1/200 of the DNA of a single parasite gave a positive result. Studies with mice indicated clearly that this PCR-based assay is much more sensitive than microscopic examination of blood throughout the course of *T. cruzi* infection (67). Russomando et al. (104) confirmed this sensitivity in a study of acutely and chronically infected patients, and other investigators have obtained similarly encouraging results.

In a second PCR-based assay, first described by Sturm and coworkers (115), a 330-bp segment of the *T. cruzi* kinetoplast minicircle is amplified. Each parasite has ~120,000 copies of this sequence, and in mixing experiments the investigators were able to detect 1/1,000 of a parasite genome. Results obtained in subsequent studies with humans suggest that this test may be useful for the definitive diagnosis of *T. cruzi* infection (8, 17, 43, 44). In view of the results obtained by these two approaches, it appears that there may be a useful role for PCR-based assays for the diagnosis of *T. cruzi* infection. Problems that may limit their widespread use, however, include the occurrence of false-positive results due to contamination of reaction mixtures, as well as the complexity of the technology that may not be appropriate for the developing countries in which Chagas' disease is endemic. Presently, no PCR-based assay for the detection of *T. cruzi* is available commercially.

EPIDEMIOLOGY

Epizootiology of *T. cruzi*

Infection with *T. cruzi* is a zoonosis, and human involvement in the cycle of transmission is not necessary for persistence of the parasite in nature. *T. cruzi* is found only in the Americas, where it infects triatomine insect vectors as well as many species of wild and domestic mammals. Triatomine vectors that transmit *T. cruzi* are found from the southern half of the United States to central Argentina. Burrows, hollow trees, palm trees, and other animal shelters are places where *T. cruzi* transmission takes place among nonhuman mammalian hosts and infected vectors. Piles of old vegetation, roof tiles, and wood near houses have also been found to harbor large numbers of triatomines (114). Insect-borne transmission to humans occurs only in areas inhabited by triatomines that defecate during or immediately after blood meals. This restriction does not apply to transmission to nonhuman mammalian hosts, however, as they can become infected by eating infected insects (105). *T. cruzi* has been found in more than 100 species of wild and domestic mammals (41) in areas that correspond to the distribution of its triatomine vectors (11, 57, 123, 124, 126). Armadillos, opossums, wood rats, raccoons, cats, and dogs are typical hosts, but *T. cruzi* is not a problem in livestock. This lack of species specificity and the fact that infected mammals have lifelong parasitemias result in enormous domestic and sylvatic reservoirs in areas where the disease is enzootic.

Numerous descriptions of *T. cruzi* infection in mammals in the United States have appeared over the years. Raccoons and dogs in Virginia (11), armadillos in Louisiana (126), coyotes in Texas (46), and more recently, dogs in Texas and Oklahoma (15, 85) have all been reported to be infected with *T. cruzi*. Most of the dogs infected with the parasite are used in hunting, and they may acquire *T. cruzi* orally when they capture and eat infected prey. *T. cruzi* infection in insect vectors in the southern United States has been reported as well. In my view the sylvatic cycle of *T. cruzi* infection in this geographic region long predates the arrival of humans, and the peridomestic cycle was established as human populations first spread through the continent.

Epidemiology of Chagas' Disease in Latin America

Humans become involved in the cycle of *T. cruzi* transmission when land is opened up for farming or other activities in areas where the disease is enzootic and where vector species adaptable to living in human dwellings, such as *Triatoma infestans* and *Rhodnius prolixus*, are prevalent. As the natural environment of the vectors and mammalian hosts is disrupted, the insects take up residence in the nooks and crannies of the settlers' primitive mud, wood, and stone houses. In this manner infected triatomines become domiciliary, and a domestic cycle of transmission that includes domestic animals such as cats and dogs, as well as humans, is established (47, 114). Thus, Chagas' disease is for the most part a public health problem among poor people who live in rural areas. The average age of initial infection in areas of intense transmission is thought to be about 4 years, and in one survey 85% of acute cases occurred in children less than 10 years old (72). The case fatality rate for acute Chagas' disease was 12% in that study of hospitalized patients, but the fatality rate for all new infections is probably less than 1%.

Early reports indicated that most cases of acute *T. cruzi* infection that came to medical attention were in children (72). Prevalence data support this perspective, but few age-specific incidence data have been available because the vast majority of cases of the acute illness go undetected because of its mild nature and a lack of access to medical care among those at high risk.

The Pan American Health Organization estimated recently that 16 million to 18 million persons are infected with *T. cruzi* and that about 45,000 deaths attributable to Chagas' disease occur each year (6). In recent years the epidemiology of *T. cruzi* infection has been improving in several countries where the disease is endemic, however, as vector and blood bank control programs have been implemented successfully. As a result of these efforts, prevalence rates in younger age groups have decreased in many areas. The framework for much of the progress achieved to date has been the major international control program in the "southern cone" nations of South America (Uruguay, Chile, Argentina, Bolivia, Brazil, and Paraguay) that was initiated in 1991. It is thought that if current trends continue, transmission will be essentially eliminated in much of the range of endemicity by the year 2003 (87, 111). Only economic and political barriers stand in the way of the elimination of *T. cruzi* infection from humans, and no technical advances, such as a vaccine, are necessary for its completion.

The epidemiology of symptomatic chronic Chagas' disease merits comment. At most about 10 to 30% of patients with chronic *T. cruzi* infections will develop symptoms of Chagas' disease (89), and there is considerable geographic variability in the prevalence of symptomatic chronic Chagas' disease among chronically infected patients (42). For example, the prevalence of cardiac disease in persons chronically infected with *T. cruzi* is lower in Colombia, Venezuela, Central America, and Mexico than in the rest of the range of endemicity. Interestingly, moreover, megaesophagus and megacolon in association with *T. cruzi* infection are virtually unknown in the regions of endemicity where cardiac disease is relatively low, whereas it is about 15 to 20% in the southern regions of endemicity. It is not known whether parasite strain differences or host genetic factors are the determinants of this geographic variation in the patterns of clinical disease (33, 100).

Epidemiology of Chagas' Disease in the United States

Even though *T. cruzi*-infected triatomine insects are present in many parts of the western and southern United States, only four autochthonous cases of acute Chagas' disease have been reported. Three of these occurred in Texas, and one occurred in California (91, 109). The rarity of acquisition of *T. cruzi* by humans in the United States most likely results from the low overall vector density and the relatively high housing standards in the United States. Other forms of acute Chagas' disease are also uncommon. In the last 26 years, nine imported cases of acute *T. cruzi* infection and seven confirmed laboratory-acquired infections have been reported to the Centers for Disease Control and Prevention (CDC). Importantly, none of the imported cases occurred in tourists returning to the United States, but two such instances have been reported in Europe (16, 30). Although the number of imported and autochthonous cases of acute Chagas' disease that go unrecognized may be several times the number described, the fact is that acute *T. cruzi* infection is rare in the United States, and there is no reason to expect that this situation will change.

In contrast, in recent decades the number of persons in the United States with chronic *T. cruzi* infections has grown enormously due to the immigration of people from Latin American countries where the disease is endemic. Between 1972 and 1994, approximately 9 million persons emigrated legally from Latin America to the United States (19), and several million more may have entered the United States illegally. A large percentage of these immigrants have come from Central America, where the prevalence of *T. cruzi* infection is high (101, 110). In a study of Nicaraguan and Salvadoran immigrants living in Washington, D.C., the prevalence of *T. cruzi* infection was 5% (64). Seroprevalence studies done with blood donors in Los Angeles, 50% of whom were Hispanic, showed that between 1 in 1,000 and 1 in 500 donors were infected with *T. cruzi* (7, 58, 113). In another investigation, done in seven blood banks in three southwestern states, 1 of 603 blood donors with Hispanic surnames was found to be infected (122). Most recently, in a study of 300,000 donors in Miami, Fla., and Los Angeles, Calif., the prevalence of *T. cruzi* infection was found to be 1 in 8,800 in the general donor population and 1 in 710 among donors who had spent at least a month in an area in which Chagas' disease is endemic (74). In all epidemiologic studies done to date in the United States, confirmatory testing has been done by radioimmunoprecipitation assay, and thus, the rates of chronic *T. cruzi* infection reported are likely to reflect the actual prevalences. When taken together, these findings and census data indicate that 50,000 to 100,000 *T. cruzi*-infected individuals now live in the United States.

This emergence of Chagas' disease in the United States merits attention for a number of reasons. In my view, because of the possible serious consequences of chronic *T. cruzi* infection, all immigrants from regions where *T. cruzi* is endemic should be screened serologically. Identification of infected persons is important because it is currently recommended that they be treated with benznidazole, even though its efficacy is less than optimal. Moreover, cardiac pacemakers have been shown to benefit some infected patients who develop rhythm disturbances (25). The possibility of congenital transmission is another justification for screening since newborns who harbor *T. cruzi* need to be treated with specific therapy (40, 73).

The presence of *T. cruzi*-infected immigrants poses a risk of transfusion-associated transmission of *T. cruzi* in North America (59), and six such cases have been reported in the United States and Canada (26, 45, 90). The courses of acute Chagas' disease in these transfusion recipients were particularly severe because of immunosuppressive treatments that they were receiving, and no doubt this contributed to the specific diagnosis. Most transfusions are given to immunocompetent persons in whom acute Chagas' disease would be a mild illness, and thus, it is reasonable to infer that many other instances of transfusion-associated transmission of *T. cruzi* have occurred in North America but have not been recognized.

The question of how best to avoid transfusion-associated transmission of *T. cruzi* is not easily answered. Since no test has been cleared by FDA for use in U.S. blood banks, serologic screening currently is not a possibility. An alternative method for reducing the risk of transmission by transfusion is to defer from donation prospective donors whose answers to a questionnaire indicate that they are at high risk for *T. cruzi* infection. In a recent study in a Los Angeles blood bank where 50% of donors are Hispanic, my coworkers and I assessed the usefulness of such a questionnaire for identifying high-risk donors and the impact of their deferral on the blood supply (7). We found that by deferring donors judged to be at high risk because of prolonged residence in areas of endemicity under conditions that favor exposure to insect vectors or a history of transfusion or seroreactivity there, the blood supply would be reduced by only 2.0%. Moreover, the prevalence of *T. cruzi* infection in the deferred group was consistent with our previous estimate of the prevalence among donors in that blood bank ($\sim$1:1,000) (58). These findings suggest that a questionnaire-based approach may effectively reduce the risk of transfusion-associated transmission of *T. cruzi* and not reduce the blood supply intolerably. Several years ago, to deal with the risk posed by the presence of *T. cruzi*-infected immigrants, FDA recommended that prospective blood donors be screened with questions relating to residence in countries where Chagas' disease is endemic. This may have reduced the number of incidents of transmission, but it is important to bear in mind that preventive methods based solely on questionnaires have not been entirely successful at eliminating transfusion-associated transmission of other infectious agents (7, 39).

TREATMENT AND PROGNOSIS

Antiparasitic Drugs

Two drugs are available for the treatment of patients infected with *T. cruzi* (29, 76, 83). The first is the nitrofuran derivative nifurtimox (Lampit; Bayer 2502), which has been used widely for more than two decades. In patients with acute Chagas' disease, nifurtimox markedly reduces the duration and severity of the illness and decreases the rate of mortality. Unfortunately, however, it results in parasitologic cure in only about 70% of patients treated during the acute phase of the illness, can cause bothersome side effects, and must be taken for an extended period (35, 98). Cure rates with nifurtimox are higher in Chile and Argentina than in Brazil and some of the other countries where the disease is endemic. A sizable percentage of patients treated with nifurtimox experience adverse side effects. Gastrointestinal complaints include nausea, vomiting, abdominal pain, anorexia, and weight loss. Possible neurologic symptoms include insomnia, restlessness, twitching, paresthesias, and seizures. Symptoms usually disappear when the dosage is reduced or therapy is discontinued.

Nifurtimox is available in 30- and 120-mg tablets. The recommended oral dosage for adults is 8 to 10 mg/kg of body weight/day. For adolescents the dosage is 12.5 to 15 mg/kg/day, and for children 1 to 10 years of age it is 15 to 20 mg/kg/day. Nifurtimox should be given in four divided doses each day, and treatment should be continued for 90 to 120 days. Nifurtimox is available from the Drug Service of CDC [(770) 639-3670 (business hours), (770) 639-2888 (other times)].

Benznidazole (Rochagan; Roche 7-1051), a nitroimidazole derivative, is the second agent used to treat patients with *T. cruzi* infection. The efficacy of this drug is similar to that of nifurtimox, with the exception that geographic differences in its efficacy have not been reported (35). Common side effects include rash, granulocytopenia, and peripheral neuropathy. The recommended dosage of benznidazole is 5 mg/kg/day by mouth for 60 days. This drug is used widely in countries where the disease is endemic, where it is viewed as the drug of choice by many experts. It also is available from the CDC Drug Service.

The question of whether patients in the indeterminate or chronic symptomatic phases of Chagas' disease should be treated with nifurtimox or benznidazole has been debated for decades. Recent evidence from studies with *T. cruzi*-infected humans and laboratory animals indicates that the presence of parasites in cardiac muscle is specifically associated with inflammation, thus implicating the organisms in the chronic pathogenesis (3, 13, 56). In addition, in a number of long-term follow-up studies the rates of appearance of and/or progression of heart pathology in treated patients were significantly lower than those in untreated controls (2, 36, 121). After reviewing these findings, an international panel of experts recently recommended that all patients with Chagas' disease be treated with either benznidazole or nifurtimox, regardless of their clinical status or the time that has elapsed since infection (97a).

The use of two drugs, which were developed for other purposes, for the treatment of acute *T. cruzi* infection merits discussion. Over a decade ago Reed (99) showed that the severity of acute *T. cruzi* infection in mice was reduced by injection of recombinant gamma interferon (IFN-γ). To my knowledge recombinant IFN-γ has been given to two patients with acute Chagas' disease. The first was an immunosuppressed patient who acquired the parasite from a contaminated transfusion (45), and the other patient became infected through laboratory work with *T. cruzi* (115a). Both patients received IFN-γ as well as nifurtimox and recovered. Serologic and PCR-based studies done with one of these patients 8 years after treatment indicate that the treatment was curative, but this issue has not been addressed with the second patient. Additional studies need to be done before a recommendation regarding the use of IFN-γ in patients with acute Chagas' disease can be made.

The usefulness of allopurinol, fluconazole, and itraconazole has been examined extensively in studies with laboratory animals and to a lesser extent with persons with *T. cruzi* infections. The results obtained do not justify the use of any of these drugs in *T. cruzi*-infected patients. Finally, an antifungal agent, bis-triazole (D0807), was recently reported to cure acute *T. cruzi* infections in mice (79, 118), but it is still in the early stages of development.

Treatment of Clinical Chagas' Disease

Most patients with acute Chagas' disease require no therapy other than nifurtimox or benznidazole since this phase of the illness generally resolves spontaneously, even in the absence of specific treatment. Management of the occasional severely ill patient with chagasic meningoencephalitis or myocarditis is for the most part supportive. The treatment of patients with symptomatic chronic chagasic heart disease is also supportive. Persons with chronic *T. cruzi* infections should have electrocardiograms done approximately every 6 months because pacemakers have been shown to be useful in managing the rhythm disturbances of chronic Chagas' disease (25). Congestive heart failure associated with cardiomyopathic Chagas' disease is generally treated with measures used for patients with cardiomyopathies caused by other processes (49, 50).

Megaesophagus associated with Chagas' disease should be treated in the same way as idiopathic achalasia. Balloon dilation of the lower esophageal sphincter is the first approach to relieving symptoms (107). Patients with megaesophagus who do not respond to repeated dilations should be treated surgically (93, 94). The procedure most often used is wide esophagocardiomyectomy of the anterior gastroesophageal junction, combined with valvuloplasty for reduction of reflux. In developed countries the use of laparoscopic myotomy for the treatment of idiopathic achalasia is becoming common. This relatively simple procedure may become the treatment of choice for idiopathic achalasia and chagasic megaesophagus if the encouraging results achieved to date continue.

Patients in the early stages of chagasic colonic dysfunction can be managed with a high-fiber diet and occasional laxatives and enemas. Fecal impaction requiring manual disimpaction can occur, as can toxic megacolon, which requires surgical treatment (68). Another complication of megacolon that requires surgical intervention is volvulus. Endoscopic emptying can be done initially for patients without clinical, radiographic, or endoscopic signs of ischemia in the affected segment. Complicated cases require surgical decompression. In either event surgical treatment of the megacolon eventually becomes necessary because recurrence of the volvulus is highly likely. Several surgical procedures have been used to treat advanced chagasic megacolon, all of which include resection of the sigmoid colon and removal of part of the rectum. The latter is done to avoid development of megacolon in the remaining segment that is anastomosed to the rectum. The Haddad et al. (48) modification of the procedure described by Duhamel (34) has successfully been used in many patients.

Heart Transplantation in Patients with Chagas' Disease

Cardiac transplantation is an option for patients with end-stage chagasic heart disease. Several dozen *T. cruzi*-infected persons have undergone cardiac transplantation in Brazil, and a dozen or so persons have had the procedure in the United States (14, 60, 78). Reactivated acute *T. cruzi* infections developed in a majority of the transplanted Brazilian patients due to the postoperative immunosuppression. This was thought to have contributed to the deaths of several patients who died despite benznidazole treatment. Three of the patients who received transplants in the United States were given nifurtimox postoperatively and did not develop reactivated acute Chagas' disease. Two of three patients not treated prophylactically developed skin lesions caused by *T. cruzi*, but these resolved when nifurtimox was given. The frequency of reactivation in the Brazilian patients may have resulted from the relatively high doses of immunosuppressive drugs that they were given. Less aggressive immunosuppressive protocols along with prophylactic antiparasitic treatment may reduce the incidence of reactivation, and recent experience in Brazil has been consistent with this approach. It is noteworthy, however, that the efficacy and side effects of long-term administration of benznidazole or nifurtimox have not been studied.

PREVENTION

Persons traveling in areas where Chagas' disease is endemic should avoid sleeping in primitive or dilapidated structures and should use insect repellent and mosquito nets to reduce exposure to vectors. No vaccine for the prevention of transmission of *T. cruzi* is available. Special precautions for hunters, campers, and others engaging in outdoor activities in the United States cannot be justified. Laboratory personnel should use eye protection and should wear gloves when working with *T. cruzi*, and suitable containment should be used when infected insects are handled (55).

CONCLUSIONS

Chagas' disease (American trypanosomiasis) is a zoonosis caused by *T. cruzi*, a flagellated protozoan parasite found only in the Americas. *T. cruzi* is usually spread among its mammalian hosts by insect vectors, but it can also be transmitted by transfusion of blood donated by persons chronically infected with the parasite. Acute *T. cruzi* infection generally is a mild illness, but chronic Chagas' disease, which can involve cardiac and gastrointestinal problems, is a major cause of morbidity and death in Latin America. It is estimated that 16 million to 18 million people are infected with *T. cruzi* and that about 45,000 deaths attributable to Chagas' disease occur each year. In recent decades the number of persons in the United States with chronic *T. cruzi* infections has grown enormously due to immigration from Latin America. Results of epidemiologic studies and census data indicate that 50,000 to 100,000 *T. cruzi*-infected persons now live in the United States. This emergence of Chagas' disease in the United States poses a risk of transfusion-associated transmission of *T. cruzi*, and six such cases have been reported in the United States and Canada. Most transfusions are given to immunocompetent persons in whom acute Chagas' disease would not be diagnosed because of its mild nature, and thus, it is reasonable to infer that many other instances of transfusion-associated transmission of *T. cruzi* have occurred in the United States but have not been recognized. Although the questions relating to risk for *T. cruzi* infection currently asked in U.S. blood banks have the potential to reduce the rate of transmission of the parasite, serologic testing of donated blood should be considered.

REFERENCES

1. **Amorim, D. S.** 1979. Chagas' disease. *Prog. Cardiol.* **8**:235–279.
2. **Andrade, A. L. S. S., F. Zicker, R. M. Oliveira, S. A. Silva, A. Luquetti, L. R. Travassos, I. C. Almeida, S. S. Andrade, and J. G. Andrade.** 1996. Randomised trial of efficacy of benznidazole in treatment of early *Trypanosoma cruzi* infection. *Lancet* **348**:1413.
3. **Andrade, S. G., S. Stocker-Guerret, A. S. Pimentel, and J. A. Grimaud.** 1991. Reversibility of cardiac fibrosis in mice chronically infected with *Trypanosoma cruzi*, under specific chemotherapy. *Mem. Inst. Oswaldo Cruz* **86**:200.
4. **Andrade, Z. A., and S. G. Andrade.** 1979. Patologia, p. 199–248. *In* Z. Brener and Z. A. Andrade (ed.), *Trypanosoma cruzi e Doença de Chagas*. Guanabara Koogan, Rio de Janeiro, Brazil.
5. **Andrade, Z. A., S. G. Andrade, G. B. Oliveira, and D. R. Alonso.** 1978. Histopathology of the conducting tissue of the heart in Chagas' myocarditis. *Am. Heart J.* **95**:316–324.
6. **Anonymous.** 1997. Chagas disease—interruption of transmission, Brazil. *Weekly Epidemiol. Rec.* **72**:1–8.
7. **Appleman, M. D., I. A. Shulman, S. Saxena, and L. V. Kirchhoff.** 1993. Use of a questionnaire to identify potential donors at risk for infection with *Trypanosoma cruzi*. *Transfusion* **33**:61–64.
8. **Avila, H. A., J. B. Pereira, O. Thiemann, E. de Paiva, W. Degrave, C. M. Morel, and L. Simpson.** 1993. Detection of *Trypanosoma cruzi* in blood specimens of chronic chagasic patients by polymerase chain reaction amplification of kinetoplast minicircle DNA: comparison with serology and xenodiagnosis. *J. Clin. Microbiol.* **31**:2421–2426.
9. **Azogue, E., C. La Fuente, and C. H. Darras.** 1985. Congenital Chagas' disease in Bolivia: epidemiological aspects and pathological findings. *Trans. R. Soc. Trop. Med. Hyg.* **79**:176–180.
10. **Barousse, A. P., J. A. Costa, M. Esposto, H. Laplume, and E. L. Segura.** 1980. Enfermedad de Chagas e inmunosupresión. *Medicina (B Aires)* **40**(Suppl. 1):17–26.
11. **Barr, S. C., O. Van Beek, M. S. Carlisle-Nowak, J. W. Lopez, L. V. Kirchhoff, A. Zajac, and A. de Lahunta.** 1995. *Trypanosoma cruzi* infection in Walker hounds in Virginia. *Am. J. Vet. Res.* **56**:1037–1044.
12. **Barrett, V. J., D. A. Leiby, J. L. Odom, M. M. Otani, J. D. Rowe, J. T. Roote, K. F. Cox, K. R. Brown, J. A. Hoiles, A. Saez-Alquezar, and J. F. Turrens.** 1997. Negligible prevalence of antibodies against Trypanosoma cruzi among blood donors in the southeastern United States. *Am. J. Clin. Pathol.* **108**:499–503.
13. **Bellotti, G., E. A. Bocchi, A. V. de Moraes, M. L. Higuchi, M. Barbero-Marcial, E. Sosa, A. Esteves-Filho, R. Kalil, R. Weiss, A. Jatene, and F. Pileggi.** 1996. In vivo detection of Trypanosoma cruzi antigens in hearts of patients with chronic Chagas' heart disease. *Am. Heart J.* **131**:301–307.
14. **Bocchi, E. A., G. Bellotti, D. Uip, J. Kalil, M. D. Higuchi, A. Fiorelli, N. Stolf, A. Jatene, and F. Pileggi.** 1993. Long-term follow-up after heart transplantation in Chagas' disease. *Transplant. Proc.* **25**:1329–1330.
15. **Bradley, K. K.** 1997. American trypanosomiasis: Chagas disease an emerging zoonotic threat in Oklahoma? *J. Okla. State Med. Assoc.* **90**:253–255.
16. **Brisseau, J. M., J. P. Cebron, T. Petit, M. Marjolet, P. Cuilliere, J. Godin, and J. Y. Grolleau.** 1988. Chagas' myocarditis imported into France. *Lancet* **i**:1046.
17. **Britto, C., M. A. Cardoso, C. M. Monteiro Vanni, A. Hasslocher-Moreno, S. S. Xavier, W. Oelemann, A. Santoro, C. Pirmez, C. M. Morel, and P. Wincker.** 1995. Polymerase chain reaction detection of *Trypanosoma cruzi* in human blood samples as a tool for diagnosis and treatment evaluation. *Parasitology* **110**:241–247.

18. **Buckner, F. S., A. J. Wilson, and W. C. Van Voorhis.** 1997. Tissues of mice chronically infected with *Trypanosoma cruzi* have demonstrable parasites in inflammatory infiltrates. *J. Invest. Med.* **45:**123A.

19. **Bureau of the Census.** 1996. *Statistical Abstract of the United States. The National Data Book*, p. 11. U.S. Department of Commerce, Washington, D.C.

20. **Burns, J. M., Jr., W. G. Shreffler, D. E. Rosman, P. R. Sleath, C. J. March, and S. G. Reed.** 1992. Identification and synthesis of a major conserved antigenic epitope of *Trypanosoma cruzi. Proc. Natl. Acad. Sci. USA* **89:**1239–1243.

21. **Carrasco, R., H. Miguez, C. Camacho, L. Echalar, S. Revollo, T. Ampuero, and J.-P. Dedet.** 1990. Prevalence of *Trypanosoma cruzi* infection in blood banks of seven departments of Bolivia. *Mem. Inst. Oswaldo Cruz* **85:**69–73.

22. **Carvalho, M. R., M. A. Krieger, E. Almeida, W. Oelemann, M. A. Shikanai-Yasuda, A. W. Ferreira, J. B. Pereira, A. Saez-Alquezar, P. E. Dorlhiac-Llacer, D. F. Chamone, and S. Goldenberg.** 1993. Chagas' disease diagnosis: evaluation of several tests in blood bank screening. *Transfusion* **33:**830–834.

23. **Chagas, C.** 1909. Nova tripanozomiase humana. Estudos sobre a morfologia e o ciclo evolutivo do *Schizotrypanum cruzi* n. gen., n. sp., agente etiológico de nova entidade mórbida do homem. *Mem. Inst. Oswaldo Cruz* **1:**159–218.

24. **Chiari, E., J. C. P. Dias, M. Lana, and C. A. Chiari.** 1989. Hemocultures for the parasitological diagnosis of human chronic Chagas disease. *Rev. Soc. Bras. Med. Trop.* **22:**19–23.

25. **Chuster, M.** 1985. Implante de marcapasso nas bradiarritmias chagásicas, p. 289–297. *In* J. R. Cançado and M. Chuster (ed.), *Cardiopatia Chagásica.* Fundação Carlos Chagas, Belo Horizonte, Brazil.

26. **Cimo, P. L., W. E. Luper, and M. A. Scouros.** 1993. Transfusion-associated Chagas' disease in Texas: report of a case. *Texas Med.* **89:**48–50.

27. **Cossio, P. M., C. Diez, and A. Szarfman.** 1974. Chagasic cardiopathy—demonstration of a serum gamma globulin factor which reacts with endocardium and vascular structures. *Circulation* **49:**13–21.

28. **Costa, R. B., and F. G. Alcantara.** 1965. Gastropatia chagásica crônica. *Rev. Bras. Med.* **22:**667–671.

29. **Coura, J. R.** 1996. Current prospects of specific treatment of Chagas' disease. *Bol. Chil. Parasitol.* **51:**69–75. (In Spanish.)

30. **Crovato, F., and A. Rebora.** 1997. Chagas' disease: a potential problem for Europe? *Dermatology* **195:**184–185.

31. **Cunha-Neto, E., M. Duranti, A. Gruber, B. Zingales, I. de Messias, N. Stolf, G. Bellotti, M. E. Patarroyo, F. Pilleggi, and J. Kalil.** 1995. Autoimmunity in Chagas disease cardiopathy: biological relevance of a cardiac myosin-specific epitope crossreactive to an immunodominant *Trypanosoma cruzi* antigen. *Proc. Natl. Acad. Sci. USA* **92:**3541–3545.

32. **de Arteaga, J., P. U. Massari, B. Galli, F. Garzon Maceda, and J. C. Zlocowsky.** 1992. Renal transplantation and Chagas' disease. *Transplant. Proc.* **24:**1900–1901.

33. **de Diego, J. A., M. T. Palau, C. Gamallo, and P. Penin.** 1998. Are genotypes of Trypanosoma cruzi involved in the challenge of chagasic cardiomyopathy? *Parasitol. Res.* **84:**147–152.

34. **Duhamel, B.** 1956. Une nouvelle opération de mégacôlon congénital. *Presse Med.* **64:**2249–2250.

35. **Ferreira, H. O.** 1988. Tratamento específico na fase aguda da doença de Chagas. *J. Pediatria* **64:**1–3.

36. **Fragata Filho, A. A., E. Boianain, M. A. D. Silva, E. B. Correia, R. Borges Filho, C. Martins, V. Salene, M. Batlouni, and E. Sousa.** 1995. Validade do tratamento etiológico da fase crônica da doença de Chagas com benznidazol. *Arq. Bras. Cardiol.* **65**(Suppl. 1):71.

37. **Frasch, A. C. C., and M. B. Reyes.** 1990. Diagnosis of Chagas' disease using recombinant DNA technology. *Parasitol. Today* **6:**137–139.

38. **Freilij, H., and J. Altcheh.** 1995. Congenital Chagas' disease: diagnostic and clinical aspects. *Clin. Infect. Dis.* **21:**551–555.

39. **Galel, S., S. Wolles, and R. Stumpf.** 1997. Evaluation of a selective donor testing strategy for T. cruzi. *Transfusion* **37:**74S. (Abstract.)

40. **Gilson, G. J., K. A. Harner, J. Abrams, L. A. Izquierdo, and L. B. Curet.** 1995. Chagas disease in pregnancy. *Obstet. Gynecol.* **86:**646–647.

41. **Goble, F. C.** 1970. South American trypanosomes, p. 597–689. *In* G. J. Jackson, R. Herman, and I. Singer (ed.), *Immunity to Parasitic Diseases in Animals.* Appleton-Century-Crofts, New York, N.Y.

42. **Goldsmith, R. S., R. J. Zarate, L. G. Zarate, G. Morales, I. Kagan, R. Drickey, and L. B. Jacobson.** 1992. Clinical and epidemiologic studies of Chagas' disease in rural communities of Oaxaca, Mexico, and an eight-year followup. II. Chila. *Bull. Pan. Am. Health Organ.* **26:**47–59.

43. **Gomes, M. L., L. M. C. Galvao, A. M. Macedo, S. D. J. Pena, and E. Chiari.** 1999. Chagas' disease diagnosis: comparative analysis of parasitologic, molecular, and serologic methods. *Am. J. Trop. Med. Hyg.* **60:**205–210.

44. **Gomes, M. L., A. M. Macedo, A. R. Vago, S. D. Pena, L. M. Galvao, and E. Chiari.** 1998. *Trypanosoma cruzi:* optimization of polymerase chain reaction for detection in human blood. *Exp. Parasitol.* **88:**28–33.

45. **Grant, I. H., J. W. M. Gold, M. Wittner, H. B. Tanowitz, C. Nathan, K. Mayer, L. Reich, N. Wollner, L. Steinherz, F. Ghavimi, R. J. O'Reilly, and D. Armstrong.** 1989. Transfusion-associated acute Chagas disease acquired in the United States. *Ann. Intern. Med.* **111:**849–851.

46. **Grogl, M., R. E. Kuhn, D. S. Davis, and G. E. Green.** 1984. Antibodies to *Trypanosoma cruzi* in coyotes in Texas. *J. Parasitol.* **70:**189–191.

47. **Gurtler, R. E., J. E. Cohen, M. C. Cecere, M. A. Lauricela, R. Chuit, and E. L. Segura.** 1998. Influence of humans and domestic animals on the household prevalence of *Trypanosoma cruzi* in *Triatoma infestans* populations in northwest Argentina. *J. Med. Entomol.* **35:**99–103.

48. **Haddad, J., A. Raia, and A. Correa Neto.** 1965. Abaixamento retroretal do colon com colostomia perineal no tratamento do megacólon adqurido: operação de Duhamel modificada. *Rev. Assoc. Med. Bras.* **11:**83–88.

49. **Hagar, J. M., and S. H. Rahimtoola.** 1991. Chagas' heart disease in the United States. *N. Engl. J. Med.* **325:**763–768.

50. **Hagar, J. M. and S. H. Rahimtoola.** 1995. Chagas' heart disease. *Curr. Probl. Cardiol.* **20:**825–924.

51. **Herwaldt, B. L., and D. D. Juranek.** 1993. Laboratory-acquired malaria, leishmaniasis, trypanosomiasis, and toxoplasmosis. *Am. J. Trop. Med. Hyg.* **48:**313–323.

52. **Hoff, R., R. S. Teixeira, J. S. Carvalho, and K. E. Mott.** 1978. *Trypanosoma cruzi* in the cerebrospinal fluid during the acute stage of Chagas' disease. *N. Engl. J. Med.* **298:**604–606.

53. **Hofflin, J. M., R. H. Sadler, and F. G. Araujo.** 1987. Laboratory-acquired Chagas' disease. *Trans. R. Soc. Trop. Med. Hyg.* **81:**437–440.

54. **Houghton, R. L., D. R. Benson, L. D. Reynolds, P. D. McNeill, P. R. Sleath, M. J. Lodes, Y. A. W. Skeiky, D. A. Leiby, and S. G. Reed.** 1999. A multiepitope synthetic peptide and recombinant protein for the detection of antibodies to *Trypanosoma cruzi* in radioimmunoprecipitation-confirmed and consensus-positive sera. *J. Infect. Dis.* **179:**1226–1234.

55. **Hudson, L., F. Grover, W. E. Gutteridge, R. A. Klein, W. Peters, R. A. Neal, M. A. Miles, J. E. Williams, M. T. Scott, R. Nourish, and B. P. Ager.** 1983. Suggested guidelines for work with live *Trypanosoma cruzi. Trans. R. Soc. Trop. Med. Hyg.* **77:**416–419.

56. **Jones, E. M., D. G. Colley, S. Tostes, E. R. Lopes, C. L. Vnencak-Jones, and T. L. McCurley.** 1993. Amplification of a *Trypanosoma cruzi* DNA sequence from inflammatory lesions in human Chagasic cardiomyopathy. *Am. J. Trop. Med. Hyg.* **48:**348–357.

57. **Karsten, V., C. Davis, and R. Kuhn.** 1992. *Trypanosoma cruzi* in wild raccoons and opossums in North Carolina. *J. Parasitol.* **78:**547–549.

58. **Kerndt, P. R., H. A. Waskin, L. V. Kirchhoff, F. Steurer, S. H. Waterman, J. M. Nelson, G. A. Gellert, and I. A. Shulman.** 1991. Prevalence of antibody to *Trypanosoma cruzi* among blood donors in Los Angeles, California. *Transfusion* **31:**814–818.

59. **Kirchhoff, L. V.** 1989. Is *Trypanosoma cruzi* a new threat to our blood supply? *Ann. Intern. Med.* **111:**773–775.

60. **Kirchhoff, L. V.** 1993. American trypanosomiasis (Chagas' disease)—a tropical disease now in the United States. *N. Engl. J. Med.* **329:**639–644.

61. **Kirchhoff, L. V.** 1993. Chagas disease. American trypanosomiasis. *Infect. Dis. Clin. N. Am.* **7:**487–502.

62. **Kirchhoff, L. V.** 1996. American trypanosomiasis (Chagas' disease). *Gastroenterol Clin. N. Am.* **25:** 517–533.

63. **Kirchhoff, L. V., and J. E. Donelson.** 1993. PCR detection of *Trypanosoma cruzi*, African trypanosomes, and *Leishmania* species, p. 443–455. *In* D. H. Persing, T. F. Smith, F. C. Tenover, and T. J. White (ed.), *Diagnostic Molecular Microbiology: Principles and Applications.* American Society for Microbiology, Washington, D.C.

64. **Kirchhoff, L. V., A. A. Gam, and F. C. Gilliam.** 1987. American trypanosomiasis (Chagas' disease) in Central American immigrants. *Am. J. Med.* **82:**915–920.

65. **Kirchhoff, L. V., A. A. Gam, R. D. Gusmao, R. S. Goldsmith, J. M. Rezende, and A. Rassi.** 1987. Increased specificity of serodiagnosis of Chagas' disease by detection of antibody to the 72- and 90-kilodalton glycoproteins of *Trypanosoma cruzi*. *J. Infect. Dis.* **155:**561–564.

66. **Kirchhoff, L. V., and F. A. Neva.** 1985. Chagas' disease in Latin American immigrants. *JAMA* **254:** 3058–3060.

67. **Kirchhoff, L. V., J. R. Votava, D. E. Ochs, and D. R. Moser.** 1996. Comparison of PCR and microscopic methods for detecting *Trypanosoma cruzi*. *J. Clin. Microbiol.* **34:**1171–1175.

68. **Kobayasi, S., E. F. Mendes, M. A. M. Rodrigues, and M. F. Franco.** 1992. Toxic dilatation of the colon in Chagas' disease. *Br. J. Surg.* **79:**1202–1203.

69. **Koberle, F.** 1968. Chagas' disease and Chagas' syndromes: the pathology of American trypanosomiasis. *Adv. Parasitol.* **6:**63–116.

70. **Koberle, F., and E. Nador.** 1955. Etiologia e patogenia do megaesófago no Brasil. *Rev. Paulista Med.* **47:**643–661.

71. **Kohl, S., L. K. Pickering, L. S. Frankel, and R. G. Yaeger.** 1982. Reactivation of Chagas' disease during therapy of acute lymphocytic leukemia. *Cancer* **50:**827–828.

72. **Laranja, F. S., E. Dias, G. Nobrega, and A. Miranda.** 1956. Chagas' disease: a clinical, epidemiologic, and pathologic study. *Circulation* **14:**1035–1060.

73. **Leiby, D. A., M. H. Fucci, and R. J. Stumpf.** 1999. *Trypanosoma cruzi* in a low- to moderate-risk blood donor population: seroprevalence and possible congenital transmission. *Transfusion* **39:**310–315.

74. **Leiby, D. A., E. J. Read, B. A. Lenes, A. J. Yund, R. J. Stumpf, L. V. Kirchhoff, and R. Y. Dodd.** 1997. Seroepidemiology of *Trypanosoma cruzi*, etiologic agent of Chagas' disease, in U.S. blood donors. *J. Infect. Dis.* **176:**1047–1052.

75. **Leiguarda, R., A. Roncoroni, A. L. Taratuto, L. Jost, M. Berthier, M. Nogues, and H. Freilij.** 1990. Acute CNS infection by *Trypanosoma cruzi* (Chagas' disease) in immunosuppressed patients. *Neurology* **40:**850–851.

76. **Levi, G. C., I. M. Lobo, E. G. Kallas, and V. Amato Neto.** 1996. Etiological drug treatment of human infection by *Trypanosoma cruzi*. *Rev. Inst. Med. Trop. Sao Paulo* **38:**35–38.

77. **Levine, N. D., J. O. Corliss, F. E. G. Cox, G. Deroux, J. Grain, G. F. Leedale, A. R. I. Loeblich, J. Lom, D. Lynn, E. G. Merinfeld, F. C. Page, G. Poljansky, J. Vavra, and F. G. Wallace.** 1980. A newly revised classification of the protozoa. *J. Protozool.* **27:**37–58.

78. **Libow, L. F., V. P. Beltrani, D. N. Silvers, and M. E. Grossman.** 1991. Post-cardiac transplant reactivation of Chagas' disease diagnosed by skin biopsy. *Cutis* **48:**37–40.

79. **Liendo, A., K. Lazardi, and J. A. Urbina.** 1998. In-vitro antiproliferative effects and mechanism of action of the bis-triazole D0870 and its S(−) enantiomer against *Trypanosoma cruzi*. *J. Antimicrob. Chemother.* **41:**197–205.

80. **Lopez-Blanco, O. A., N. H. Cavalli, A. Jasovich, D. Gotlieb, and S. Gonzalez-Cappa.** 1992. Chagas' disease and kidney transplantation—follow-up of nine patients for 11 years. *Transplant. Proc.* **24:**3089–3090.

81. **Luders, C., M. A. Caetano, L. E. Ianhez, J. A. Fonseca, and E. Sabbaga.** 1992. Renal transplantation in patients with Chagas' disease: a long-term follow-up. *Transplant. Proc.* **24:**1878–1879.

82. **Luquetti, A. O.** 1990. Use of *Trypanosoma cruzi* defined proteins for diagnosis—multicentre trial serological and technical aspects. *Mem. Inst. Oswaldo Cruz* **85:**497–505.

83. **Marr, J. J., and R. Docampo.** 1986. Chemotherapy for Chagas' disease: a perspective on current therapy and considerations for future research. *Rev. Infect. Dis.* **8:**884–903.

84. **Marsden, P. D., A. C. Barreto, C. C. Cuba, M. B. Gama, and J. Ackers.** 1979. Improvements in routine xenodiagnosis with first instar *Dipetalogaster maximus* (Uhler 1894) (Triatominae). *Am. J. Trop. Med. Hyg.* **28:**649–652.

85. **Meurs, K. M., M. A. Anthony, M. Slater, and M. W. Miller.** 1998. Chronic *Trypanosoma cruzi* infection in dogs: 11 cases (1987–1996). *J. Am. Vet. Med.* **213:**497–500.

86. **Mocelin, A. J., L. Brandina, P. A. Gordon, J. L. S. Baldy, and P. P. Chieffi.** 1977. Immuno-suppression and circulating *Trypanosoma cruzi* in a kidney transplant recipient. *Transplantation* **23:**163.

87. **Moncayo, A.** 1997. Progress toward elimination of transmission of Chagas disease in Latin America. *World Health Stat. Q.* **50:**195–198.

88. **Moser, D. R., L. V. Kirchhoff, and J. E. Donelson.** 1989. Detection of *Trypanosoma cruzi* by polymerase chain reaction gene amplification. *J. Clin. Microbiol.* **27:**1744–1749.

89. **Mota, E. A., A. C. Guimaraes, O. O. Santana, I. Sherlock, R. Hoff, and T. H. Weller.** 1990. A nine year prospective study of Chagas' disease in a defined rural population in Northeast Brazil. *Am. J. Trop. Med. Hyg.* **42:**429–440.

89a. **Neva, F. A., and H. W. Brown.** 1994. *Basic Clinical Parasitology*, 6th ed. Appleton & Lange, Norwalk, Conn.

90. **Nickerson, P., P. Orr, M.-L. Schroeder, L. Sekla, and J. B. Johnston.** 1989. Transfusion-associated *Trypanosoma cruzi* infection in a non-endemic area. *Ann. Intern. Med.* **111:**851–853.

91. **Ochs, D. E., V. Hnilica, D. R. Moser, J. H. Smith, and L.V. Kirchhoff.** 1996. Postmortem diagnosis of autochthonous acute chagasic myocarditis by polymerase chain reaction amplification of a species-specific DNA sequence of *Trypanosoma cruzi. Am. J. Trop. Med. Hyg.* **34:**526–529.

92. **Pan, A. A., G. B. Rosenberg, M. K. Hurley, G. J. Schock, V. P. Chu, and A. Aiyappa.** 1992. Clinical evaluation of an EIA for the sensitive and specific detection of serum antibody to *Trypanosoma cruzi* (Chagas' disease). *J. Infect. Dis.* **165:**585–588.

93. **Pinotti, H. W., V. N. Felix, B. Zilberstein, and I. Cecconello.** 1991. Surgical complications of Chagas' disease: megaesophagus, achalasia of the pylorus, and cholelithiasis. *World J. Surg.* **15:**198–204.

94. **Pinotti, H. W., A. Habr-Gama, I. Cecconello, V. N. Felix, and B. Zilberstein.** 1993. The surgical treatment of megaesophagus and megacolon. *Dig. Dis.* **11:**206–215.

95. **Pizzi, T. P., V. A. De Criozret, G. Smok, and M. Diaz.** 1982. Enfermedad de Chagas en un paciente con transplante renal y tratamiento inmunosupresor. *Rev. Med. Chile* **110:**1207–1211.

96. **Prata, A., E. R. Lopes, and E. Chapadeiro.** 1985. Morte súbita, p. 114–120. *In* J. R. Cançado and M. Chuster (ed.), *Cardiopatia Chagásica*. Fundaçao Carlos Chagas, Belo Horizonte, Brazil.

97. **Rassi, A.** 1979. Clínica: fase aguda, p. 249–264. *In* Z. Brener and Z. A. Andrade (ed.), *Trypanosoma cruzi e Doença de Chagas*. Guanabara Koogan, Rio de Janeiro, Brazil.

97a. **Rassi, A.** Personal communication.

98. **Rassi, A., and H. O. Ferreira.** 1971. Tentativas de tratamento específico da fase aguda da doença de Chagas com nitrofuranos em esquemas de duração prolongada. *Rev. Soc. Bras. Med. Trop.* **5:**235–262.

99. **Reed, S. G.** 1988. In vivo administration of recombinant IFN-gamma induces macrophage activation, and prevents acute disease, immune suppression, and death in experimental *Trypanosoma cruzi* infections. *J. Immunol.* **140:**4342–4347.

100. **Reis, D. D., E. M. Jones, S. Tostes, E. R. Lopes, E. Chapadeiro, G. Gazzinelli, D. G. Colley, and T. L. McCurley.** 1993. Expression of major histocompatibility complex antigens and adhesion molecules in hearts of patients with chronic Chagas' disease. *Am. J. Trop. Med. Hyg.* **49:**192–200.

101. **Rivera, T., R. Palma-Guzman, and W. Morales.** 1995. Seroepidemiological and clinical study of Chagas' disease in Nicaragua. *Rev. Inst. Med. Trop. Sao Paulo* **37:**207–213.

102. **Rivero, I., M. Moravenik, J. Morales, M. Gomez, and J. M. De Rosas.** 1974. Chagas' disease—another hazard in acute leukemia. *N. Engl. J. Med.* **290:**285.

103. **Rocha, A., A. C. Oliveira de Meneses, A. M. da Silva, M. S. Ferreira, S. A. Nishioka, M. K. N. Burgarelli, E. Almeida, G. Turcato, Jr., K. Metze, and E. R. Lopes.** 1994. Pathology of patients with Chagas' disease and acquired immunodeficiency syndrome. *Am. J. Trop. Med. Hyg.* **50:**261–268.

104. **Russomando, G., A. Figueredo, M. Almiron, M. Sakamoto, and K. Morita.** 1992. Polymerase chain reaction-based detection of *Trypanosoma cruzi* DNA in serum. *J. Clin. Microbiol.* **30:** 2864–2868.

105. **Ryckman, R. E., and L. E. Olsen.** 1965. Epizootiology of *Trypanosoma cruzi* in Southwestern North America. Part VI. Insectivorous hosts of Triatominae—the perizootiological relationship to *Trypanosoma cruzi. J. Med. Entomol.* **2:**99–106.

106. **Salgado, P. R., A. G. Gorski, A. R. Aleixo, and E. O. M. de Barros.** 1996. Tumor-like lesion due to Chagas' disease in a patient with lymphocytic leukemia. *Rev. Inst. Med. Trop. Sao Paulo* **38:**285–288.

107. **Salis, G. B., J. C. Chiocca, E. Perisse, E. Acosta, and P. A. Mazure.** 1991. Acalasia del esófago: veinte años de experiencia en el tratamiento no quirúrgico. *Acta Gastroenterol. Latinoam.* **21:**11–16.

108. **Sartori, A. M., M. A. Shikanai-Yasuda, V. Mato Neto, and M. H. Lopes.** 1998. Follow-up of 18 patients with human immunodeficiency virus infection and chronic Chagas' disease, with reactivation of Chagas' disease causing cardiac disease in three patients. *Clin. Infect. Dis.* **26:**177–179.

109. **Schiffler, R. J., G. P. Mansur, T. R. Navin, and K. Limpakarnjanarat.** 1984. Indigenous Chagas' disease (American trypanosomiasis) in California. *JAMA* **251:**2983–2984.

110. **Schmunis, G. A.** 1991. *Trypanosoma cruzi*, the etiologic agent of Chagas' disease: status in the blood supply in endemic and nonendemic countries. *Transfusion* **31:**547–557.

111. **Schmunis, G. A., F. Zicker, and A. Moncayo.** 1996. Interruption of Chagas' disease transmission through vector elimination. *Lancet* **348:**1171–1172.

112. **Shikanai-Yasuda, M. A., M. H. Lopes, J. E. Tolezano, E. Umezawa, V. Amato Neto, A. C. Pereira Barreto, Y. Higaki, A. A. B. Moreira, G. Funayama, A. A. Barone, A. Duarte, V. Odone, G. C. Cerri, M. Sato, D. Possi, and M. Shiroma.** 1990. Doença de Chagas aguda: vias de transmissao, aspectos clínicos e resposta à terapêutica específica em casos diagnosticados em um centro urbano. *Rev. Inst. Med. Trop. Sao Paulo* **32:**16–27.

113. **Shulman, I. A., M. D. Appleman, S. Saxena, A. L. Hiti, and L. V. Kirchhoff.** 1997. Specific antibodies to Trypanosoma cruzi among blood donors in Los Angeles, California. *Transfusion* **37:**727–731.

114. **Starr, M. D., J. C. Rojas, R. Zeledon, D. W. Hird, and T. E. Carpenter.** 1991. Chagas' disease: risk factors for house infestation by *Triatoma dimidiata*, the major vector of *Trypanosoma cruzi* in Costa Rica. *Am. J. Epidemiol.* **133:**740–747.

115. **Sturm, N. R., W. Degrave, C. Morel, and L. Simpson.** 1989. Sensitive detection and schizodeme classification of *Trypanosoma cruzi* cells by amplification of kinetoplast minicircle DNA sequences: use in diagnosis of Chagas' disease. *Mol. Biochem. Parasitol.* **33:**205–214.

115a.**Tanowitz, H. B.** Personal communication.

116. **Teixeira, A. R. L., and C. A. Santos-Buch.** 1975. The immunology of experimental Chagas' disease. *Immunology* **28:**401–410.

117. **Troncon, L. E. A., R. B. Oliveira, L. M. F. Romanello, L. Rosa-E-Silva, M. C. C. Pinto, and N. Iazigi.** 1993. Abnormal progression of a liquid meal through the stomach and small intestine in patients with Chagas' disease. *Dig. Dis. Sci.* **38:**1511–1517.

118. **Urbina, J. A., G. Payares, J. Molina, C. Sanoja, A. Liendo, K. Lazardi, M. M. Piras, N. Perez, P. Wincker, and J. F. Ryley.** 1996. Cure of short- and long-term experimental Chagas' disease using D0870. *Science* **273:**969–971.

119. **Van Voorhis, W. C., L. Schlekewy, and H. L. Trong.** 1991. Molecular mimicry by *Trypanosoma cruzi*: the F1-160 epitope that mimics mammalian nerve can be mapped to a 12-amino acid peptide. *Proc. Natl. Acad. Sci. USA* **88:**5993–5997.

120. **Villanueva, M. S.** 1993. Trypanosomiasis of the central nervous system. *Semin. Neurol.* **13:**209–218.

121. **Viotti, R., C. Vigliano, H. Armenti, and E. Segura.** 1994. Treatment of chronic Chagas' disease with benznidazole: clinical and serologic evolution of patients with long-term follow-up. *Am. Heart J.* **127:**151–162.

122. **Winkler, M. A., R. J. Brashear, H. J. Hall, J. D. Schur, and A. A. Pan.** 1995. Detection of antibodies to *Trypanosoma cruzi* among blood donors in the southwestern and western United

States. II. Evaluation of a supplemental enzyme immunoassay and radioimmunoprecipitation assay for confirmation of seroreactivity. *Transfusion* **35:**219–225.

123. **Wisnivesky-Colli, C., R. E. Gurtler, N. D. Solarz, M. A. Lauricella, and E. L. Segura.** 1985. Epidemiological role of humans, dogs, and cats in the transmission of *Trypanosoma cruzi* in a central area of Argentina. *Rev. Inst. Med. Trop. Sao Paulo* **27:**346–352.

124. **Wisnivesky-Colli, C., N. J. Schweigmann, A. Alberti, S. M. Pietrokovsky, O. Conti, S. Montoya, A. Riarte, and C. Rivas.** 1992. Sylvatic American trypanosomiasis in Argentina. *Trypanosoma cruzi* infection in mammals from the Chaco Forest in Santiago del Estero. *Trans. R. Soc. Trop. Med. Hyg.* **86:**38–41.

125. **Wood, J. N., L. Hudson, T. M. Jessell, and M. Yamamoto.** 1982. A monoclonal antibody defining antigenic determinants on subpopulations of mammalian neurones and *Trypanosoma cruzi* parasites. *Nature* **296:**34–38.

126. **Yaeger, R. G.** 1988. The prevalence of *Trypanosoma cruzi* infection in armadillos collected at a site near New Orleans, Louisiana. *Am. J. Trop. Med. Hyg.* **38:**323–326.

Emerging Infections 3
Edited by W. M. Scheld, W. A. Craig, and J. M. Hughes
© 1999 ASM Press, Washington, D.C.

Chapter 9

Pfiesteria piscicida and Human Health

David W. Oldach, Lynn M. Grattan, and J. Glenn Morris

Of the thousands of species of microalgae (including heterotrophic dinoflagellates) which form the base of the marine food chain, about 60 are believed to be toxic or harmful. However, when these species proliferate, they may cause massive kills of fish and shellfish, alterations of marine habitats, and human illness and death. While data are limited, there is clear evidence that the frequency of such "harmful algal blooms" (HAB) is increasing, as are the ranges of recognized toxin-producing species (2, 15, 24). This emergent trend has been linked to global climate change and other ecologic disturbances associated with humans.

Presumptive exposure to toxins produced by *Pfiesteria piscicida*, a small dinoflagellate found in mid-Atlantic estuarine waters, emerged as the cause of a novel human health syndrome of impaired cognition associated with skin rash, headache, gastrointestinal symptoms, and respiratory complaints following fish-kill events in Maryland's Chesapeake Bay in 1997 (22). The association was recognized among these individuals (predominantly Maryland watermen) because members of this community were aware of *Pfiesteria*'s previous environmental, political, and potential human health impact in North Carolina and pressed for a governmental response when unexplained health problems emerged after fish-kill events in Maryland waters. Thus was initiated a new chapter in the history of this "emergent" dinoflagellate.

DINOFLAGELLATES

Dinoflagellates are unicellular eukaryotic organisms (protists) found in most aquatic habitats. Their name derives from the Greek word *deinos* for whirling or turning, an apt description of the mobility produced by their two dimorphic flagella (in *Pfiesteria*, these flagella comprise a transverse flagellum located within a transverse groove, the cingulum, and a longitudinal flagellum that extends in whip-like

David W. Oldach • Department of Medicine and Institute of Human Virology, University of Maryland School of Medicine, Baltimore, MD 21201. *Lynn M. Grattan* • Department of Neurology, University of Maryland School of Medicine, Baltimore, MD 21201. *J. Glenn Morris* • Department of Medicine, University of Maryland School of Medicine, Baltimore, MD 21201.

fashion from a longitudinal groove, the sulcus) (Fig. 1) (5, 7, 54). Dinoflagellates meet their nutritional needs either by photosynthesis (autotrophy), phagocytosis of food sources (heterotrophy), or combinations of these strategies (mixotrophy). It is not surprising, then, that these organisms have been claimed by both botanists (as algae) and protozoologists (as protozoa). They are cosmopolitan (the majority of species are marine or estuarine), and representatives may be found in extremely diverse niches ranging from pelagic plankton to endosymbionts within corals and tridacnid clams; some are intracellular parasites of other dinoflagellates. Dinoflagellates have a nuclear membrane, with permanently condensed chromosomes. They reproduce asexually through binary fission, although sexual reproduction has also been described for a few species. Toxin production, including water- and lipid-soluble substances with cytotoxic, neurotoxic, or hemolytic activity, has been described for approximately 60 of the roughly 2,000 extant dinoflagellate species (10, 55). The dinoflagellates are not alone among single-celled aquatic plants and animals in their capacity to produce toxic substances that cause disease in humans; microcystins and anabaena toxin production by blue-green algae (cyanobacteria) (*Microcystis aeruginosa* and *Anabaena flos-aquae*) (29) and domoic acid production by *Pseudonitzschia* diatoms (49, 56) are two well-recognized examples. Blooms of populations of these and other organisms that affect environmental quality and, at times, human health are often considered collectively under the general topic of HAB.

DINOFLAGELLATE-ASSOCIATED HUMAN ILLNESS

Toxin production by marine and estuarine dinoflagellates is responsible for four previously described human health syndromes. Paralytic shellfish poisoning (PSP) occurs following consumption of shellfish containing high concentrations of the sodium channel blocker saxitoxin (a broad grouping of toxins that includes at least 12 distinct toxin structures); in the United States blooms of the dinoflagellates *Alexandrium tamarensis* and *Alexandrium catenella* are most frequently implicated (18, 19, 52). Symptoms, including paresthesias, ataxia, dysarthria, and confusion, are primarily neurologic and typically ensue within an hour of consumption of the contaminated shellfish. In severe cases, death due to respiratory paralysis may occur. Human health problems occur as a result of ingestion of bioaccumulated toxin in shellfish; to our knowledge, illness related to environmental exposure to waters during blooms of these organisms has never been described. In the United States, PSP occurs primarily in the New England states of the East Coast and in Alaska, California, and Washington on the West Coast. Algal blooms responsible for PSP occur primarily from April through October, but their occurrence cannot be predicted. Prevention relies, therefore, upon surveillance of shellfish for toxicity by health departments in at-risk states and closure of shellfish beds for harvesting when toxin levels exceed threshold levels.

Neurotoxic shellfish poisoning (NSP) is attributed to brevetoxins, linear polycyclic ether compounds produced during blooms of the organism *Gymnodinium breve*, which occur in the Gulf of Mexico and along the Atlantic coasts of Florida, Georgia, and North Carolina (42, 44, 52). As with PSP, NSP occurs most commonly

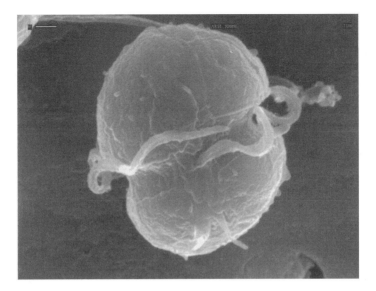

Figure 1. Scanning electron micrograph of *P. piscicida* (toxic zoospore, ventral view). Bar, 1 μm. From H. Glasgow and J. Burkholder, North Carolina State University.

following consumption of bioaccumulated toxins in shellfish and is characterized by neurological illness including paresthesias, dizziness, and ataxia. Prominent gastrointestinal symptoms including abdominal cramping, nausea, diarrhea, and vomiting occur. Recovery is complete, and there are no reports of chronic neurological symptoms as a consequence of intoxication. The causative organism is an unarmored dinoflagellate (one that lacks thecal plates) and may lyse with agitation, releasing its toxic metabolites. Aerosolization of the toxin(s) may occur and can result in illness through inhalation, with prominent respiratory symptoms and eye irritation (44). Thus, there is a well-described precedent for human illness attributable to environmental exposure to dinoflagellate toxins through inhalation, a finding of possible relevance to ongoing studies of *Pfiesteria*-related illness.

Ciguatera, or ciguatera fish poisoning, occurs following consumption of predatory coral reef fish such as barracuda, snapper, and grouper that have accumulated toxins produced by coral reef-associated dinoflagellates (*Gambierdiscus toxicus*, among others) (16, 20, 30, 39–41). The toxins bioaccumulate, and levels in tissue are amplified at higher levels of the food chain; thus, larger predatory fish are most toxic. A clinical syndrome with characteristic gastrointestinal and neurologic symptoms develops within 24 h of consumption of toxin (a heat-stable compound that is not inactivated by cooking)-containing fish. Gastrointestinal symptoms are prominent and include nausea, vomiting, diarrhea, and abdominal pain. Neurologic symptoms may develop later or concomitantly and include paresthesias, pain and weakness in the extremities, and unusual features such as paradoxical temperature dysesthesia (cold feels hot) and "aching teeth." Acute intoxication may be severe, with hypotension, coma, and, in rare cases, death. Some patients develop chronic or recrudescent illnesses, which may be particularly debilitating. A number of toxins associated with ciguatera have been identified, including ciguatoxins (small, lipid-soluble polyethers that interfere with sodium channels), scaritoxins (lipid-soluble neurotoxins that induce membrane depolarization); and maitotoxins (water-soluble toxins that activate membrane calcium channels) (52). Prevention of ciguatera rests on the use of commonsense measures, with avoidance of consumption of predatory reef fish in at-risk areas being the most significant.

Diarrheic shellfish poisoning is a more limited disease caused by consumption of shellfish-bioaccumulated okadaic acid produced by algal blooms of *Dinophysis* and *Prorocentrum* species (10, 39). Illness is acute following consumption of contaminated shellfish and includes diarrhea, nausea, vomiting, and abdominal pain. No chronic illness has been described, although chronic okadaic acid exposure has been associated in the laboratory setting with immunosuppression and malignancy (10).

While not a dinoflagellate-associated human illness, amnesic shellfish poisoning (ASP) is a prominent syndrome among the human illnesses linked to harmful algal blooms. First described in Prince Edward Island, Canada, in 1987, ASP occurs following consumption of shellfish, particularly mussels, that have accumulated domoic acid (a prenylated amino acid) produced by strains of the diatom *Pseudonitzschia* (49, 52, 56). Patients with acute illness present with gastrointestinal symptoms, including nausea, diarrhea and abdominal pain, and headache. As the name suggests, memory disturbance may occur; in patients with severe illness, neuronal necrosis (primarily in the hippocampus and amygdala), seizure, and death may occur. Survivors of severe illness may suffer profound loss of anterograde memory. Prevention of this intoxication syndrome relies upon monitoring of both shellfish domoic acid concentrations and diatom populations.

P. PISCICIDA

P. piscicida was first observed as an aquaculture dinoflagellate contaminant responsible for fish death in 1988 (7, 53). The organism was subsequently identified in North Carolina estuarine waters, was linked with fish kills there in 1992 (7), and was formally described as a new species (*P. piscicida*) in a new family (Pfiesteriaceae) within the order Dinamoebales in 1996 (54). Among the dinoflagellates, the organism is relatively nondescript, is small, and does not have a distinctive armor structure that could be seen through a light microscope and that might have led to an earlier description. As a result, phycologists must resort to membrane-stripping or suture-swelling procedures followed by meticulous tabulation of the thecal plate arrangement by electron microscopy to confidently identify the organism. By light microscopy, trained observers can identify the organism only to the level of "pfiesteria-like organisms," among which are represented several genera of dinoflagellates. However, the organism appears to be remarkable in many other regards. A polymorphic and multiphasic life cycle has been described, with flagellate, amoeboid, and cyst stages (8). Such complex life cycles were described among freshwater dinoflagellates by the phycologist Lois Pfiester (50, 51), in whose honor the genus *Pfiesteria* was named (5, 54). The organism is identified in its typical dinoflagellate biflagellate stage (haploid, ca. 7 to 12 μm), at which time it is motile and can be found in the water column. Motile, flagellate forms in the water column, all unicellular, may include smaller biflagellate gametes (haploid, ca. 5 to 8 μm) and larger, triflagellate cells (diploid, ca. 25 to 60 μm) called planozygotes (5, 7). The amoeboid forms that have been described vary in size and morphology, and the cysts are small ($\sim$5 μm).

P. piscicida, the only species in the genus that has been formally described (54), is a heterotrophic dinoflagellate that can sometimes be mixotrophic by retaining "kleptochloroplasts" from algal prey (34). That is, it is not capable of photosynthesis without chloroplasts retained from other organisms, and it generally subsists on bacteria, algae, microfauna, and sloughed organic materials from fish prey (4, 5, 8). The cells are capable of phagocytosis in both the amoeboid and flagellate forms.

On the basis of many laboratory experiments as well as field data, the dominant niche for the organism is found at the sediment-water column interface, where amoeboid and cyst forms are believed to predominate; however, zoospore counts found in the water column during bloom and fish-kill events rise to levels as high as 1,000 to 35,000 organisms/ml (4, 5, 7). Counts in surface waters may rapidly drop to undetectable levels (by light microscopy) following fish-kill events, which led to the description of *Pfiesteria* as ephemeral and phantom-like (4, 5, 7).

The trophic factors controlling *Pfiesteria* growth and survival are complex, for the organism apparently adapts to available prey. In the absence of fish prey, under appropriate physical conditions (temperature, salinity, and flushing), the growth of *Pfiesteria* can be stimulated by the addition of organic and inorganic nitrogen and phosphorus (5, 7, 8, 9). These laboratory experiments and field data underlie the hypothesis that *Pfiesteria* blooms are linked to enrichment of those waters by agricultural runoff, human sewage, poorly treated wastes from industrialized concentrated animal operations, and other nutrient-rich sources (5, 6). Nutrient enrichment supports phytoplankton blooms and may thus indirectly support the growth of grazing dinoflagellates such as *Pfiesteria* (5, 9). In the presence of fish prey, under appropriate physical conditions, *Pfiesteria* may be induced to produce toxins that result in fish death and epidermal sloughing (5, 11, 46). However, it is important to note that during most of an annual cycle and under most conditions, *Pfiesteria* exists in a benign (non-toxicity-associated) state; hence, to implicate this dinoflagellate in fish-kill or disease events, the presence of actively toxic populations in water samples taken during the events must be verified (until assays for direct detection of *Pfiesteria*-related toxins are developed). The specific chemical signals that induce toxin production are as yet unidentified substances in fish excrement, secretions, and tissues (5). Observations in North Carolina suggest that the optimal conditions for *Pfiesteria* toxin production that result in fish-kill or distress events include (i) calm, shallow waters with poor flushing, presumably permitting accumulation of sufficient toxin concentrations, (ii) brackish conditions (i.e., salinity of 2 to 20 ppt), (iii) warm temperatures (about 25°C or higher), and (iv) abundant prey that produce the appropriate stimulus for toxin production (4–13). Schooling fish may therefore create the ideal stimulus for toxin production, and in Maryland and North Carolina waters, the Atlantic menhaden (*Brevoortia tyrannus*) has been the most heavily affected in fish-kill events (6, 7, 10).

P. piscicida and Fish Health

Any number of environmental stressors may induce fish mortality, including infection (fungal, bacterial, viral, parasitic), chemical exposure (pollutants, toxins, suboptimal water quality), or physical factors (low dissolved oxygen concentrations, rapid water temperature change, trauma). When large numbers of diseased or dying fish are observed in association with "blooms" of a particular dinoflagellate (or algal) species, injury may have occurred through direct mechanisms (toxin or toxic metabolite production) or through indirect effects such as low dissolved oxygen levels. Thus, direct attribution of a fish-kill event to a particular dinoflagellate or dinoflagellate-derived toxin is, at best, difficult (11, 27). However, a great deal of evidence implicating *P. piscicida* with such events has accumulated.

As stated above, *Pfiesteria* was first described when it was linked with unexpected fish mortality in a laboratory setting after addition of freshly collected estuarine water to the aquaria (7, 53). Similar events have occurred repeatedly in laboratories in North Carolina and Maryland (6, 7, 27, 46, 47) and have been routinely observed for 8 years in *P. piscicida* cultures with fish at the Aquatic Botany Laboratory at North Carolina State University. The linkage in the laboratory between *Pfiesteria* cultures and ichthyotoxicity is well established.

Pfiesteria was detected in bloom during a fish kill in the Pamlico River (North Carolina) in 1991 that resulted in the death of an estimated 1 million Atlantic menhaden (*B. tyrannus*) (7). *Pfiesteria* cell counts at this and subsequent fish-kill events observed later that year on the Neuse and Pamlico Estuaries (North Carolina) ranged from 400 to ~35,000 zoospores/ml (7, 8, 21). The organism was counted and tentatively identified by light microscopy, with subsequent verification of toxicity by fish bioassays with water samples from the kills, followed by species identification by scanning electron microscopy of suture-swollen cells (5, 7, 11). No other explanation for the observed fish mortality during these events was evident. Subsequently, *P. piscicida* was identified at 21 field-kill events in North Carolina waters from 1991 to 1993, and the organism was implicated in ~50% of all fish-kill events that occurred annually in these estuaries (6). Since that time, *Pfiesteria* has been linked with repeated fish-kill events in North Carolina waters, including an event that affected 500,000 fish in the Neuse Estuary in the summer of 1998 (12).

P. piscicida was first detected in Chesapeake Bay waters in 1993 (Jenkins Creek in the Choptank River drainage) (33). The organism was subsequently identified in water samples collected during a striped bass mortality event that occurred at an outdoor aquaculture facility on the Manokin River in August 1996 (13). In the late summer and early fall of 1997, several fish-kill events occurred in estuarine tributaries of the Chesapeake Bay on Maryland's Eastern Shore (the Pocomoke, Manokin, and Chicamacomico Rivers) (Fig. 2) (36). *P. piscicida* was isolated from water samples collected at each of these events, and *Pfiesteria*-like organisms were present in water samples at counts ranging from 300 to 1,400 zoospores/ml in water

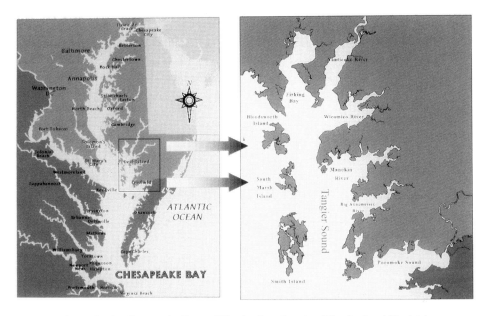

Figure 2. The Chesapeake Bay and Tangier Sound region (Maryland and Virginia). Fish-kill events associated with human health problems occurred on the Pocomoke, Manokin, and Chicamacomico Rivers during the late summer and fall of 1997. The Chicamacomico River is a small tributary of Fishing Bay.

samples collected during these events (13, 36). Fish bioassays demonstrating ichthyotoxicity yielded *P. piscicida* as the dominant species (13) as well as fivefold-lower densities of a second toxic *Pfiesteria*-like species ("species B," which has not yet been formally named and has also been found in North Carolina estuaries [5]). A number of other heterotrophic dinoflagellates were isolated from the water samples collected during these events, including two *Gyrodinium* spp., two *Cryptoperidiniopsis* (gen. nov.) spp., one scripsielloid species, and five gymnodinioid species (13, 36). None of these other dinoflagellate isolates caused fish distress, disease, or death when tested separately (13).

Many fish collected during *Pfiesteria*-related fish-kill events display aberrant swimming behavior and have diffuse epithelial injury, with hemorrhage and necrosis. These effects are attributed to the toxins produced by *Pfiesteria* and have been reproduced in the laboratory setting (7, 37, 46, 47). In addition, fish collected during fish-kill events attributed to *Pfiesteria* and at other times in these same bodies of water have been noted to have characteristic deep ulcers. For menhaden, these body sores are commonly observed near the anus of the fish (Color Plate 1). Microbiological evaluation of these lesioned fish has revealed a variety of bacterial pathogens (including *Vibrio* spp., *Aeromonas* spp., and *Pseudomonas fluorescens*) (22). On histologic examination, granulomatous disease with prominent fungal hyphae is common, and species of the fungal genus *Aphanomyces* have been commonly isolated (3, 11, 14, 45). Thus, some fish lesions initially associated with *Pfiesteria*-related fish kills appear to be a consequence of invasive chronic fungal infection,

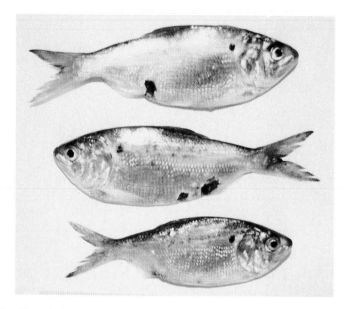

Color Plate 1. Characteristic external lesions observed in Atlantic menhaden (*B. tyrannus*) collected from the Chicamacomico River during a fish-kill event associated with the toxin-producing dinoflagellate *P. piscicida*. Fish with similar external lesions were observed throughout this region (Fig. 2) during 1997. As noted in the text, histologic evaluation of such lesions has frequently revealed the presence of opportunistic bacterial and fungal pathogens in granuloma formations. Photo courtesy of Ernest Brown.

with secondary and variable bacterial superinfection. In the field, during most seasons and under most circumstances, actively toxic populations of *P. piscicida* have not been linked with such lesions; however, under certain conditions (i.e., during warm seasons in poorly flushed brackish waters with large schools of menhaden), the presence of such lesions in 20% or more of sampled fish has been used successfully as an indicator of the presence of actively toxic populations of *P. piscicida* and species B (11). A current hypothesis holds that the precipitating event that permits opportunistic fungal infection is exposure to *Pfiesteria* toxins.

Pfiesteria and *Pfiesteria*-like organisms have been isolated from estuarine waters from Delaware Bay to Mobile Bay on the Gulf Coast (5, 6), and recent sampling of sediments from multiple estuarine sites in Maryland (Chesapeake Bay and coastal bays) indicates that *P. piscicida* is relatively ubiquitous in estuarine waters in this region (13). Evaluation of *Pfiesteria*'s impact on environmental quality and human health must therefore include an assessment of organism numbers (i.e., is an algal bloom under way?) and (presumed) toxin production; assays designed to provide such data are under development.

P. piscicida Toxins

In laboratory cultures, *P. piscicida* has been associated with profound effects on fish health. Fish placed in active, toxicity-associated cultures (hereafter referred to as "toxic cultures") rapidly develop aberrant behavior (described as "narcotized," with aberrant fright responses and swimming behavior) and epithelial hemorrhage (5–7). Culture filtrate (0.22-μm-pore-size filters) derived from active toxic cultures containing >250 flagellated cells/ml induces the same effect (4, 5). In contrast, fish placed in *Pfiesteria* cultures raised on algal prey to similar concentrations (or in filtrates derived from these cultures) do not suffer immediate injury (however, toxin production can be induced in this fashion). Suspensions of cells and water from active toxic *Pfiesteria* cultures were injected intraperitoneally into rats (at inocula ranging from 30,000 to 100,000 cells/kg of body weight) and produced no discernible symptomatic disease (the animals appeared to be normal by observation), but the rats had impaired radial maze-learning behavior (31, 32). Although the inocula in these experiments were sometimes crude (i.e., dinoflagellates, their presumed toxins, bacteria, and products of dying fish), the observations suggest that substances present during *Pfiesteria*-related fish killing may have neurobehavioral effects upon mammals as well.

Toxic *Pfiesteria* culture filtrates and water- and lipid-soluble extracts of this material have demonstrated cytotoxicity against a variety of cells (including mouse neuroblastoma (Neuro 2A) and hypothalamic (GT1-7) cell lines, rat pituitary cells (GH$_4$C$_1$), and human hepatoma cells (HepG2) by the 3-(4,5-dimethylthiazol-2-yl)-2,5-diphenyltetrazolium bromide (MTT) assay (a measure of mitochondrial dehydrogenase activity) (17). In toxicological investigations, an extension of the cytotoxicity assay is the reporter gene assay. Reporter gene assays depend upon binding of toxins with cell surface receptors and can be used even if the specific cell surface receptor is unknown, so long as internal secondary events can be recognized. Fairey and colleagues (17) have developed such an assay for detection of putative *Pfiesteria* toxins. In this case, a reporter, the luciferase gene, is linked downstream of the binding sites for fos, an inducible regulatory protein of the cellular AP-1 transcription complex. When an appropriate stimulus is presented to the cell (i.e., binding of toxins to specific receptors), production of the targeted regulatory protein (fos, in this case) occurs, which results in (measurable) reporter gene (luciferase gene) expression. Toxic *Pfiesteria* culture water filtrates and extracts were found to induce c-*fos* expression (measured by luciferase activity) in this reporter gene assay (in GH$_4$C$_1$ cells), while the well-characterized algal toxins brevetoxin, ciguatoxin, saxitoxin, and domoic acid did not (13). In addition, chromatographically separated fractions with reporter gene assay activity also retained (at comparable or enhanced levels) fish-killing toxicity. These assays are being used to guide efforts to concentrate and purify the *Pfiesteria* toxin(s) for physical and chemical characterization. It is also possible that the reporter assay will be of use in screening for the presence of the *Pfiesteria* toxin(s) in environmental water samples or human biological specimens (sera or urine) in the future. If specific toxin receptors are recognized, it will then become possible to perform specific receptor-ligand assays; it is anticipated that this will be the next significant advance in the characterization of the *Pfiesteria* toxin(s).

Thus, there is now considerable evidence that cultures of the dinoflagellate *P. piscicida* are associated with toxic factors that (i) induce behavioral changes and death in fish bioassays, (ii) are cytotoxic to fish and mammalian cell lines in vitro when present at sufficient concentrations, (iii) interact with specific cell surface receptors on particular cell lines, inducing measurable changes in transcriptional regulatory proteins (fos), and (iv) result in neurobehavioral change in a mammalian model (rat maze-learning behavior). Although the association of this toxicity with *P. piscicida* cultures has been established, it should be pointed out that the actual existence of a specific toxin, its physical characteristics, and the mechanisms of such toxin production and activity remain unproven. It is possible that a family of related toxin structures are generated, as has been described for saxitoxins and toxins associated with ciguatera (52). For instance, lipid- and water-soluble fractions derived from toxic cultures display distinct cytotoxicity and reporter gene activity (17). These preliminary data suggest that more than one form of the putative toxin(s) exists or that completely distinct toxins are present.

Detection of *P. piscicida* in Environmental Samples

The Burkholder and Glasgow research team (Aquatic Botany Laboratory, North Carolina State University, Raleigh) developed a three-tiered evaluation strategy for evaluation of suspected *Pfiesteria* blooms or fish-kill events that was used by several mid-Atlantic states in 1997 and 1998. The first level is an assessment by light microscopy of the number of *Pfiesteria*-like dinoflagellates in fixed (acid Lugol's iodine solution-treated) water samples (5–7). Keeping in mind that the organism cannot be positively identified by light microscopy alone, this first screen simply informs the investigator as to the likelihood that *Pfiesteria* or a *Pfiesteria*-like dinoflagellate is contributing to an observed event (at the Aquatic Botany Laboratory, North Carolina State University, cell counts of >100 cells/ml are implicated in fish disease and counts of >250 cells/ml are implicated in fish kills) (13). If organisms consistent with *Pfiesteria* are present at concentrations believed to be capable of inducing disease, the next stage of analysis is performance of the fish-kill bioassay. If organisms in culture are associated with the ability to kill fish within defined time parameters, this is taken as strong evidence that the same organisms were present, actively toxic, and responsible for the observed event in the environment. This assay was developed by the Burkholder lab and has been cross-corroborated by independent laboratories as an effective technique for detection of toxic *Pfiesteria* and *Pfiesteria*-like dinoflagellates (33, 37, 46). The final stage of analysis has been amplification of cultures with live fish to concentrations sufficient for evaluation by scanning electron microscopy. The outer membranes of the organism must be stripped or the sutures between thecal plates must be swollen to permit tabulation of the cellulose plates (thecal plates or "armor") for species identification. This is a very tedious and detailed process that provides definitive morphologic data, but it requires weeks to perform and may be complicated by overgrowth of competing dinoflagellate species during the culture amplification phase.

The small-subunit (18S) rRNA gene sequences of *P. piscicida* and a number of related heterotrophic dinoflagellates have been determined, and species-specific PCR and in situ hybridization assays that permit detection of the organism have been developed (28, 48). These assays are being validated, and it is expected that they will enhance ecological studies of the organism and public health-based monitoring on the basis of the ability of sequence-based methods to provide (i) species-specific amplification, (ii) relatively rapid, high-throughput screening, and (iii) quantitative data (48). However, detection of the organism alone does not inform the investigator regarding the presence or absence of (putative) toxin production. Thus, multiple modalities including fish-kill bioassay, light and scanning electron microscopy, sequence-based organism detection, and newly developed toxin detection assays are all being used in ongoing studies of the organism.

P. piscicida and Human Health

The first indication that toxins produced by *Pfiesteria* could cause human illness came when investigators working with the organism in Burkholder's laboratory in North Carolina experienced problems with respiratory and eye irritation, skin rashes, gastroenteritis (stomach cramps, nausea, vomiting), and, of particular concern, cognition and personality changes (21). These symptoms occurred following recurrent or chronic exposure to toxin-producing *P. piscicida* cultures. One individual who experienced dramatic symptoms of cognitive impairment (including short-term memory loss, reading difficulty, and emotional lability) underwent formal neuropyschological evaluation, and it was thought that there was objective evidence of an organic amnesia syndrome; electroencephalogram, cerebral magnetic resonance imaging, and positron emission tomography were normal (21). Other individuals in the laboratory developed similar symptoms (headaches, malaise, confusion, and disorientation) in temporal association with exposure to *P. piscicida* cultures. While most symptoms appear to have resolved, concerns about subtle persistent effects 6 to 7 years after the acute incident remain among the affected individuals. In addition, there have been many anecdotal accounts of health problems among commercial and recreational fishermen, including skin lesions and confusional states, following exposure to North Carolina waters with prior or concurrent fish-kill events (21, 43). These reports have appeared in the lay media, in newspaper and magazine accounts, and in a book that generated considerable controversy in North Carolina (1).

An epidemiological evaluation of persons exposed to three *Pfiesteria*-related fish-kill events occurring in the Neuse and Pamlico River estuaries (North Carolina) in 1995 was performed by the North Carolina Department of Environment, Health, and Natural Resources (43). A total of 51 individuals with potential exposure (physical contact with affected waters during the fish-kill event or time spent in a boat on those waters during the event) were evaluated. At the Pamlico River event, only one of seven individuals interviewed complained of new health problems (skin rash, burning). Among 12 individuals present at a fish kill on Goose Creek, N.C. (a tributary of the Neuse River), 4 complained of eye irritation and 3 complained of headache during and following exposure. Thirty-two individuals exposed to a fish kill that occurred on the Neuse River were interviewed, and 14 of 32 (44%) reported new symptoms associated with exposure. Among the symptoms reported, eye irritation (16%), skin rash or irritation (22%), gastroenteritis (13%), word-finding difficulties (22%), concentration difficulties (16%), and fatigue (19%) were the most prominent. Five individuals present at this event reported persistent cognitive difficulty which lasted for several weeks; three underwent neuropsychological evaluation approximately 2 months following exposure (a significant delay, on the basis of later observations of the neuropsychological effects of exposure [22]). Testing revealed deficits in learning in two of three individuals, but the results were potentially confounded by underlying depression in one individual and the marked delay between the onset of symptoms and the time of evaluation. The investigators were unable to confirm a causal relationship between environmental exposure during *Pfiesteria*-related fish-kill events and reported symptoms and noted a number of factors that confounded their investigation. Prominent among them were the absence of baseline data, selection bias in cohort identification, the subjective and nonspecific nature of the reported symptoms, difficulty gauging exposure, and the absence of a specific diagnostic assay for the detection of a toxin or toxicity. Collective observations from North Carolina were nonetheless extremely important in laying the groundwork for subsequent evaluations performed in Maryland in 1997 and for ongoing multistate Centers for Disease Control and Prevention-sponsored cohort studies (in Maryland, North Carolina, and Virginia).

In the fall of 1996 through the spring and summer of 1997, Maryland watermen working along the Pocomoke and other small rivers emptying into Tangier Sound on the Eastern Shore of the Chesapeake Bay reported increasing numbers of fish with "punched-out" skin lesions. Some watermen reported problems with fatigue, headaches, respiratory irritation, and memory disturbances. Preliminary studies performed in Burkholder's laboratory indicated that *P. piscicida* was present in the Pocomoke River (13, 36), and after the occurrence of a fish-kill event there in August 1997, the Maryland Department of Health and Mental Hygiene asked investigators from the medical schools of the University of Maryland and Johns Hopkins University to evaluate health complaints among these watermen.

Twenty-four individuals were evaluated, including 13 with high levels of exposure (6 to 8 h/day on affected waterways, with significant direct exposure to water and aerosols) to the fish-kill area (22). Seven individuals had moderate levels of exposure (8 to 20 h/week on affected waterways); four had low levels of exposure (they spent time on boats in the affected area but had little or no direct skin contact with affected waters and a limited overall duration of exposure). Commonly reported symptoms included acute confusion, forgetfulness, episodes of disorientation, and difficulty concentrating. Other symptoms included headaches, skin lesions and "burning" on contact with affected waters, and gastroenteritis (nausea, vomiting, abdominal cramping). In a comparison of the group with a high level of exposure with control watermen who worked on the Atlantic Ocean, the occurrence of neuropsychological symptoms, headache, and complaints of skin lesions and burning differed significantly.

No consistent or unexpected abnormalities were found on physical examination (see discussion of dermatologic findings below). Detailed laboratory assessments, including complete blood counts and differentials and serum electrolyte, creatinine, transaminase, serum albumin, and bilirubin concentration determinations, did not reveal consistent abnormalities. Study participants had normal (intact) delayed-type hypersensitivity responses to common antigens (candida and mumps virus), and peripheral blood T-lymphocyte subset percentages and absolute counts were normal. Chest radiographs and pulmonary function tests, which were performed for most subjects, were normal in the absence of a heavy smoking history and chronic obstructive pulmonary disease.

A variety of dermatologic conditions were observed, including common findings such as tinea and lamellar dyshidrosis ("dish pan hands") which were unrelated to exposure. Four individuals with high levels of exposure had unexplained or suspicious lesions that comprised erythematous papules or scaling patches. Biopsy of these lesions revealed an inflammatory response with eosinophils in two individuals, and these were possibly consistent with an allergic or toxic reaction (35). However, no definitive *Pfiesteria*-related skin lesion was identified.

Participants underwent detailed evaluations by neuropsychological testing, and significant associations between the degree of exposure to *Pfiesteria*-affected Maryland waterways and deficiencies in learning, memory, and higher-order cognitive function (divided attention) were found (Fig. 3). Results were most striking on the Rey auditory, verbal, learning, and memory test, on which 75% of persons with high levels of exposure to affected waterways scored below the 2nd percentile compared with appropriately matched national norms; this reflects a profound and potentially disabling deficit (22). The primary deficit appeared to be in the ability of patients to place new observations into memory (i.e., to learn); in contrast, material which had already been learned could be recalled without difficulty. The range of affected cognitive domains (new learning, capacity for divided-attention activities, concentration) was entirely consistent with the reported cognitive complaints of the exposed individuals. When patients (and controls) were retested 3 and 6 months after their initial evaluation, test scores among affected individuals increased significantly, returning in all instances to the normal range. While deficits

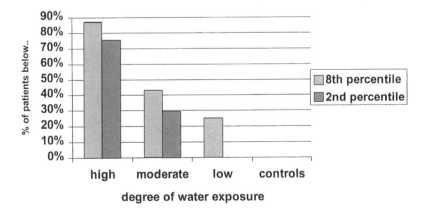

Figure 3. Percentage of study participants with exposure to *Pfiesteria*-related fish-kill events scoring below the 8th and 2nd percentiles (in comparison with age- and education-matched national normative data) on the Rey auditory, verbal, learning, and memory test, grouped by degree of exposure to waterways with *Pfiesteria* activity. Controls were watermen who worked on ocean waters without potential *Pfiesteria* exposure. Data are from reference 22.

in most instances appear to have resolved completely, some individuals continue to feel that they are not back to normal.

Patients in the Maryland studies tended to be young, male, self-employed, and otherwise healthy; on tests of mood state, most ranked as vigorous. Findings were not consistent with a hysterical reaction (23), and persons with any suggestion of malingering or symptom exaggeration or who had any other possible explanation for the observed deficits were excluded from analyses in the published report (22).

A subsequent *Pfiesteria*-related fish-kill event occurred on a second Maryland river, the Chicamacomico, in September 1997 (36). On the basis of the medical findings linked with the August fish kill on the Pocomoke River, Maryland State health authorities closed the river to public access. An acute influenza-like illness characterized by headache, gastrointestinal symptoms (crampy abdominal pain, nausea, vomiting), and malaise was reported by a number of individuals charged with maintaining closure of the river. Neuropsychological testing performed 2 weeks postexposure (and follow-up 3 months later) did not reveal a pattern of depressed test scores among exposed workers compared with those among nonexposed workers. When compared with the experience of the Pocomoke River watermen evaluated 1 month earlier, the exposure in these cases was more limited both in intensity and in duration. This has led to the hypothesis that graded responses to exposure may occur (flu-like illness with prominent headache, with or without an associated confusional state following mild to moderate levels of exposure, with more severe illness and associated measurable cognitive deficits occurring following intense exposure).

In a case-control study performed in North Carolina, persons exposed to estuarine waterways had significant deficiencies in visual contrast sensitivity, an indicator of impairment in human visual system function (25). The visual deficits were similar to those observed in workers following exposures to organic solvents, although cases in the North Carolina study (individuals with exposure to estuarine waters with potential for *Pfiesteria* exposure) and controls (persons working on the ocean with no possibility of *Pfiesteria* exposure) did not differ in their history of exposure to such compounds. Contrast sensitivity testing was not performed during the 1997 Maryland evaluation, and further evaluation of the clinical utility of these tests is under way.

As with the North Carolina evaluations, the 1997 investigation of individuals in Maryland with exposure to *Pfiesteria*-related fish-kill events suffered from an absence of baseline (preexposure) data for participants, an unavoidable circumstance that was addressed in part by follow-up testing at later time points. With funding from the Centers for Disease Control and Prevention, long-term cohort studies are under way in Maryland, Virginia, and North Carolina. The latter studies include collection of baseline neurocognitive data, regular follow-up of cohort members, and linkage of neurocognitive findings with data on exposure to estuarine waterways and the presence of *Pfiesteria* in the environment. As these data become available, we should have a much better understanding of clinical syndromes which may be associated with exposure to putative *Pfiesteria* (and other estuarine dinoflagellate) toxins during work and recreation on estuarine waters.

CONCLUSIONS

P. piscicida is a recently described toxic dinoflagellate that has been implicated as a causative agent of fish-kill events in the environment. As outlined in this chapter, much remains to be learned about the organism, its presumed toxins, the environmental conditions which promote toxin expression, and the mechanisms by which these toxins might cause disease in humans. At the same time, there is an increasing convergence of data which support the idea of a link between exposure to toxins produced by this and related dinoflagellates and the occurrence of illness in humans. The emergence of this "new" pathogen underscores the complexity of the ecosystems of which we are a part and the ever present potential for the appearance of new diseases as these ecosystems change and evolve.

Acknowledgments. We acknowledge the pioneering efforts, support, and collaboration of JoAnn Burkholder and Howard Glasgow of the Aquatic Botany Laboratory at North Carolina State University. John Ramsdell (National Oceanic and Atmospheric Administration) generously shared preliminary observations and insights for this publication. Donald Schmechel (Duke University) provided invaluable advice as preparations were made for the initial evaluation of affected Pocomoke River watermen. This is Ecology and Oceanography of Harmful Algal Blooms (ECOHAB), National Oceanic and Atmospheric Administration, publication 002.

REFERENCES

1. **Barker, R.** 1998. *And the Waters Turned to Blood: the Ultimate Biological Threat.* Touchstone Books, New York, N.Y.
2. **Boesch, D. E., D. M. Anderson, R. A. Horner, S. E. Shumway, P. A. Tester, and T. E. Whitledge.** 1996. *Harmful Algal Blooms in Coastal Waters: Options for Prevention, Control, and Mitigation.* NOAA Coastal Oceans Program Decision Analysis Series no. 10. Coastal Oceans Office, National Oceanic and Atmospheric Administration, Silver Spring, Md.
3. **Boesch, D. E.** 1999. *Special Report of the Technical Advisory Committee on Harmful Algal Outbreaks in Maryland: Causes and Significance of Menhaden Lesions.* Horn Point Environmental Laboratory, University of Maryland, Cambridge.
4. **Burkholder, J. M., and H. B. Glasgow, Jr.** 1997. Trophic controls on stage transformations of a toxic ambush-predator dinoflagellate. *J. Eukaryot. Microbiol.* **44:**200–205.
5. **Burkholder, J. M., and H. B. Glasgow, Jr.** 1997. *Pfiesteria piscicida* and other toxic *Pfiesteria*-like dinoflagellates: behavior, impacts, and environmental controls. *Limnol. Oceanogr.* **42:**1052–1074.
6. **Burkholder, J. M., H. B. Glasgow, Jr., and C. W. Hobbs.** 1995. Distribution and environmental conditions for fish kills linked to a toxic ambush-predator dinoflagellate. *Mar. Ecol. Prog. Ser.* **124:**43–61.
7. **Burkholder, J. M., E. J. Noga, C. W. Hobbs, H. B. Glasgow, Jr., and S. A. Smith.** 1992. New "phantom" dinoflagellate is the causative agent of major fish estuarine fish kills. *Nature* **358:**407–410. (Erratum, **360:**768.)
8. **Burkholder, J. M., and H. B. Glasgow, Jr.** 1995. Interactions of a toxic estuarine dinoflagellate with microbial predators and prey. *Arch. Protistenkd.* **145:**177–188.
9. **Burkholder, J. M., H. B. Glasgow, Jr., and A. J. Lewitus.** 1998. Physiological ecology of *Pfiesteria piscicida,* with general comments on 'ambush-predator' dinoflagellates. *NATO ASI Ser. Ser. G* **44:**175–191.
10. **Burkholder, J. M.** 1998. Implications of harmful microalgae and heterotrophic dinoflagellates in management of sustainable marine fisheries. *Ecol. Appl.* **8**(Suppl.)**:**S37–S62.
11. **Burkholder, J. M., M. A. Mallin, and H. B. Glasgow, Jr.** 1999. Fish kills, bottom-water hypoxia, and the toxic *Pfiesteria* complex in the Neuse River and Estuary. *Mar. Ecol. Prog. Ser.* **179:**301–310.

12. **Burkholder, J. M., H. B. Glasgow, Jr., N. J. Deamer-Melia, and E. K. Hannon.** 1999. The 1998 fish kill season: tracking a toxic Pfiesteria outbreak in the Neuse Estuary, North Carolina, USA. *In Proceedings of the Winter Meeting of the American Society of Limnology and Oceanography.* (Abstract.)

13. **Burkholder, J. M., and H. B. Glasgow, Jr.** Unpublished data.

14. **Dykstra, M. J., J. F. Levine, and E. J. Noga.** 1989. Ulcerative mycosis: a serious menhaden disease of the southeastern coastal fisheries of the United States. *J. Fish Dis.* **12:**175–178.

15. **ECOHAB.** 1994. The ecology and oceanography of harmful algal blooms: a national research agenda. Report of a workshop held at Snow Mountain Ranch, Colo., 23 to 28 August 1994. [Online.] http://www.redtide.whoi.edu/hab/nationplan/ECOHAB. [12 July 1999, last date accessed.]

16. **Engleberg, N. C., J. G. Morris, Jr., J. Lewis, J. P. McMillan, R. A. Pollard, and P. A. Blake.** 1983. Ciguatera fish poisoning: a major common source outbreak in the U.S. Virgin Islands. *Ann. Intern. Med.* **98:**336–337.

17. **Fairey, E. R., J. S. Edmunds, N. J. Deamer-Melia, H. B. Glasgow, Jr., F. M. Johnson, P. R. Moeller, J. M. Burkholder, and J. S. Ramsdell.** Reporter gene assay for fish-killing activity produced by *Pfiesteria piscicida. Environ. Health Perspect.,* in press.

18. **Gessner, B. D., P. Bell, G. J. Doucette, E. Moczydlowski, M. A. Poli, F. Van Dolah, and S. Hall.** 1997. Hypertension and identification of toxin in human urine and serum following a cluster of mussel-associated paralytic shellfish poisoning outbreaks. *Toxicon* **35:**711–722.

19. **Gessner, B. D., and J. P. Middaugh.** 1995. Paralytic shellfish poisoning in Alaska: a 20-year retrospective analysis. *Am. J. Epidemiol.* **141:**766–770.

20. **Gillespie, N. C., R. J. Lewis, J. H. Pearn, A. T. C. Bourke, M. J. Holmes, J. B. Bourke, and W. J. Shields.** 1986. Ciguatera in Australia: occurrence, clinical features, pathophysiology and management. *Med. J. Aust.* **145:**584–590.

21. **Glasgow, H. B., Jr., J. M. Burkholder, D. E. Schmechel, P. A. Rublee, and P. A. Tester.** 1995. Insidious effects of a toxic estuarine dinoflagellate on fish survival and human health. *J. Toxicol. Environ. Health* **46:**501–522.

22. **Grattan, L. M., D. Oldach, T. M. Perl, M. H. Lowitt, D. L. Matuszak, C. Dickson, C. Parrott, R. C. Shoemaker, C. L. Kauffman, M. P. Wasserman, J. R. Hebel, P. Charache, and J. G. Morris, Jr.** 1998. Learning and memory difficulties after environmental exposure to waterways containing toxin-producing *Pfiesteria* or *Pfiesteria*-like dinoflagellates. *Lancet* **352:**532–539.

23. **Greenberg, D. R., J. K. Tracy, and L. M. Grattan.** 1998. A critical review of the *Pfiesteria* hysteria hypothesis. *Md. Med. J.* **47:**133–136.

24. **Halegraeff, G. M.** 1993. A review of harmful algal blooms and their apparent global increase. *Phycologia* **32:**79–99.

25. **Hudnell, H. K.** 1998. Human visual function in the North Carolina clinical study on *Pfiesteria piscicida. In Abstracts of the Ceres Forum on* Pfiesteria *and the Environment.*

26. **Jordan, S. J., and E. B. May.** 1998. *Histological and Microbiological Study Findings on Fish Taken from the Pocomoke River and Adjacent Tributaries.* Cooperative Oxford Laboratory, Maryland State Department of Natural Resources, Oxford.

27. **Kane, A. S., D. Oldach, and R. Reimschuessel.** 1998. Fish lesions in the Chesapeake Bay: *Pfiesteria*-like dinoflagellates and other etiologies. *Md. Med. J.* **47:**106–112.

28. **Kempton, J. W.** 1999. PCR and FISH assays for the detection of *P. piscicida.* M.S. thesis. University of North Carolina, Greensboro.

29. **Krishnamurthy, T., W. W. Carmichael, and E. W. Sarver.** 1986. Toxic peptides from freshwater cyanobacteria (blue-green algae). I. Isolation, purification and characterization of peptides from *Microcystis aeruginosa* and *Anabaena flos-aquae. Toxicon* **24:**865–873.

30. **Lange, W. R., F. R. Snyder, and P. J. Fudala.** 1992. Travel and ciguatera fish poisoning. *Arch. Intern. Med.* **152:**2049–2053.

31. **Levin, E. D., D. E. Schmechel, J. M. Burkholder, H. B. Glasgow, Jr., N. J. Deamer-Melia, V. C. Moser, and G. J. Harry.** 1998. Persisting learning deficits in rats after exposure to *Pfiesteria piscicida. Environ. Health Perspect.* **105:**1320–1325.

32. **Levin, E. D., B. B. Simon, D. E. Schmechel, H. B. Glasgow, Jr., N. J. Deamer-Melia, J. M. Burkholder, V. C. Moser, K. Jensen, and G. J. Harry.** 1999. Pfiesteria toxin and learning performance. *Neurotoxicol. Teratol.* **21:**215–221.

33. **Lewitus, A. J., R. V. Jesien, T. M. Kana, J. M. Burkholder, H. B. Glasgow, Jr., and E. May.** 1995. Discovery of the "phantom" dinoflagellate in Chesapeake Bay. *Estuaries* **18:**373–378.
34. **Lewitus, A. J., H. B. Glasgow, Jr., and J. M. Burkholder.** 1999. Kleptoplastidy in the toxic dinoflagellate Pfiesteria piscicida (Dinophyceae). *J. Phycol.* **35:**303–312.
35. **Lowitt, M. H., and L. Kauffman.** 1998. *Pfiesteria* and the skin: a practical update for clinicians. *Md. Med. J.* **47:**124–126.
36. **Magnien, R. E., J. M. Burkholder, and H. B. Glasgow, Jr.** 1998. *Pfiesteria* in Chesapeake Bay in 1997. *In Proceedings, Annual Summer Meeting, American Society of Limnology and Oceanography.* (Abstract.)
37. **Marshall, H. (Old Dominion University, Norfolk, Va.).** Personal communication.
38. **Morris, J. G., Jr.** Harmful algal blooms: a model for emergence of pathogenic microorganisms under conditions of ecologic stress. *Annu. Rev. Energy Environ.*, in press.
39. **Morris, J. G., Jr.** 1995. Natural toxins associated with fish and shellfish, p. 251–256. *In* M. J. Blaser, P. D. Smith, J. I. Ravdin, H. B. Greenberg, and R. L. Guerrant (ed.), *Infections of the Gastrointestinal Tract.* Raven Press, New York, N.Y.
40. **Morris, J. G., Jr., P. Lewin, N. T. Hargrett, C. W. Smith, P. A. Blake, and R. Schneider.** 1982. Clinical features of ciguatera fish poisoning: a study of the disease in the US Virgin Islands. *Arch. Intern. Med.* **142:**1090–1092.
41. **Morris, J. G., Jr., P. Lewin, C. W. Smith, P. A. Blake, and R. Schneider.** 1982. Ciguatera fish poisoning: epidemiology of the disease on St. Thomas, U.S. Virgin Islands. *Am. J. Trop. Med. Hyg.* **31:**574–578.
42. **Morris, P. D., D. S. Campbell, T. H. Taylor, and J. I. Freeman.** 1991. Clinical and epidemiological features of neurotoxic shellfish poisoning in North Carolina. *Am. J. Public Health* **81:**471–474.
43. **Morris, P. D.** 1996. *Acute Symptoms Reported by Persons Exposed to Fish Kills Associated with Pfiesteria piscicida.* Occupational and Environmental Epidemiology Section, Division of Epidemiology, North Carolina State Department of Environment, Health, and Natural Resources, Raleigh.
44. **Music, S. I., J. T. Howell, and C. L. Brumback.** 1973. Red tide: its public health implications. *J. Fla. Med. Assoc.* **60:**27–29.
45. **Noga, E. J., and M. J. Dykstra.** 1986. Oomycete fungi associated with ulcerative mycosis in menhaden, *Brevoortia tyrannus* (Latrobe). *J. Fish Dis.* **9:**47–53.
46. **Noga, E. J., L. Khoo, J. B. Stevens, Z. Fan, and J. M. Burkholder.** 1995. Novel toxic dinoflagellate causes epidemic disease in estuarine fish. *Mar. Pollut. Bull.* **32:**219–224.
47. **Noga, E. J., S. A. Smith, J. M. Burkholder, C. Hobbs, and R. A. Bullis.** 1993. A new ichthyotoxic dinoflagellate: cause of acute mortality in aquarium fishes. *Vet. Rec.* **133:**96–97.
48. **Oldach, D. W., E. Brown, and P. Rublee.** 1998. Strategies for environmental monitoring of toxin producing phantom dinoflagellates in the Chesapeake. *Md. Med. J.* **47:**113–119.
49. **Perl, T. M., L. Bedard, T. Kosatsky, J. C. Hockin, E. C. D. Todd, and R. S. Remis.** 1990. An outbreak of toxic encephalopathy caused by eating mussels contaminated with domoic acid. *N. Engl. J. Med.* **322:**1775–1780.
50. **Pfiester, L. A., and J. Popovsky.** 1979. Parasitic, amoeboid dinoflagellates. *Nature* **279:**421–424.
51. **Popovsky, J., and L. A. Pfiester.** 1990. Dinophyceae (Dinoflagellida). Gustav Fischer Verlag, Jena, Germany.
52. **Shimizu, Y.** 1996. Microalgal metabolites: a new perspective. *Annu. Rev. Microbiol.* **50:**431–465.
53. **Smith, S. A., E. J. Noga, and R. A. Bullis.** 1998. Mortality in *Tilapia aurea* due to a toxic dinoflagellate bloom, p. 167–168. *In Proceedings of the Third International Colloquium on the Pathology of Marine Aquaculture.*
54. **Steidinger, K. A., J. M. Burkholder, H. B. Glasgow, Jr., C. W. Hobbs, J. K. Garrett, E. W. Truby, E. J. Noga, and S. A. Smith.** 1996. *Pfiesteria piscicida* (Pfiesteriaceae), a new toxic dinoflagellate with a complex life cycle and behavior. *J. Phycol.* **32:**157–164.
55. **Steidinger, K. A., and K. Tangen.** 1996. Dinoflagellates, p. 387–584. *In* C. R. Tomas (ed.), *Identifying Marine Phytoplankton.* Academic Press, Inc., New York, N.Y.
56. **Teitelbaum, J. S., R. J. Zatorre, S. Carpenter, D. Gendreon, A. C. Evans, A. Gjedde, and N. R. Cashman.** 1990. Neurologic sequelae of domoic acid intoxication due to ingestion of contaminated mussels. *N. Engl. J. Med.* **322:**1781–1787.
57. **Tester, P. A.** 1994. Harmful marine phytoplankton and shellfish toxicity. Potential consequences of climate change. *Ann. N. Y. Acad. Sci.* **740:**69–76.
58. **Todd, E. C. D.** 1994. Emerging diseases associated with seafood toxins and other water-borne agents. *Ann. N. Y. Acad. Sci.* **740:**77–94.

Emerging Infections 3
Edited by W. M. Scheld, W. A. Craig, and J. M. Hughes
© 1999 ASM Press, Washington, D.C.

Chapter 10

Emerging Diseases of Animals

Corrie Brown

Emerging diseases of humans have certainly captured the fascination of medical communities and the general public throughout the world. Apocalyptic visions of Andromeda strains and other doomsday bugs not only have been visible on the fiction bookshelves and the silver screen but also have been the focus of serious discussions within all sectors of human biomedicine. There is no doubt that new infectious diseases of humans are arising at an alarming rate and that the consciousness of both the public and regulators has been raised.

However, a lesser-known phenomenon is occurring at the same time in animals. The last 10 years has witnessed an exponential increase in new diseases of various animal species, creating havoc in agriculture and the natural world. The potential impact that these new diseases could have on both animal and human populations deserves to be addressed.

The increase in animal disease occurrence is basically due to the same factors that have been described for human disease emergence. These factors include movement to a susceptible population, environmental disruption, crossing of species boundaries, and lifestyle changes (or, perhaps better put in the case of animals, husbandry changes). Interestingly, almost all emerging diseases of animals are the result of some manipulation by humans.

MOVEMENT TO A SUSCEPTIBLE POPULATION

Movement to a susceptible population has been a reason for emerged diseases of animals for centuries. Genghis Khan, Attila the Hun, and Napoleon all spread cattle diseases in their wake as draft animals subclinically harboring rinderpest (cattle plague) and contagious bovine pleuropneumonia were taken to new areas where cattle populations had no immunity (37). There are many modern examples as well. After the Persian Gulf War, the Kurds fleeing Iraq into Turkey took rinderpest with them in their goats and cattle, engendering outbreaks in Turkey, which,

Corrie Brown • Department of Pathology, College of Veterinary Medicine, University of Georgia, Athens, GA 30602-7388.

like the rest of Europe, had been free of the disease for some decades. The European Union responded by sending 1,000 teams of vaccinators to Turkey to help stem the spread of this emergent problem in a close neighbor.

Foot-and-mouth disease (FMD) is a reemerging disease of significant proportions in terms of regulatory effects. This disease, caused by a picornavirus, is the most feared disease of livestock and spreads in an uncontrollable way through highly infectious aerosols. Vesicles form in oral and pedal epithelia, making infected animals reluctant to eat, drink, or nurse. There is a drastic drop in production, which may last as long as a month. The presence of this disease spells economic ruin in any area of the world where intensive agriculture is practiced, which today means all except the most undeveloped regions. Consequently, the international regulatory community spends a great deal of effort tracking the movements of various strains of this virus.

In 1993, FMD surfaced in Italy, engendering the destruction of 8,000 head of cattle to control the spread (40). Entrance into the country was via a chronically and subclinically infected cow sold to an Italian by a Croatian cattle producer seeking to liquidate assets in order to purchase arms for the civil strife there.

In 1997, a huge outbreak of FMD emerged in Taiwan. Although the source of the outbreak was never confirmed, there were strong suspicions that it resulted from illegal importation of infected animals. The rapid spread of the disease within Taiwan necessitated the slaughter of 8 million hogs and cost the Taiwanese government over US$8 billion in lost production and export restrictions (48).

Hog cholera, also known as classical swine fever (CSF), caused by a pestivirus, also reemerges periodically in CSF-free areas, with devastating results. This disease was first described in pigs in the Ohio River Valley in the 1830s and subsequently was disseminated to many parts of the world through trading of pigs and pork products. The disease presents as either a severe, acute, viremic illness that culminates in death or a chronic infection characterized by a variety of reproductive failure syndromes. CSF was eradicated from the United States in 1974, and the United States continues to maintain stringent regulatory programs to prevent its introduction, as do many countries. The Netherlands is a country with a sizeable and very intensive swine industry and also strives to remain free of CSF through border controls. In the winter of 1997, however, there was a very severe cold snap, and wash water used to decontaminate livestock lorries entering The Netherlands from Germany froze as it hit the slats inside the truck, effectively preserving manure clods deposited earlier by CSF-infected German pigs. Later in the day, after some Dutch pigs were loaded into the truck, sun warmed the frozen bits of manure, and the pigs, ever curious, nosed around, allowing the virus easy access to susceptible animals. Once CSF gained hold in The Netherlands, it quickly spread over wide areas, decimating an economically vital industry and necessitating the destruction of 8 million hogs (20).

However, it is not only live animals moving from country to country that can take disease to susceptible populations. Animal products can be just as effective. African swine fever (ASF), caused by a poxvirus-like agent, is a disease of hogs associated with various rates of mortality that depend on the infecting strain. This virus was spread to many parts of the world in the 1960s largely through the disposal of uncooked airline garbage, which ended up as food for swine (26). Hogs can be chronically infected with the viral agent that causes ASF, and the virus can survive in uncooked but cured meat for as long as 1 year. When ASF-infected meat is part of the garbage fed to pigs, the virus gains entry to a new host and can spread rapidly within a swine herd. This was the case in the Iberian peninsula in the 1960s and then in the Caribbean in the 1970s and 1980s. Eradication efforts, which were eventually successful, were costly and prolonged.

All of these large-scale outbreaks of diseases emergent in countries that have been free of them usually result in massive depopulation of herds or flocks. This depopulation in and of itself can have significant impacts on humans. First, for each food-producing animal that is killed (and not consumed), there is considerable resource wastage; that is, all of the materials required to grow the animal are never recovered in the form of consumable protein. Second, there can be major environmental problems associated with the disposal of carcasses. For instance, in the Taiwanese FMD outbreak, approximately 500,000 metric tons of dead pigs had to be discarded. In many, if not most, parts of the world, the use of landfills is not an acceptable solution, and more and more, there is only a limited opportunity for burning. Environmental pollution created from the discarding of carcasses is a factor that needs to be considered in emerging animal diseases, especially with respect to livestock.

There is currently a sizeable international trade of animals and animal products that will only continue to grow with global increases in human population and the expansion of free trade. In general, the animals and animal products that cross borders are subject to stringent regulatory controls related to those diseases with which the scientific agricultural community is already familiar. Wildlife, as well, are increasingly mobile. It is not uncommon to fly reproductively active individuals of endangered species to another continent to help facilitate increases in the population. Free-ranging populations are on the move, and humans destroy habitat and force outmigrations. All of this increased movement guarantees that animal diseases will continue to emerge as infectious agents are taken to susceptible populations.

ENVIRONMENTAL DISRUPTION

Environmental disruption is a factor that is frequently cited for its ability to cause emerging disease in humans. In animals there are numerous examples of alterations in ecology that have resulted in new diseases.

Massive die-offs of seals in the North Sea gained the attention of scientists in the late 1980s. Animal carcasses with lesions reminiscent of canine distemper were washing ashore. Viral isolation yielded a morbillivirus that had never been recognized previously and that was quickly dubbed phocine distemper. Serologic examination of seals on the North American Atlantic coastline revealed that many had antibodies to the virus, but there was no clinical illness. This led some investigators to hypothesize that overfishing on the North American side of the Atlantic forced some seals to migrate across the Arctic in search of more fish, ending up in the North Sea and inadvertently taking what had been an old, familiar virus to which they were thoroughly adapted to a naive and very susceptible population

(14, 15). Recently, this virus has spread even farther, to other susceptible populations, and threatens the existence of the very endangered monk seal population in the Mediterranean and off the coast of Mauritania (32). A cetacean morbillivirus has surfaced as well and has killed striped dolphins (*Stenella coeruleoalba*) in the Mediterranean and bottle-nosed dolphins (*Tursiops truncatus*) along the eastern coast of the United States and in the Gulf of Mexico (23). The reasons for the emergence of these new diseases are unclear, but it is believed that the underlying reason for all of these recent epizootics is the transfer of virus to immunologically naive populations, probably secondary to habitat disruption (23).

North American wild waterfowl populations have witnessed huge outbreaks of infectious disease in recent years, with tens of thousands of birds dying of Newcastle disease, caused by an avian paramyxovirus, in northern Canada and the Great Lakes (4, 24); fowl cholera, caused by *Pasteurella multocida*, in the Chesapeake Bay (3, 6); and duck plague, caused by a herpesvirus, in Texas and California (5). There is general agreement that the decreasing availability of wetlands has led to crowding of these birds and a resultant critical mass for facilitation and maintenance of an outbreak (19).

Rift Valley fever, caused by a phlebovirus in the family *Bunyaviridae*, is transmitted by mosquitoes and affects a wide range of species. It tends to emerge following periods of heavy rainfall, which allow proliferation of the mosquito vector (34). The disease is particularly pathogenic for ruminants, in which it causes acute and severe hepatic failure, and is strongly associated with abortion. The disease can also be transmitted to humans, in which it appears as a flu-like illness, often with hemorrhagic complications and retinitis. The disease broke out in eastern Africa in early 1997, after periods of exceptionally heavy rains (2). In addition to the human losses, thousands of livestock succumbed, and there was a significant toll on wildlife as well.

Environmental disruption not only makes it possible for a disease to move to a new species but also creates tremendous potential for new microbes to evolve. The ability of viruses, especially RNA viruses, to evolve to adapt to a new environment is tremendous (13). Since RNA viruses lack the proofreading function, their error rate in replication is approximately a million times higher than that of any eukaryote. As a result, replication of a single purified virion can, within a matter of hours, become a "quasispecies" or, perhaps less scientifically stated, a "mutant viral swarm" (16). When that quasispecies is placed in a new environment, only those versions that are compatible with the new environment will survive, and this can result in an entirely new phenotype. Charles Darwin, writing over a century ago, described the process of evolution as "wedging into any gaps in the economy of nature" (10). Although he was referring to vertebrates, it is probably even more applicable to microbes, and investigators should pay close attention to all the attendant potentials of new environments and to the resulting "gaps" that are created and into which new variants may wedge. When dealing with animal populations, the possibilities and probabilities that new gaps will arise increase exponentially, just because of the number of species and the complex environmental interconnectedness, especially of the free-ranging populations.

The status of endogenous flora and how these microorganisms may cause disease if given the opportunity should be mentioned. Recently, attention has been paid to the status of knowledge regarding the endogenous flora of humans. The discovery of human herpesvirus 8 and of its link with Kaposi's sarcoma underscores the need for society to have humility regarding knowledge of endogenous organisms. Even with bacteria, which are more readily identifiable, the ones that we can recognize are only the tip of the iceberg compared to the oceans of unknowns (36). Certainly, even fewer of the flora endogenous to animals are known. As animals are moved around and grouped in new ways, as their environments are modified, and as technological advances to increase production are promoted, there is tremendous potential for that endogenous flora to wedge into new gaps, as alluded to above.

CROSSING OF SPECIES BOUNDARIES

Crossing of species boundaries is a time-honored way of creating new disease. Humans have become alarmed, and rightfully so in recent years, about the potential of bovine spongiform encephalopathy to cross into humans and create a progressive unrelenting dementia (7, 22, 44). Similarly, the AIDS virus, which has done so much to change the face of biomedicine, is believed to have adapted to humans from an original simian host. However, these are examples of diseases that have crossed from animals into a single species, *Homo sapiens*. If one considers just the numbers of animal species, it is obvious that the permutations and combinations of diseases that cross species boundaries increase logarithmically. Numerous examples illustrate the fact that this is indeed happening.

Canine distemper is caused by a morbillivirus that normally affects only dogs and some of their close relatives, e.g., wolves, foxes, and raccoons. Under routine conditions, canine distemper is not infectious for any members of the cat family. However, in 1995, a large number of lions in the Serengeti ecosystem began behaving in a strange manner, dying after a protracted period of grand mal seizures and ataxia (28). Examination of postmortem tissues revealed that they were dying from an infection with the virus that causes canine distemper. Epidemiologic investigation showed that the lions had contracted the virus from hyenas, which traverse between the dog population on the exterior of the Serengeti National Park and the lions within the park. Increasing human population pressures had increased the number of dogs at the edge of the park, and with enough chances, the virus successfully moved from dogs to hyenas and was eventually detected when it fully adapted to lions, with devastating results (8).

Since 1994, house finches up and down the eastern seaboard of the United States have become affected by a syndrome characterized by grossly swollen and inflamed conjunctivae. Effectively blinded, the birds are unable to forage and they die (11). Culturing of conjunctival lesions yields *Mycoplasma gallisepticum*, an important upper respiratory pathogen of domestic poultry. Molecular studies indicate distinctions between the strains from finches and the strains from poultry, suggesting either a separate source or, more likely, significant evolution as a result of adaptation to a new host. The gregarious behavior of house finches, specifically as a result of the practice of using bird feeders, is facilitating spread of the disease. In addition, the mycoplasmal conjunctivitis has also spread to American goldfinches (17).

Several new diseases have emerged in Australia over the last few years as the result of the movement of endemic viruses into new species. The first to arise was discovered when a group of horses kept at a racing stable succumbed to a syndrome of acute severe pulmonary edema and death. The trainer caring for these horses also became ill and died. A previously undescribed paramyxovirus was isolated from the tissues of both the horses and the trainer and was eventually named Hendra virus, for the property where the disease was first seen (30a, 31). A thorough search of both domestic and wild animals in the area revealed a significant seroprevalence rate among *Pteropus* spp., also known as fruit bats or flying foxes (49). Studies with experimental animals indicated that the virus is carried subclinically by the bats and is shed in the uterine secretions at the time of parturition (47). During the period of intensive investigation of fruit bats and infection with this virus, individuals handling the bats were closely scrutinized. A bat rehabilitator was found to be seriously ill with central nervous system signs, and another new virus, this one a lyssavirus, was also isolated and was found to be carried by the bats and to have the capability of crossing species and causing infections in humans (18, 21). Yet another virus was incriminated when a group of pigs was found to have various reproductive problems, with two of the animal caretakers also experiencing a flu-like illness. A paramyxovirus that was isolated was found to have a high serologic prevalence among the fruit bat population (33).

Highly pathogenic avian influenza virus is a well-recognized emerging and re-emerging pathogen for the poultry industry. The last major outbreak in the United States, in 1983, resulted in the destruction of 17 million chickens and US$56 million in eradication costs (25). Outbreaks of this lethal disease of chickens occur sporadically throughout the world. One of the most recent outbreaks, in Hong Kong in 1997, delivered a big surprise, when the virus jumped species to infect and kill some humans (39). Previously, the hemagglutinin type for this virus, H5, was thought to be infectious only for avian species.

Crossing of species boundaries will continue to be a problem in the creation of new diseases among human and animal populations. As animals are moved around and their environments are disrupted, humans are at risk of contracting new diseases. The ever increasing popularity of keeping exotic animals, whether it be iguanas as pets in the family room or llamas as pack animals in the Rocky Mountains, guarantees that evolutionarily incompatible species will be placed in proximity to humans. Zoos and game parks are wonderful breeding grounds for new disease, and we need to keep a very watchful eye on these artificial situations for the emergence of disease. Xenotransplantation (see chapter 11) is an issue that deserves careful scrutiny because of the possibilities of placing endogenous viruses from one species into intimate contact with another species. Ecotourism, as well, while engendering hope in that it signifies a heightened level of awareness of the natural environment, has the potential to take endogenous agents to isolated and immunologically naive populations, with devastating results.

HUSBANDRY CHANGES

Husbandry changes, the correlate of which in human medicine would be lifestyle changes, are responsible for a number of emerging diseases in animals. As producers strive to increase the efficiency and economic vitality of animal industries to feed the ever growing number of humans, technological changes are inevitably instituted, often with totally unexpected results.

Certainly, the best-known example of this is bovine spongiform encephalopathy. This disease, which was first recognized in England in the late 1980s as a syndrome of adult dairy cattle characterized by progressive ataxia and behavioral changes, was the subject of intense epidemiologic investigations. A point source was suspected, and the recycling of ruminant-origin protein to cattle was incriminated. Evidently, a change in the rendering process initiated in the early 1980s resulted in the survival of the prion agent through the process and the effective oral reinoculation of the agent (43). Whether the initial prion came from sheep with scrapie, a transmissible spongiform encephalopathy recognized for centuries, or whether it came from a bovine animal with spontaneous spongiform encephalopathy is still unresolved. In either case, the prion agent was effectively amplified through feeding of subtotally inactivated recycled ruminant protein.

With the resulting circumstantial link with new-variant Creutzfeldt-Jakob disease in humans in 1996 (36a), bovine spongiform encephalopathy and all the other spongiform encephalopathies came under increased scrutiny. Chronic wasting disease of mule deer and elk was described in the early 1980s in limited areas of Colorado and Wyoming where such animals are held captive (45, 46). In light of heightened awareness, increased surveillance efforts to monitor this disease have recently been undertaken. As a result, several cases have been found in free-ranging mule deer, white-tailed deer, and elk (38). The transmission potential of this disease to species other than members of the deer family (*Cervidae*) is unknown.

Bovine tuberculosis, caused by *Mycobacterium bovis*, has been recognized as a serious disease problem in cattle and causes the formation of caseating granulomas in a number of visceral organs. The zoonotic disease potential of this organism is also well recognized, and human clinical disease due to *M. bovis* is indistinguishable from that due to *Mycobacterium tuberculosis* (9). Although it continues to be a significant problem among cattle in underdeveloped countries, bovine tuberculosis has largely been eradicated from the United States, with stringent regulatory controls imposed whenever the disease surfaces in cattle. However, *M. bovis* does occur with some regularity in captive cervids. Deer are quite susceptible to infection with this organism, and when they are kept in close quarters, such as on game ranches or through the practice of winter feeding, *M. bovis* spreads rapidly through a large number of animals. Consequently, this has become an emerging disease problem in captive or group-fed deer. Unfortunately, instances in which free-ranging deer are succumbing to the infection are now occurring, and in some cases, the infection has spread back to the livestock population, from which *M. bovis* had been presumed to be eradicated (42). The resulting regulatory controls spark ample conflict between wildlife enthusiasts and agricultural producers. As a sidebar in the whole story of tuberculosis crossing species boundaries, a group of elephants and their caretakers were recently found to be positive for *M. tuberculosis*, with a chicken-and-egg question as to who infected whom (27).

DISEASES ATTRIBUTED TO OTHER FACTORS

In addition, a number of emerging diseases of animals cannot be attributed primarily to any one of the factors listed above. For instance, papillomatous digital dermatitis of cattle, a disease characterized by wart-like proliferations on the caudal interdigital space, has emerged in many parts of the world and is causing considerable economic losses, especially in the dairy industry (35). This disease is thought to be caused by a treponeme, but the reasons for its emergence are unclear. Postweaning multisystemic wasting syndrome in pigs, first identified in Canada in 1991, has now been seen in all swine-producing areas of the world and presents as pneumonia, lymphadenopathy, nephritis, and ill thrift. A novel viral agent, named porcine circovirus, has been demonstrated in tissues (1). Although a porcine circovirus had been identified in cell culture over a decade ago, the virus that causes the disease has some very distinct differences and the origin is unknown (29). Porcine intestinal spirochetosis, caused by *Serpulina pilosicoli*, has been documented as a growing cause of colitis in swine in intensive operations, especially when excellent management has ensured the absence of salmonellosis and swine dysentery (41). Isolates have been retrieved from humans and dogs as well as pigs, but the association has yet to be clarified (30). Poult enteritis and mortality syndrome is a disease of turkeys that causes severe runting and chronic diarrhea (12). Numerous etiologies have been proposed but have not yet been confirmed. For all of these emerging diseases, there has been a significant unanticipated impact on the respective industries but no solid knowledge as to where each disease came from or how its emergence could have been prevented.

CONCLUSIONS

There are a variety of emerging diseases of animals, and they are caused by many of the same factors that are at play in human diseases. Most of the emerging diseases of animals are due to some alterations engendered by the human stewards of the planet. In addition, most, if not all, of the emerging diseases of animals will have significant impacts on human health through the jeopardization of food sources, the creation of zoonotic hazards, or the alteration of ecosystems. In fact, the two fields of human and animal health are very intertwined. Rudolf Virchow, considered to be the father of modern pathology, first underscored the importance of a "one-medicine" theme over a century ago, as his work on trichinosis led him to the conclusion that disease in one species cannot be studied in isolation. Perhaps now more than ever this one-medicine theme needs to be rigorously adopted as humans face the myriad of new diseases and the intricate interconnections among all living beings.

REFERENCES

1. **Allan, G. M., F. McNeilly, S. Kennedy, B. Daft, E. G. Clarke, J. A. Ellis, D. M. Haines, B. M. Meehan, and B. M. Adair.** 1998. Isolation of porcine circovirus-like viruses from pigs with a wasting disease in the USA and Europe. *J. Vet. Diagn. Invest.* **10:**3–10.
2. **Anonymous.** 1998. Rift Valley Fever—East Africa, 1997–1998. *Morbid. Mortal. Weekly Rep.* **47:** 261–264.
3. **Ban, B. D.** 1994. Avian cholera hits Chesapeake Bay. *J. Am. Vet. Med. Assoc.* **204:**1121.
4. **Bannerjee, M., W. M. Reed, S. D. Fitzgerald, and B. Panigrahy.** 1994. Neurotropic velogenic Newcastle disease in cormorants in Michigan: pathology and virus characterization. *Avian Dis.* **38:** 873–878.
5. **Barr, B. C., D. A. Jessup, D. E. Docherty, and L. J. Lowenstine.** 1992. Epithelial intracytoplasmic herpes viral inclusions associated with an outbreak of duck virus enteritis. *Avian Dis.* **36:**164–168.
6. **Botzler, R. G.** 1991. Epizootiology of avian cholera in wildfowl. *J. Wildl. Dis.* **27:**367–395.
7. **Bruce, M. E., R. G. Will, J. W. Ironside, I. McConnell, D. Drummond, A. Suttie, L. McCardle, A. Chree, J. Hope, C. Birkett, S. Cousens, H. Fraser, and C. J. Bostock.** 1997. Transmission to mice indicates that "new variant" CJD is caused by the BSE agent. *Nature* **389:**498–501.
8. **Carpenter, M. A., M. J. Appel, M. E. Roelke-Parker, L. Munson, H. Hofer, M. East, and S. J. O'Brien.** 1998. Genetic characterization of canine distemper virus in Serengeti carnivores. *Vet. Immunol. Immunopathol.* **65:**259–266.
9. **Cosivi, O., J. M. Grange, D. J. Daborn, M. C. Raviglione, T. Fujikura, D. Cousins, R. A. Robinson, H. F. A. K. Huchzermeyer, I. deKantor, and F.-X. Meslin.** 1998. Zoonotic tuberculosis due to *Mycobacterium bovis* in developing countries. *Emerg. Infect. Dis.* **4:**59–70.
10. **Darwin, C.** 1859. *The Origin of Species by Means of Natural Selection or the Preservation of Favoured Races in the Struggle for Life.* Penguin, New York, N.Y. [Reprint, 1958.]
11. **Dhondt, A. A., D. L. Tessaglia, and R. L. Slothower.** 1998. Epidemic mycoplasmal conjunctivitis in house finches from eastern North America. *J. Wildl. Dis.* **34:**265–280.
12. **Doerfler, R. E., F. W. Edens, C. R. Parkhurst, G. B. Havenstein, and M. A. Qureshi.** 1998. Hypothermia, hypoglycemia, and hypothyrosis associated with poult enteritis and mortality syndrome. *Poult. Sci.* **77:**1103–1109.
13. **Domingo, E., E. Baranowski, C. M. Ruiz-Jarabo, A. M. Martin-Hernández, J. C. Sáiz, and C. Escarmis.** 1998. Quasispecies structure and persistence of RNA viruses. *Emerg. Infect Dis.* **4:** 521–527.
14. **Duignan, P. J., J. T. Saliki, D. J. St. Aubin, G. Early, S. Sadove, J. A. House, K. Kovacs, and J. R. Geraci.** 1995. Epizootiology of morbillivirus infection in North American harbor seals (*Phoca vitulina*) and gray seals (*Halichoerus grypus*). *J. Wildl. Dis.* **31:**491–501.
15. **Duignan, P. J., O. Nielsen, C. House, K. M. Kovacs, N. Duffy, G. Early, S. Sadove, D. J. St. Aubin, B. K. Rima, and J. R. Geraci.** 1997. Epizootiology of morbillivirus infection in harp, hooded, and ringed seals from the Canadian Arctic and western Atlantic. *J. Wildl. Dis.* **33:**7–19.
16. **Eigen, M., and P. Schuster,** 1979. *The Hypercycle: a Principle of Natural Self-Organization.* Springer, Berlin, Germany.
17. **Fischer, J. R., D. E. Stallknecht, M. P. Luttrell, A. D. Dhondt, and K. A. Converse.** 1997. Mycoplasmal conjunctivitis in wild songbirds: the spread of a new disease in a contagious population. *Emerg. Infect. Dis.* **3:**69–72.
18. **Fraser, G. C., P. T. Hooper, R. A. Lunt, A. R. Gould, L. J. Gleeson, A. D. Hyatt, G. M. Russell, and J. A. Kattenbelt.** 1996. Encephalitis caused by a lyssavirus in fruit bats in Australia. *Emerg. Infect. Dis.* **2:**327–331.
19. **Friend, M.** 1995. Increased avian diseases with habitat change, p. 401–405. *In* E. T. LaRoe, G. S. Farris, C. E. Puckett, et al. (ed.), *Our Living Resources—a Report to the Nation on the Distribution, Abundance, and Health of U.S. Plants, Animals, and Ecosystems.* National Biological Service, U.S. Department of the Interior, Washington, D.C.
20. **Gaele, D. (Agriculture Canada).** Personal communication.
21. **Gould, A. R., A. D. Hyatt, R. Lung, J. A. Kattenbelt, S. Hengstberger, and S. D. Blacksell.** 1998. Characterisation of a novel lyssavirus isolated from Pteropid bats in Australia. *Virus Res.* **54:**165–187.

22. **Hill, A. F., M. Desbruslais, S. Joiner, K. C. L. Sidle, L. J. Doey, P. Lantos, I. Gowland, and J. Collinge.** 1997. The same prion strain causes vCJD and BSE. *Nature* **389:**448–450.

23. **Kennedy, S.** 1998. Morbillivirus infections in aquatic animals. *J. Comp. Pathol.* **119:**201–225.

24. **Kuiken, T., F. A. Leighton, G. Wobeser, K. L. Danesik, J. Riva, and R. A. Heckert.** 1998. An epidemic of Newcastle disease in double-crested cormorants from Saskatchewan. *J. Wildl. Dis.* **34:** 457–471.

25. **Lasley, F. A., S. D. Short, and W. L. Henson.** 1985. *Economic Assessment of the 1983–84 Avian Influenza Eradication Program.* ERS staff report no. AGES841212. National Economics Division, Economic Research Service, U.S. Department of Agriculture, Washington, D.C.

26. **Mebus, C. A.** 1992. African swine fever, p. 65–73. *In* W. W. Buisch, J. L. Hyde, and C. A. Mebus (ed.), *Foreign Animal Diseases.* U.S. Animal Health Association, Richmond, Va.

27. **Michalak, K., C. Austin, S. Diesel, J. M. Bacon, P. Zimmerman, and J. N. Maslow.** 1998. *Mycobacterium tuberculosis* infection as a zoonotic disease: transmission between humans and elephants. *Emerg. Infect. Dis.* **4:**283–287.

28. **Morell, V.** 1994. Canine distemper virus. Serengeti's big cats going to the dogs. *Science* **264:**1664.

29. **Morozov, I., T. Sirinarumitr, S. D. Sorden, P. G. Halbur, M. K. Morgan, K. H. Yoon, and P. S. Paul.** 1998. Detection of a novel strain of porcine circovirus in pigs with postweaning multisystemic wasting syndrome. *J. Clin. Microbiol.* **36:**2535–2541.

30. **Muniappa, N., and G. E. Duhamel.** 1997. Phenotypic and genotypic profiles of human, canine, and porcine spirochetes associated with colonic spirochetosis correlates with in vivo brush border attachment. *Adv. Exp. Med. Biol.* **412:**159–166.

30a.**Murray, K., B. Eaton, P. Hooper, L. Wang, M. Williamson, and P. Young.** 1998. Flying foxes, horses, and humans: a zoonosis caused by a new member of the *Paramyxoviridae*, p. 43–58. *In* W. M. Scheld, D. Armstrong, and J. M. Hughes (ed.), *Emerging Infections 1.* ASM Press, Washington, D.C.

31. **Murray, K., P. Selleck, P. Hooper, A. Hyatt, A. Gould, L. Gleeson, H. Westbury, L. Hiley, L. Selvey, B. Rodwell, et al.** 1995. A morbillivirus that caused fatal disease in horses and humans. *Science* **268:**94–97.

32. **Osterhaus, A., J. Groen, H. Niesters, M. van de Bildt, B. Martina, L. Vedder J. Vos, H. van Egmond, B. Abou-Sidi, and M. E. Barham.** 1997. Morbillivirus in monk seal mass mortality. *Nature* **388:**838–839.

33. **Philbey, A. W., P. D. Kirkland, A. D. Ross, R. J. Davis, A. B. Gleeson, R. J. Love, P. W. Daniels, A. R. Gould, and A. D. Hyatt.** 1998. An apparently new virus (family *Paramyxoviridae*) infectious for pigs, humans, and fruit bats. *Emerg. Infect. Dis.* **4:**269–271.

34. **Pretorius, A., M. J. Oelofsen, M. S. Smith, and E. van deer Ryst.** 1997. Rift Valley fever virus: a seroepidemiologic study of small terrestrial vertebrates in South Africa. *Am. J. Trop. Med. Hyg.* **57:**693–698.

35. **Read, D. H., and R. L. Walker.** 1998. Papillomatous digital dermatitis (footwarts) in California dairy cattle: clinical and gross pathologic findings. *J. Vet. Diagn. Invest.* **10:**67–76.

36. **Relman, D. A.** 1998. Detection and identification of previously unrecognized microbial pathogens. *Emerg. Infect. Dis.* **4:**382–389.

36a.**Schonberger, L. B.** 1998. New-variant Creutzfeldt-Jakob disease and bovine spongiform encephalopathy: the strengthening etiologic link between two emerging diseases, p. 1–15. *In* W. M. Scheld, W. A. Craig, and J. M. Hughes (ed.), *Emerging Infections 2.* ASM Press, Washington, D.C.

37. **Schwabe, C. S.** 1984. *Veterinary Medicine and Human Health,* 3rd ed. The Williams & Wilkins Co., Baltimore, Md.

38. **Spraker, T. R., M. W. Miller, E. S. Williams, D. M. Getzy, W. J. Adrian, G. G. Schoonveld, R. A. Spowart, K. I. O'Rourke, J. M. Miller, and P. A. Merz.** 1997. Spongiform encephalopathy in free-ranging mule deer (*Odocoileus hemionus*), white-tailed deer (*Odocoileus virginianus*), and Rocky Mountain elk (*Cervus elaphus nelsoni*) in northcentral Colorado. *J. Wildl. Dis.* **331:**1–6.

39. **Subbarao, K., A. Klimov, J. Katz, H. Regnery, W. Lim, H. Hall, M. Perdue, D. Swayne, C. Bender, J. Huang, M. Hemphill, T. Rowe, M. Shaw, X. Xu, K. Fukuda, and N. Cox.** 1998. Characterization of an avian influenza A (H5N1) virus isolated from a child with fatal respiratory illness. *Science* **279:**393–396.

40. **Tanaka, R.** 1993. Foot-and-mouth disease in Italy, p. 8–9. *In Foreign Animal Disease Report*, vol. 21, issue 213. Animal and Plant Health Inspection Service, U.S. Department of Agriculture, Washington, D.C.

41. **Trott, D. J., T. B. Stanton, N. S. Jensen, G. E. Duhamel, J. L. Johnson, and D. J. Hampson.** 1996. *Serpulina pilosicoli* sp. nov., the agent of porcine intestinal spirochetosis. *Int. J. Syst. Bacteriol.* **46:**206–215.

42. **Whipple, D. L., R. M. Meyer, D. F. Berry, J. L. Jarnagin, and J. B. Payeur.** 1997. Molecular epidemiology of tuberculosis in wild white-tailed deer in Michigan and elephants, p. 543–546. *In Proceedings of the 101st Annual Meeting of the U.S. Animal Health Association.* U.S. Animal Health Association, Richmond, Va.

43. **Wilesmith, J. W., G. A. H. Wells, M. P. Cranwell, and J. B. M. Ryan.** 1988. Bovine spongiform encephalopathy: epidemiologic studies on the origin. *Vet. Rec.* **128:**199–203.

44. **Will, R. G., J. W. Ironside, M. Zeidler, S. Cousens, K. Estebeiro, A. Alperovitch, S. Poser, M. Pocchiari, A. Hofman, and P. G. Smith.** 1996. A new variant of Creutzfeldt-Jakob disease in the UK. *Lancet* **347:**921–925.

45. **Williams, E. S., and S. Young.** 1980. Chronic wasting disease of captive mule deer: a spongiform encephalopathy. *J. Wildl. Dis.* **16:**89–98.

46. **Williams, E. S., and S. Young.** 1982. Spongiform encephalopathy of Rocky Mountain elk. *J. Wildl. Dis.* **18:**465–472.

47. **Williamson, M. M., and P. T. Hooper (Australian Animal Health Laboratory).** Personal communication.

48. **Wilson, T. M., and C. Tuszynski.** 1997. Foot-and-mouth disease in Taiwan—1997 overview, p. 114–124. *In Proceedings of the 101st Annual Meeting of the U.S. Animal Health Association.* U.S. Animal Health Association, Richmond, Va.

49. **Young, P. L., K. Halpin, P. W. Selleck, H. Field, J. L. Gravel, M. A. Kelly, and J. S. Mackenzie.** 1996. Serologic evidence for the presence in *Pteropus* bats of a paramyxovirus related to equine morbillivirus. *Emerg. Infect. Dis.* **2:**239–240.

Emerging Infections 3
Edited by W. M. Scheld, W. A. Craig, and J. M. Hughes
© 1999 ASM Press, Washington, D.C.

Chapter 11

Infectious Disease Issues in Xenotransplantation

Louisa E. Chapman, William M. Switzer, Paul A. Sandstrom, Salvatore T. Butera, Walid Heneine, and Thomas M. Folks

BACKGROUND: WHAT IS XENOTRANSPLANTATION?

Xenotransplantation refers to the therapeutic use of living animal tissue in humans (7). Before and during the early 20th century "heterografting," as it was then called, was intermittently reported, most commonly as an attempt to cure Bright's disease (renal failure), which was universally fatal at that time. Transplantation of kidneys from goats, sheep, rabbits, or other species into humans with renal insufficiency invariably failed, and the frequency of heterografting declined as an understanding of the immune basis of organ rejection developed.

In the latter half of the 20th century, advances in immunology and the advent of immunosuppressive drugs introduced the era of allotransplantation (transplantation of tissues and organs between humans). As with all advances in knowledge, the success of allotransplantation simultaneously solved and created problems. The number of people benefiting from lifesaving allotransplantation procedures has steadily increased. Approximately 13,000 solid-organ allotransplant procedures were performed in 1988, whereas approximately 20,000 were performed in 1996 (41). However, the number of people on waiting lists for transplantation has also sharply increased (Fig. 1) (41). At the end of 1996, an estimated 50,000 persons were awaiting organ donations (41). Between 1988 and 1996, the annual death rate among the incidence cohort of patients on the waiting list to receive transplantable organs in the United States fluctuated between 167.8 and 125.5 deaths per 1,000 patient years at risk, with no evident downward trend. Thus, the shortage of available human donor organs contributes substantially to the risk of death associated with the existence of a medical condition potentially curable by allotransplantation. Most authoritative estimates suggest that attempts to increase participation in the human donor pool or to develop artificial organs may decrease but will not close

Louisa E. Chapman, William M. Switzer, Paul A. Sandstrom, Salvatore T. Butera, Walid Heneine, and Thomas M. Folks • HIV/AIDS and Retrovirology Branch, Division of AIDS, STD, and TB Laboratory Research, National Center for Infectious Diseases, Centers for Disease Control and Prevention, Mail Stop G-19, 1600 Clifton Rd., Atlanta, GA 30333.

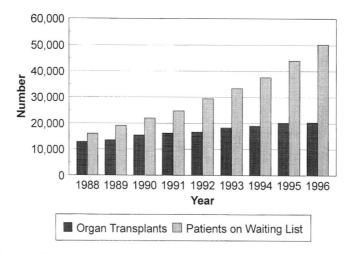

Figure 1. Number of U.S. organ transplants compared to number of patients on waiting list at year's end, 1988 to 1996 (41).

the gap between supply and demand. This continual disparity between the number of people who could benefit from allotransplantation and the number of human donor organs available for transplantation is the driving force behind the revived interest in xenotransplantation.

Most people date the beginning of the modern xenotransplantation era in the United States to 1963 or 1964, when a surgical team at Tulane University transplanted chimpanzee kidneys into six humans with renal failure who lacked access to hemodialysis or appropriate living related donors. One of the recipients survived for 9 months with the functioning chimpanzee kidney (34). These experiments were discontinued as hemodialysis became universally available and the use of cadaver donors increased the number of human kidneys available for transplantation.

Public impressions of xenotransplantation have been shaped largely by media attention to intermittent dramatic attempts at whole-organ transplantation, such as the transplantation of chimpanzee kidneys described above or of a baboon heart into an infant ("Baby Fae") in 1984 (11, 34). Indeed, before the last decade, the U.S. clinical experience with xenotransplantation largely consisted of rare, whole-organ transplants. Recipient survival after the xenograft was generally measured in days or weeks. Outside of the public eye, however, a quiet progression away from whole-organ xenografting toward the development of promising cellular applications was occurring. More recently, the majority of proposed clinical xenotransplantation trials are using cellular preparations that are often immunoprotected in some manner. As a result, increasing numbers of xenograft recipients are surviving for months to years after receiving cellular preparations that have functioned for prolonged periods of time.

In the United States, clinical trials of xenotransplantation are proposed or in progress. These trials use porcine neurologic, pancreatic, and hepatic cells to treat degenerative neurologic disorders (such as Parkinson's disease), diabetes, and hepatic failure (10, 12, 17); bovine adrenal preparations to ameliorate intractable pain in cancer patients (7); and baboon hearts as bridges for pediatric patients with heart failure (30). The recognition that baboons are refractory to infection with human immunodeficiency virus (HIV) and hepatitis B virus (HBV), both of which form persistent destructive infections in humans, has resulted in attempts to use this species differential to advantage by transplanting baboon bone marrow in an attempt to reconstitute the immune systems of patients with AIDS and baboon livers into persons with catastrophic liver failure due to dual infection with HBV and HIV (3, 29).

XENOTRANSPLANTATION AS A PUBLIC HEALTH CONCERN

Why is xenotransplantation a public health concern? Succinctly, allotransplantation is known to transmit infections endemic in humans from donors to recipients. Xenotransplantation has the potential to infect human recipients with agents that are not endemic in human populations, thereby introducing new infections to the human community (xenogeneic infections). By juxtaposing animal tissue and its microbiologic flora with human tissue in ways that bypass most or all of the normal host defense systems, xenotransplantation creates intimate and prolonged contact that may facilitate transmission of infections. Manipulations intended to circumvent the immunologic barriers to xenograft acceptance may also facilitate the transmission of agents that rarely or never infect humans under natural circumstances. Zoonoses (diseases transmitted between humans and animals under natural conditions) have been shown to cause widespread disease (e.g., the 1918 swine influenza pandemic and the current HIV-AIDS pandemic). Therefore, clinical trials of xenotransplantation combine a potential benefit for individual recipients with a potential risk to the human community that is unquantifiable (4, 9).

PHS GUIDELINE ON INFECTIOUS DISEASE ISSUES IN XENOTRANSPLANTATION

In response to the concerns outlined above, the Centers for Disease Control and Prevention (CDC), the Food and Drug Administration (FDA), the Health Resources and Services Administration, and the National Institutes of Health collaborated to develop a U.S. Public Health Service (PHS) draft guideline on infectious disease issues in xenotransplantation. A draft of this guideline was published in the *Federal Register* for public comment in September 1996 (42). The guideline is under revision in response to both comments received from the public and interim advances in science and international policy development (14). Publication of the final guideline is anticipated in 1999.

The PHS Draft Guideline on Infectious Disease Issues in Xenotransplantation emphasizes the importance of including experts in human and veterinary infectious diseases and microbiology on the xenotransplantation team. The guideline also emphasizes the importance of the informed-consent and education processes, which extend beyond the individual recipient to include close contacts and health care workers, and adequate protocol review. The guideline specifies that all U.S. clinical trials of xenotransplantation proceed under FDA regulation and discusses the creation of the Secretary's Advisory Committee on Xenotransplantation. The guideline particularly emphasizes the importance of safety monitoring, which is built around two key concepts: pretransplantation screening and posttransplantation surveillance (14, 42).

In addition to this guideline, other national and international organizations have developed or are developing guidance documents on public health issues in xenotransplantation (1, 5, 13, 23, 25, 35, 44, 48).

PRETRANSPLANTATION SCREENING AND POSTTRANSPLANTATION SURVEILLANCE

The concept of pretransplantation screening is nested in animal-husbandry techniques that limit and define the lifelong exposure histories of the source animals (14, 42). The goal of pretransplantation screening is to eliminate known problematic infectious agents from the xenograft prior to transplantation. Problematic infectious agents include recognized zoonotic agents, as well as agents with suspected or unexplored zoonotic potential. Animal blood, tissues, or organs that are infected with recognized exogenous retroviruses or other persistent infectious agents would not be considered suitable xenografts.

Ideally, pretransplantation screening would eliminate the need for posttransplantation surveillance. However, our knowledge of the microbiology of source animals used for xenografts remains incomplete. Posttransplantation surveillance is necessary to identify infectious agents that were transplanted with the xenograft because either they were not known to exist, they were known to exist but our diagnostic tools were inadequate to detect them (for example, prions), or they could not be removed from the xenograft (e.g., endogenous retroviruses). At present, for example, FDA requires that all U.S. recipients of porcine xenografts be monitored for porcine endogenous retrovirus (PERV) infections.

APPROACHES TO SURVEILLANCE FOR XENOGENEIC INFECTIONS

Development of an approach to posttransplantation surveillance of xenograft recipients is difficult. Surveillance for clinical episodes compatible with xenogeneic infections is the major posttransplantation tool available for the detection of infections with agents that are not yet recognized or for which adequate diagnostic tools do not exist. Lifelong clinical surveillance is recommended for xenograft recipients (14, 42). In addition, the PHS guideline discusses the development of national registries that would enable epidemiologic surveillance of populations of xenograft recipients and thus enhance our ability to detect rare clinical events. A pilot registry involving xenograft recipients at three clinical centers is under development by PHS (46). Clinical surveillance can be augmented by laboratory-based surveillance for infectious agents that can be identified but not removed from the xenograft, such as endogenous retroviruses.

ENDOGENOUS RETROVIRUSES AND XENOTRANSPLANTATION

The origin of endogenous retroviruses is unclear. Since all retroviruses intercalate into the genome of the infected cell, endogenous retroviruses are thought to represent the germ-line fixation of previously infectious (or exogenous) retroviruses. The genomes of most, if not all, mammalian species contain multiple endogenous retroviral sequences which are transmitted from parent to child through Mendelian inheritance. Most endogenous retroviral sequences are defective and incapable of expressing infectious viruses. However, some endogenous retroviral sequences can express replication-competent virus. While these are usually incapable of forming an active infection in their host species, they can infect cells from other species in vitro (so-called xenotropic endogenous retroviruses). Therefore, the existence of endogenous retroviruses potentially complicates xenotransplantation (8).

Both pigs and baboons have been shown to have endogenous retroviruses that are capable of infecting human cells in vitro, raising concerns that transplantation of porcine or baboon xenografts into humans may enable these endogenous retroviruses to infect humans in vivo (26, 27, 33, 47). PERV is expressed by a variety of porcine tissues including spleen, kidney, heart, aortic endothelium, hepatocyte, skin, lung, and pancreatic islet cells. Three PERV variants with distinct envelope sequences (PERV-A, -B, and -C) have been partially characterized and have been demonstrated to differ in infectivity for human cells in vitro (2, 26, 27, 33, 38, 47).

TOOLS THAT ENABLE SURVEILLANCE FOR ENDOGENOUS RETROVIRAL INFECTION OF XENOGRAFT RECIPIENTS

New diagnostic assays that allow posttransplantation surveillance to assess the risk that endogenous retroviruses can infect xenograft recipients have been developed (2, 18, 19, 28, 39). The CDC diagnostic algorithms for these viruses combine virus-specific approaches with more generic assays for retroviruses (e.g., detection of reverse transcriptase activity by the Amp-RT assay, PCR amplification of highly conserved retroviral *pol* gene sequences, culture techniques, and use of electron microscopy).

The standard virus-specific approach to diagnosis is to look for serologic reactivity. Western blot serology has been developed to detect antibodies to PERV and baboon endogenous retrovirus (BaEV) (28). However, assays for serologic reactivity may be less reliable in the xenotransplantation setting, in which a portion of recipients will be immunocompromised and less able to reliably mount an antibody response to antigenic stimulus. Alternative approaches include attempts to identify the virus itself through culture, but this approach is both labor- and time-intensive. Thus, molecular approaches are assuming more importance for this patient population (18, 19, 39). PCR assays have been developed for the detection of both BaEV and PERV DNAs, and reverse transcription-PCR assays have been developed for assessment of evidence of viral expression (39).

Endogenous retroviruses are part of the genome of every cell of the host species. Therefore, in theory, endogenous genomic material should always be identifiable by PCR if source animal cells are present. As a result, algorithms for the diagnosis of human infection with endogenous retroviruses must be able to assess the presence of microchimerism, the persistent presence of source-animal cells in the human recipient. PCR assays specific for mitochondrial DNAs (mtDNAs) from pigs and baboons have been developed. These assays are used with assays for PERV and BaEV DNAs to distinguish endogenous retrovirus infection of the recipient from persistent microchimerism. Positive PCR signals for PERV accompanied by positive signals for porcine mitochondrial DNA suggest microchimerism. If true endogenous retrovirus infection of human tissue exists, persistent detection of PERV would be anticipated in the absence of detection of porcine mtDNA (Fig. 2) (18, 19, 39). If prolonged xenograft survival is achieved, it may be necessary to quantify the amount of porcine mtDNA present relative to the amount of PERV DNA present to discriminate microchimerism from infection. These virus-specific approaches are used in tandem with Amp-RT, an assay that detects the generic presence of reverse transcriptase as evidence of retroviral expression (16, 22, 49).

SURVEILLANCE FOR EVIDENCE OF IN VIVO ENDOGENOUS RETROVIRAL INFECTIONS IN XENOGRAFT RECIPIENTS

Study of BaEV in an HIV-1-Infected Recipient of a Baboon Bone Marrow Xenograft

In a collaboration between researchers at the University of Pittsburgh, the University of California, San Francisco, and CDC, these newly developed diagnostic

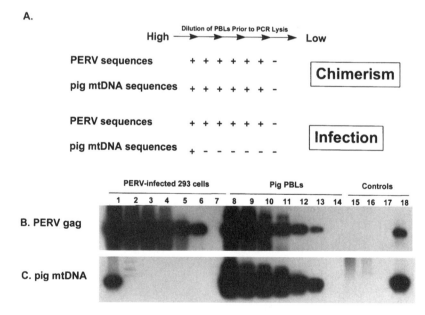

Figure 2. Distinguishing infection from microchimerism in endogenous retrovirus DNA-positive samples. (Adapted and reprinted from reference 39.)

assays and algorithms were used to monitor an HIV type 1 (HIV-1)-infected recipient of baboon bone marrow for the presence of BaEV infection (29). As anticipated, testing prior to the transplantation showed a strong presence of both BaEV and baboon mtDNA in peripheral blood lymphocytes (PBLs) from the baboon, while PBLs from the recipient were not positive for either signal. However, at 5 days posttransplantation, both signals were detectable in PBLs from the recipient, indicating microchimerism. Thirteen days after the transplantation, baboon mtDNA was persistently identifiable in the recipient, but BaEV DNA was no longer detectable; thereafter, neither signal was detected (29). The inability to detect BaEV DNA 13 days after transplantation, despite the persistence of microchimerism with baboon tissue, can be explained by the difference in the quantity of cellular DNA and the limits of detection of the assays. Baboon mtDNA is present at thousands of copies per cell, while BaEV DNA is present, at most, at hundreds of copies per cell. Thus, with low levels of microchimerism, BaEV DNA would be expected to be undetectable, while baboon mtDNA would remain identifiable.

Study of PERV in Diabetic Recipients of Renal Allografts and Porcine Fetal Pancreatic Islet Cell Xenografts

In a collaborative study, researchers at CDC and the Karolinska Institute in Stockholm, Sweden, looked for evidence of PERV infection in 10 diabetic patients, each of whom had received 2×10^5 to 1×10^6 pig fetal islet cells between 1990 and 1993 (2, 6, 15, 37, 40). Prolonged xenograft survival (more than 6 months) was documented in five patients by either urinary excretion of porcine C peptide or detection of pig mtDNA in serum, or both (Table 1) (21, 40). However, markers of PERV infection were not detected in any patient, despite extended exposure to pig cells and concomitant immunosuppressive therapy. For example, screening for two PERV sequences in PBLs collected from patients at multiple time points 4 to 7 years after the xenotransplantation was negative. Markers of PERV expression, including viral RNA and reverse transcriptase, were undetectable in sera collected both early (day 3 to day 180) and late (4 to 7 years) after xenotransplantation. Western blot analysis for PERV-reactive antibodies was also consistently negative. The methodology used in that study established a minimum standard for posttransplantation surveillance of human recipients of porcine xenografts (21).

Study of PERV in Renal Dialysis Patients Receiving Extracorporeal Perfusion through Porcine Kidneys

In a third collaborative study, researchers at The Institute of Cancer Research, Chester Beatty Laboratories, in London, and the Göteborg University in Göteborg, Sweden, assessed evidence of PERV infection in patients exposed to living porcine tissue through extracorporeal perfusion (32). Serial blood samples were collected from two renal dialysis patients whose circulation was linked extracorporeally to pig kidneys. These samples were tested for pig DNA (porcine mitochondrial cytochrome oxidase subunit II [COII] and beta-globin) and PERV DNA by nested PCR assays. The serum was also tested for neutralizing antibodies to two distinct PERV isolates. No evidence of pig or PERV DNA was found, even as early as

Table 1. PCR analysis of pig mtDNA sequences in serum samples from 10 diabetic patients who received pig islet cell xenografts between June 1990 and April 1993[a]

| Patient | Pig mtDNA | | | | | | Transplant characteristics | | |
	2–3 days	2 wk	3 wk	6 mo	1 yr	4–7 yr[b]	Evidence of xenograft islet cell survival	Site	No. of ICCs (10^3)
XIT1	+	+	+	+	−	−	C peptide +	IP	390
XIT2	+	−	−	−	NA	NA		IP	520
XIT3	−	NA	−	−	NA	NA		IP	460
XIT4	+	−	−	−	NA	−		IP	410
XIT5	+	−	−	−	NA	−		IP	330
XIT6	−	−	−	−	NA	−	C peptide +	IP	520
XIT7	+	−	−	+	+	−	C peptide +	IP	800
XIT8	+	+	−	+	−	−	C peptide +	IP	1,020
XIT9	−	−	−	−	NA	NA		RC	200
XIT10	−	+	−	+	NA	NA	Biopsy +	RC	410
Pig mtDNA	6/10	3/10	1/10	4/10	1/3	0/8			

[a]Adapted from reference 21, with permission of the publisher. Abbreviations: NA, samples not available; IP, intraportal; RC, renal capsule; ICC, islet-like cell clusters; C peptide +, urinary excretion of porcine C peptide detected; Biopsy +, detection of pig cells under the renal capsule in a biopsy specimen obtained 3 weeks posttransplantation.
[b]The results for years 4 to 7 are for samples collected in both April and August 1997.

6 h after perfusion, and neutralizing antibodies were not identified in the plasma of either patient (Table 2).

SPECTRUM OF RISK OF HUMAN INFECTION WITH XENOGENEIC ENDOGENOUS RETROVIRUSES

The risk that any xenograft recipient may become infected with PERV is likely a function of multiple factors associated with the source animal, the xenotransplantation technique, and the characteristics of the human recipient. These may include the duration of pig cell persistence in xenograft recipients, the presence of anastomosis between the host and the xenograft blood supply, the general level of PERV infectivity for human cells, the level of PERV expression by the transplanted cells, and the level of immunosuppression in the recipient. As a result, defining the overall risks of PERV infection for xenograft recipients is complex, and the extent to which the results of any individual study can be generalized to other types of exposure is limited.

One approach to overcoming the immune barriers that prevent successful xenotransplantation has been the development of pigs transgenically engineered to circumvent hyperacute rejection (HAR), a modification anticipated to facilitate graft survival but also feared to compromise lytic complement clearance of PERV (31, 33, 36, 38, 43, 45). Most mammals bear galactose-α-1-3-galactose (α-Gal) terminal sugar residues on their cell surfaces. The α-Gal epitope is absent from humans and Old World primates. Humans have circulating immunoglobulin G specific for α-Gal. Preexisting α-Gal-specific antibodies in human xenograft recipients bind to the α-Gal moieties on the surfaces of xenografts, resulting in complement activation, leading to HAR, the catastrophic destruction of the vascular endothelium of the porcine xenograft within minutes of implantation into humans (34). The HAR barrier to porcine xenograft acceptance by humans may also provide a barrier to human infection with porcine retroviruses. Retroviruses that bud from cells other than those of humans and Old World primates bear surface α-Gal residues, rendering them susceptible to lysis by the α-Gal-specific antibody and complement found in normal human sera. The sensitivity of pig cell-derived PERV to inacti-

Table 2. Analysis of DNA from patient peripheral blood mononuclear cells for porcine sequences and patient plasma for anti-PERV antibodies[a]

Time postdialysis	Result of PCR for:			Presence of anti-PERV antibodies
	PERV	COII	Beta-globin	
Predialysis	–	–	–	—
6 h	–	–	–	NT
7 days	–	–	–	NT
21/24 mo	–	–	–	NT
33/36 mo	–	–	–	—

[a]Adapted from reference 33, with permission of the publisher. In all cases, positive controls indicated that PCR assays could detect near a single copy of the target sequence. Symbols and abbreviations: –, negative PCR result; —, absence of neutralizing antibodies to either PERV variant A or PERV variant B vectors; NT, not tested.

vation and lysis by human sera has been demonstrated, and a single passage of PERV through human cells has been shown to cause the virus to become resistant to inactivation by normal human sera (33).

Recipients of xenografts from nontransgenic pigs, the only population studied and for which data have been reported to date, likely represent the lowest end of a spectrum of risk for PERV infection (21, 32). No attempts were made to remove preformed xenoantibodies or to block complement activation in any patient studied for in vivo PERV infection. Risks will need to be independently assessed for alternative xenograft applications, including the use of xenografts procured from transgenic pigs (21, 38).

SPECULATION ON NATURE OF PERV INFECTION: REASONING BY ANALOGY FROM FeLV INFECTION

Some researchers have noted that consensus sequences of PERV virions released from porcine PK-15 cells and MRK virus (2) are closely related to gibbon ape leukemia virus as well as to the feline leukemia virus (FeLV) and the murine leukemia virus (31). They reason, therefore, that FeLV infections may be more appropriate models than the human retroviruses (HIV and human T-cell leukemia virus [HTLV]) for speculation about the nature of putative PERV infections in humans.

Although abortive infection with subsequent recovery is the most frequent outcome of feline infection with FeLV, a minority of cats do become persistently infected with FeLV. These cats have high levels of viremia in plasma and shed the virus in saliva and other body fluids. Sequestered infections, in which FeLV is cleared from other anatomic sites yet continues to replicate in epithelial sites like salivary glands and mammary glands, can also occur (31).

This line of reasoning, if correct, has implications for posttransplantation surveillance, infection control practices, and preventive clinical interventions. The possibility of sequestered infections that conform to the anatomic model provided by FeLV may produce effective transmitters whose infections are unlikely to be detected by the current means of surveillance focused on PBLs. Consideration of surveillance approaches aimed at the detection of PERV in saliva may be appropriate. Because FeLV is present in the saliva of infected cats, HBV or cytomegalovirus infections may provide more appropriate models for infection control practices following human exposure to PERV than do infections with human retroviruses (HIV and HTLV), in which saliva poses a negligible risk as a means of transmission (31, 36). Transient peritransplantation prophylactic intervention with antiretroviral pharmaceuticals as well as pretransplantation vaccination may protect porcine xenograft recipients from PERV infection (31, 36). Vaccines against FeLV are in commercial use for cats, suggesting that protecting porcine xenograft recipients from PERV infection through pretransplantation vaccination may some day be possible.

IMPORTANCE OF ARCHIVES OF BIOLOGIC MATERIALS

In addition to emphasizing the importance of screening and surveillance, the PHS Draft Guideline on Infectious Disease Issues in Xenotransplantation recommends that archives of biologic specimens obtained from the xenograft source animals and human recipients both before and at intervals following the xenotransplantation be maintained (14, 42). These archives would ensure the availability of biologic materials for public health investigations that may become necessary. The draft guideline places responsibility for the archives on the principal investigators and the FDA investigational new drug (IND) sponsors and states that the materials should be archived indefinitely (42).This recommendation has been controversial (14). The formidable costs involved, the realities of underfunding for investigators, and the short life spans of many biotechnology companies preclude reliable maintenance of such archives in the private sector. The duration of archival storage of biologic materials has been defined at 50 years following the transplantation, and the advisability of creating a central PHS archive is under consideration (14).

Past experience has demonstrated the value of such archives. For example, one can contrast the outcomes of two CDC investigations of persons occupationally exposed to simian retroviruses. In the first, a laboratory worker was found to be infected with simian immunodeficiency virus (SIV) (24). The employer had regularly collected and archived sera from occupationally exposed workers. By retrospectively testing banked sera, CDC investigators were able to identify a narrow window of seroconversion between October 1988 and April 1989. This seroconversion corresponded to a time frame when the worker regularly handled the blood of SIV-infected macaque monkeys without wearing gloves, despite dermatitis of the worker's hands and arms that was severe enough to warrant therapy with oral steroids. Thus, the availability of stored sera allowed the investigators to identify both the time of seroconversion and a specific exposure that placed the worker at risk of infection.

In response to that investigation, CDC began prospective surveillance of workers exposed to nonhuman primates for evidence of infection with SIV and other simian retroviruses. In 1997, this surveillance identified four workers infected with simian foamy virus (SFV) (20). All four workers had been exposed to nonhuman primates for more than 20 years. Although the documented duration of infections ranged from 2 to 20 years, the sparse availability of stored sera allowed documentation of a window of seroconversion for only one worker, and this was based on the study of sera collected more than a decade apart. Therefore, in contrast to the SIV-infected worker, the absence of adequate banked sera and the resultant inability to pinpoint a narrow window of seroconversion for any of these four SFV-infected workers prevented the association of these SFV infections with any specific types of exposures. As a result, the exact nature of the exposures that led to infection remains unidentified.

SIGNIFICANCE OF XENOGENEIC INFECTIONS

Because infection is not always equivalent to disease, the public health significance of xenogeneic infections in xenograft recipients cannot be precisely assessed. An infection that is associated with disease is of clear importance to the infected individual, even if it is an end-point infection that does not pose a risk to other humans. As a general rule, for an infection to be of significance to the public health, it must be transmitted secondarily between humans and must be associated with disease. However, a nonpathogenic virus that infects the host persistently and that has a propensity for recombination may also have public health significance.

Rare zoonotic infection in humans can serve as a surrogate for xenogeneic infections and provide a basis for reasoning by analogy about the significance of purported xenogeneic infections.

SIGNIFICANCE OF RARE ZOONOSES IN HUMANS: SFV AS A SURROGATE FOR XENOGENEIC INFECTIONS

Retroviruses can be divided into three groups: those associated with cell proliferation (oncoviruses, such as HTLV, simian T-lymphotropic virus, and FeLV), those associated with cell death (lentiviruses, such as HIV, SIV, and feline immunodeficiency virus), and those unassociated with an identified pathogenic effect in any host (spumaviruses, also called foamy viruses, such as SFV and feline foamy virus). Although nearly ubiquitous in many mammals (cows, cats, sea lions, hamsters, and nonhuman primates), foamy virus infection has never been associated with disease in any of its natural hosts.

Although humans have been shown to be infected with foamy viruses endemic to other species, these infections have also never been associated with recognized disease. The four SFV-infected workers discussed earlier all remain in good health, without evidence of disease potentially attributable to their SFV infections. Three of the four infected workers have been in sexually active monogamous relationships for more than 20 years and deny the use of barrier contraceptives, spermicide, or other methods that might logically decrease the probability of sexual transmission. Their partners, tested by serology and PCR, remain uninfected, suggesting that SFV is not transmitted easily between humans and may represent end-point infections in humans. However, isolation of SFV from the blood of two infected workers raises concerns that secondary transmission of SFV among humans may occur through exposure to infected blood. This potential route of human-to-human transmission has not yet been investigated (20).

The significance of SFV infection in humans remains unclear. Xenogeneic infections may be similar in this regard. Demonstration of infection of humans may be easier than determination of the significance of that infection.

PERSISTENT MICROCHIMERISM WITH SFV- AND BaEV-CONTAINING CELLS IN RECIPIENTS OF BABOON LIVER XENOGRAFTS

Allan and colleagues (3) have studied human recipients of baboon livers and have documented the persistent presence of SFV and BaEV in microchimeric baboon cells, constituting potentially ongoing sources for human infection following receipt of baboon xenografts. SFV is not eliminated from persistently microchimeric baboon cells. Given that humans have been infected with SFV of baboon origin following transient occupational exposures (20), it is highly likely that this more intimate ongoing exposure would result in infection.

With rare exceptions, the high prevalence of SFV infections in all species for whom spumaviruses are endemic, including nonhuman primates, precludes the availability of foamy virus-free animals prior to the investment of substantial time and financial resources in the development of spumavirus-free colonies. For all practical purposes, these considerations eliminate the possibility of using SFV-free baboons as xenograft sources in the foreseeable future.

The absence of recognized disease attributable to foamy virus in infected animals of any species, including the small numbers of SFV-infected humans studied to date, combined with the absence of identified secondary transmission among humans, have led some experts to argue that foamy virus infections of humans are benign end-point infections of no significance to human health. These arguments may be correct. However, the limited number of observations with humans precludes confidence in the persistently benign nature of human infections with these viruses. In light of these considerations, despite the apparently benign nature of human SFV infections at present, intentional or negligent exposure of humans to foamy virus-infected xenografts is not warranted in the absence of substantially more data supporting the long-term safety of such exposures.

CONCLUSIONS

Efforts to address issues in xenotransplantation have accomplished much in a short time. Major research questions have been framed, an infrastructure for public policy has been outlined, and tools that enable the science necessary to define whether endogenous retroviruses pose a risk to human xenograft recipients have been developed and deployed. However, much remains to be done. The present challenge, to define the ability of PERV and other xenogeneic agents to infect xenograft recipients, will likely be superseded by the challenge of defining the significance of identified xenogeneic infections. Continued collaborative work between the public health, infectious diseases, and transplantation communities is needed to resolve the dilemmas posed by future clinical trials in xenotransplantation.

REFERENCES

1. **Advisory Group on the Ethics of Xenotransplantation.** 1997. *Animal Tissues into Humans.* Her Majesty's Stationery Office, London, United Kingdom.
2. **Akiyoshi, D. E., M. Denaro, H. Zhu, J. L. Greenstein, P. Banerjee, and J. A. Fishman.** 1998. Identification of a full-length cDNA for an endogenous retrovirus of miniature swine. *J. Virol.* **72:** 4503–4507.
3. **Allan, J. S., S. R. Broussard, M. G. Michaels, T. E. Starzl, K. L. Leighton, E. M. Whitehead, A. G. Comuzzie, R. E. Lanford, M. M. Leland, W. M. Switzer, and W. Heneine.** 1998. Amplification of simian retroviral sequences from human recipients of baboon liver transplants. *AIDS Res. Hum. Retroviruses* **14:**821–824.
4. **Bach, F. H., J. A. Fishman, N. Daniels, J. Proimos, B. Anderson, C. B. Carpenter, L. Forrow, S. C. Robson, and H. V. Fineberg.** 1998. Uncertainty in xenotransplantation: individual benefit versus collective risk. *Nat. Med.* **4:**141–144.
5. **Bellucci, S., A. Bondolfi, B. Husing, and A. Ruegsegger.** 1998. The Swiss Technology Assessment (TA) project on xenotransplantation. *Ann. N. Y. Acad. Sci.* **862:**155–165.

6. **Bjoersdorff, A., O. Korsgen, R. Feinstein, A. Andersson, J. Tollemar, A.-S. Malmborg, A. Ehrnst, and C. G. Groth.** 1995. Microbiological characterization of porcine fetal islet-like cell clusters for intended clinical xenografting. *Xenotransplantation* **2**:26–31.

7. **Bloom, E. T., A. D. Moulton, J. McCoy, L. E. Chapman, and A. P. Patterson.** 1999. Xenotransplantation: the potential and the challenges. *Crit. Care Nurs.* **19**:76–83.

8. **Brown, J., A. L. Matthews, P. A. Sandstrom, and L. E. Chapman.** 1998. Xenotransplantation and the risk of retroviral zoonosis. *Trends Microbiol.* **6**:411–415.

9. **Chapman, L. E., T. M. Folks, D. R. Salomon, A. P. Patterson, T. E. Eggerman, and P. D. Noguichi.** 1995. Xenotransplantation and xenogeneic infections. *N. Engl. J. Med.* **333**:1498–1501.

10. **Chari, R. S., B. H. Collins, J. C. Magee, J. M. DiMaio, A. D. Kirk, R. C. Harland, R. L. McCann, J. L. Platt, and W. C. Meyers.** 1994. Brief report: treatment of hepatic failure with ex vivo pig-liver perfusion followed by liver transplantation. *N. Engl. J. Med.* **331**:234–237.

11. **Daar, A. S.** 1999. Analysis of factors for the prediction of the response to xenotransplantation. *Ann. N. Y. Acad. Sci.* **862**:222–233.

12. **Deacon, T., J. Schumacher, J. Dinsmore, C. Thomas, P. Palmer, S. Kott, A. Edge, D. Penney, S. Kassissieh, P. Dempsey, and O. Isacon.** 1997. Histological evidence of fetal pig neural cell survival after transplantation into a patient with Parkinson's disease. *Nat. Med.* **3**:350–353.

13. **De Sola, C.** 1998. Current developments on xenotransplantation in the Council of Europe. *Ann. N. Y. Acad. Sci.* **862**:211–213.

14. **DHHS Interagency Working Group on Xenotransplantation.** 1998. The Draft US Public Health Service Guideline on Infectious Disease Issues in Xenotransplantation. *Ann. N. Y. Acad. Sci.* **862**: 166–170.

15. **Galili, U., A Tibell, B. Samuelsson, L. Rydberg, and C. G. Groth.** 1995. Increased anti-gal activity in diabetic patients transplanted with fetal porcine islet cell clusters. *Transplantation* **59**:1549–1556.

16. **Garcia Lerma, J. G., S. Yamamoto, M. Gomez-Cano, V. Soriano, T. A. Green, M. P. Busch, T. M. Folks, and W. Heneine.** 1998. Measurement of human immunodeficiency virus type 1 plasma virus load based on reverse transcriptase (RT) activity: evidence of variabilities in levels of virion-associated RT. *J. Infect. Dis.* **177**:1221–1229.

17. **Groth, C. G., O. Korsgren, A. Tibell, J. Tollemar, E. Moller, J. Bolinder, J. Ostman, F. P. Reinholt, C. Hellerstrom, and A. Andersson.** 1994. Transplantation of porcine fetal pancreas to diabetic patients. *Lancet* **344**:1402–1404.

18. **Heneine, W.** 1996. Strategies for diagnosis of xenotransplant-associated retroviral infections. *Mol. Diagn.* **1**:255–260.

19. **Heneine, W., and W. M. Switzer.** 1996. Highly sensitive and specific polymerase chain reaction assays for detection of baboon and pig cells following xenotransplantation in humans. *Transplantation* **62**:1360–1362.

20. **Heneine, W., W. M. Switzer, P. Sandstrom, J. Brown, S. Vedapuri, C. A. Schable, A. S. Khan, N. W. Lerche, M. Schweizer, D. Neumann-Haefelin, L. E. Chapman, and T. M. Folks.** 1998. Identification of a human population infected with simian foamy viruses. *Nat. Med.* **4**:391–392.

21. **Heneine, W., A. Tibell, W. M. Switzer, P. A. Sandstrom, G. Vazquez-Rosales, A. Mathews, O. Korsgren, L. E. Chapman, T. M. Folks, and C. G. Groth.** 1998. No evidence of infection with porcine endogenous retrovirus in recipients of porcine islet-cell xenografts. *Lancet* **352**:695–699.

22. **Heneine, W., S. Yamamoto, W. M. Switzer, T. J. Spira, and T. M. Folks.** 1995. Detection of reverse transcriptase by a highly sensitive assay in sera from individuals infected with the human immunodeficiency virus type 1. *J. Infect. Dis.* **171**:1210–1216.

23. **Institute of Medicine.** 1996. *Xenotransplantation: Science, Ethics, and Public Policy.* National Academy Press, Washington, D.C.

24. **Khabbaz, R. F., W. Heneine, J. R. George, B. Parekh, T. Rowe, T. Woods, W. M. Switzer, H. M. McClure, M. Murphey-Corb, and T. M. Folks.** 1994. Brief report: infection of a laboratory worker with simian immunodeficiency virus. *N. Engl. J. Med.* **330**:172–177.

25. **La Prairie, A. J. P., and D. R. Brodie.** 1998. Public confidence and government regulation. *Ann. N. Y. Acad. Sci.* **862**:171–176.

26. **Le Tissier, P., J. P. Stoye, Y. Yasuhiro, C. Patience, and R. A. Weiss.** 1997. Two sets of human-tropic pig retrovirus. *Nature* **389**:681–682.

27. **Martin, U., V. Kiessig, J. H. Blusch, A. Haverich, K. von der Helm, T. Herden, and G. Steinhoff.** 1998. Expression of pig endogenous retrovirus by primary porcine endothelial cells and infection of human cells. *Lancet* **352:**692–694.

28. **Matthews, A. L., J. Brown, W. Switzer, T. M. Folks, W. Heneine, and P. A. Sandstrom.** 1999. Development and validation of a Western immunoblot assay for detection of antibodies to porcine endogenous retrovirus. *Transplantation* **67:**939–943.

29. **Michaels, M., J. Hilliard, S. Deeks, P. Gupta, W. Heneine, D. Pardi, C. Kaufman, C. Rinaldo, K. St. George, L. Chapman, T. Folks, Y. Colson, P. Volberding, and S. Ildstat.** 1996. Institute of Human Virology. *J. Acquir. Immune Defic. Syndr. Hum. Retrovirol.* **14**(Suppl.)**:**3 (abstr. 11).

30. **Michler, R.** 1996. Xenotransplantation: risks, clinical potential, and future prospects. *Emerg. Infect. Dis.* **2:**64–70.

31. **Onions, D., D. Galbraith, D. Hart, C. Mahoney, and K. Smith.** 1998. Endogenous retroviruses and the safety of porcine xenotransplantation. *Trends Microbiol.* **6:**430–431.

32. **Patience, C., G. S. Patton, Y. Takeuchi, R. A. Weiss, M. O. McClure, L. Rydberg, and M. E. Breimer.** 1998. No evidence of pig DNA or retroviral infection in patients with short-term extracorporeal connection to pig kidneys. *Lancet* **352:**699–701.

33. **Patience, C., Y. Takeuchi, and R. A. Weiss.** 1997. Infection of human cells by an endogenous retrovirus of pigs. *Nat. Med.* **3:**282–286.

34. **Reemstma, K., et al.** 1969. Renal heterotransplantation from nonhuman primates to man. *Ann. N. Y. Acad. Sci.* **162:**412–418.

35. **Ronchi, E.** 1998. *Policy Consideration on International Issues in Transplantation Biotechnology Including the Use of Non-Human Cells, Tissues, and Organs.* Organization for Economic Cooperation and Development, Paris, France.

36. **Sandstrom, P. A. and L. E. Chapman.** 1998. Author's response. *Trends Microbiol.* **6:**432. (Letter.)

37. **Satake, M., et al.** 1994. Kinetics and character of xenoantibody formation in diabetic patients transplanted with fetal porcine islet cells clusters. *Xenotransplantation* **1:**24.

38. **Stoye, J.** 1998. No clear answers on safety of pigs as tissue donor source. *Lancet* **352:**666–667.

39. **Switzer, W. M., V. Shanmugan, L. E. Chapman, and W. Heneine.** 1999. Polymerase chain reaction assays for the diagnosis of infection with the porcine endogenous retrovirus and the detection of pig cells in human and nonhuman recipients of pig xenografts. *Transplantation* **68:**183–188.

40. **Tibell, A., F. P. Reinholt, O. Korsgren, A. Andersson, C. Hellerstrom, E. Moller, and C. G. Groth.** 1994. Morphological identification of porcine islet cells three weeks after transplantation to a diabetic patient. *Transplant. Proc.* **26:**1121.

41. **United Network for Organ Sharing.** 1997. *Data Highlights from the 1997 Annual Report: The U.S. Scientific Registry of Transplant Recipients and the Organ Procurement and Transplantation Network—Transplant data: 1988–1996.* U.S. Department of Health and Human Services, Rockville, Md.

42. **U.S. Public Health Service.** 1996. Draft guideline on infectious disease issues in xenotransplantation. *Fed. Regist.* **61:**49920–49932.

43. **Van der Kuyl, A. C., and J. Goudsmit.** 1998. Xenotransplantation: about baboon hearts and pig livers. *Trends Microbiol.* **6:**431–432.

44. **Van Rongen, E.** 1998. Xenotransplantation: perspective for The Netherlands. *Ann. N. Y. Acad. Sci.* **862:**177–183.

45. **Weiss, R.** 1998. Commentary: transgenic pigs and virus adaptation. *Nature* **391:**327–328.

46. **Whitehead, J., A. P. Patterson, and A. Moulton.** 1998. Development of databases and registries: international issues. *Ann. N. Y. Acad. Sci.* **862:**217–221.

47. **Wilson, C. A., S. Wong, J. Muller, C. E. Davidson, T. M. Rose, and P. Burd.** 1998. Type C retrovirus released from porcine primary peripheral blood mononuclear cells infects human cells. *J. Virol.* **72:**3082–3087.

48. **World Health Organization.** 1998. *Xenotransplantation: Guidance on Infectious Disease Prevention and Management.* World Health Organization, Geneva, Switzerland.

49. **Yamamoto, S., T. M. Folks, and W. Heneine.** 1996. Highly sensitive qualitative and quantitative detection of reverse transcriptase activity: optimization, validation and comparative analysis with other detection systems. *J. Virol. Methods* **61:**135–143.

Emerging Infections 3
Edited by W. M. Scheld, W. A. Craig, and J. M. Hughes
© 1999 ASM Press, Washington, D.C.

Chapter 12

The Emerging Role of Pathology in Infectious Diseases

Sherif R. Zaki and Christopher D. Paddock

BACKGROUND AND OVERVIEW

In the United States, infectious diseases continue to produce extensive mortality and morbidity. On a global scale, infectious diseases are the leading cause of death (32, 80). During the past three decades, the world has witnessed the emergence of many new infectious diseases as well as the reemergence of previously known diseases. Notable recent infectious disease challenges faced by public health professionals include Legionnaires' disease, AIDS, cat scratch disease, *Helicobacter pylori*-associated disease, ehrlichiosis, hepatitis C, hantavirus pulmonary syndrome (HPS), Ebola virus hemorrhagic fever (EHF), leptospirosis, and new-variant Creutzfeldt-Jakob disease (9, 15, 31). Effective surveillance systems are essential for the timely recognition of emerging infections before they become major public health problems. These systems require a thorough understanding of the epidemiology of infectious diseases, good communication and collaboration among health care professionals and the public health community, and very importantly, effective diagnostic capabilities. Strengthening of the capacity of various health care professionals to diagnose infectious diseases is therefore one of the critical steps in an effective response to emerging microbial threats (9, 15).

Infectious disease pathologists have a long-standing history of contributing to the diagnosis and identification of infectious disease agents. Notable early contributions include landmark studies of *Rickettsia rickettsii* by the pathologists Howard Ricketts and S. Burt Wolbach (71). More recently, because of increased awareness of infectious diseases, there has been renewed interest and revitalization in infectious disease pathology (57, 59). Table 1 provides a sample of recently described diseases for which pathologists have had an important role in identifying the causative agent or describing the pathogenetic process.

Sherif R. Zaki and Christopher D. Paddock • Division of Viral and Rickettsial Diseases, National Center for Infectious Diseases, Centers for Disease Control and Prevention, Mail Stop G-32, 1600 Clifton Rd. NE, Atlanta, GA 30333.

Table 1. Selected examples of emerging infectious diseases with significant contributions by pathology

Disease or syndrome	Agent(s)	Selected reference(s)
Cryptosporidiosis	*Cryptosporidium parvum*	29, 38
Legionellosis	*Legionella* spp.	79
Cat scratch disease	*Bartonella henselae*	1, 61, 75
Adult T-cell leukemia/ lymphoma	Human T-cell lymphotropic virus type 1	3
AIDS	Human immunodeficiency virus type 1	5, 19, 55
Gastroduodenal disease	*Helicobacter pylori*	47, 74, 81
Microsporidiosis	*Enterocytozoon bieneusi, Encephalitozoon intestinalis, Encephalitozoon hellem*	7, 43, 58
Bacillary angiomatosis	*B. henselae, Bartonella quintana*	37, 50, 66
Human ehrlichioses	*Ehrlichia chaffeensis, Ehrlichia phagocytophila*	2, 23, 24, 72
Granulomatous amebic encephalitis	*Balamuthia mandrillaris*	70
Coccidian enteritis	*Cyclospora cayetanensis*	21, 67
Hantavirus pulmonary syndrome	SNV	28, 85, 86
Leptospirosis	*Leptospira* spp.	16, 69, 91
Kaposi's sarcoma	Human herpesvirus 8	4, 20
Ebola hemorrhagic fever	Ebola virus	27, 35, 39, 90
Viral encephalitides	Hendra virus, Nipah virus	17, 18, 44, 62, 73
	Cache Valley virus	63
	Enterovirus 71	13, 65
New-variant Creutzfeldt-Jakob disease	Prion	77

Pathologists are characteristically among the first health care workers involved in the recognition of infectious disease outbreaks and are in an excellent position to discover new pathogens and infectious disease syndromes. These discoveries have been accomplished by collaborative research with colleagues from other scientific disciplines, such as epidemiology, clinical care, veterinary medicine, and microbiology.

Traditionally, anatomic pathologists have relied on routine histopathology or special stains to arrive at a diagnosis. Some pathogens, such as certain species of fungi and bacteria, are morphologically distinct and can be readily identified by microscopy or with special stains. Additionally, viral pathogens, such as rabies virus, herpesviruses, parvovirus, and measles virus, produce characteristic intracellular inclusions which may support a specific diagnosis. Observations of patterns of tissue injury and host responses are also important because tissues often react to infections in specific and predictable ways, making it possible to suspect certain infections. Nonetheless, in many cases it is impossible to identify a specific infectious agent by morphologic observations alone. Recent experience at the Centers for Disease Control and Prevention (CDC) and other institutions has shown that use of a combination of traditional morphology with immunologic and molecular pathology techniques is an extremely useful approach for the confirmation of diagnoses for patients with otherwise unexplained illnesses.

Immunologic and molecular methods, such as immunohistochemistry (IHC), in situ hybridization (ISH), and PCR, have revolutionized the ability of pathologists to diagnose and study infectious diseases (88). These techniques allow detection of microbial antigen or nucleic acid sequences in formalin-fixed, paraffin-embedded tissues. In this context, unexplained diseases may be investigated prospectively, as well as retrospectively, with archival tissue samples. Traditionally, microbial identification has relied primarily on serologic assays and culture techniques. Serologic assays characteristically require the collection of paired serum samples to demonstrate rising titers of antibody against a specific pathogen. Certain circumstances, including immunocompromised states, early therapy, or rapid death, may preclude the development of diagnostic antibody responses. Finally, serologic tests may occasionally give nonspecific results, especially if only a single sample is available for evaluation. Visualization of microbial antigens or nucleic acids in the context of pathology allows the pathologist to assess the clinical significance of serologic test results or microbial isolation.

Culture of fastidious pathogens and obligate intracellular viruses and bacteria is often labor-intensive, may require biosafety facilities not readily available, and may take weeks or months to yield results. By comparison, the use of molecular pathology techniques offers several distinct advantages over traditional microbiologic methods, including speed, sensitivity, reduced risk of exposure of laboratory personnel to the agent, and tissue localization of pathogens. The unique role of molecular pathology in the confirmation of infection in seronegative patients and the detection of fastidious or nonculturable organisms cannot be overemphasized. A prompt, specific diagnosis can prevent the use of unnecessary therapeutic regimens, reduce the need for invasive diagnostic procedures, and alert the medical community to institute appropriate therapeutic and precautionary measures that can control or halt the spread of the disease.

The use of molecular techniques in infectious disease pathology has proven to be a powerful tool in the diagnosis of previously unexplained syndromes. By using a syndrome-based approach, the pathologist can narrow the diagnostic possibilities and perform targeted molecular testing for a limited number of organisms. A syndrome-based approach to diagnosis is currently used for CDC surveillance efforts for Unexplained Deaths due to Possibly Infectious Causes. This program represents the first attempt to conduct early detection of new infectious diseases in large segments of the U.S. population (49).

Table 2 lists the IHC and ISH tests available in laboratories of the Infectious Disease Pathology Activity (IDPA), which is CDC's organizational unit that serves as a scientific and technical resource for studies of the pathology and pathogenesis of infectious diseases. Epidemiologic, clinical, and histopathologic findings enable CDC pathologists to use the most appropriate initial immunologic and molecular pathology tests. This chapter highlights some of the contributions of CDC pathologists in addressing some of the challenges posed by new, emerging, and reemerging infectious diseases.

Table 2. IHC and ISH tests used by IDPA, CDC, for diagnosis of infectious disease agents

Pathogen[a]	Test availability	
	IHC	ISH
Viruses		
Adenovirus	+	+
Crimean-Congo hemorrhagic fever virus	+	+
Dengue virus	+	
Ebola virus	+	+
Eastern equine encephalitis virus	+	
Enterovirus 71	+	+
Guanarito virus	+	
Hantaviruses (cross-reactive and serotype-specific assays)	+	+
Hendra virus	+	+
Herpesviruses		
HHV-1, HHV-2 (HSV-1, HSV-2)		+
HHV-3 (VZV)		+
HHV-4 (EBV)		+
HHV-5 (CMV)	+	+
HHV-6		+
HHV-7		+
HIV-1	+	+
HTLV-1		+
Human papillomavirus		+
Human parvovirus	+	+
Influenza and parainfluenza viruses	+	
Japanese encephalitis virus	+	
JC virus		+
Junin virus	+	
La Crosse encephalitis virus	+	
Lymphocytic choriomeningitis virus		+
Machupo virus	+	
Marburg virus	+	
Measles virus	+	+
Nipah virus	+	+
Rabies virus	+	
Respiratory syncytial virus	+	
Rift Valley fever virus	+	
SIV		+
St. Louis encephalitis virus	+	
Venezuelan equine encephalitis virus	+	
Western equine encephalitis virus	+	
Yellow fever virus	+	
Rickettsiae and ehrlichiae		
Ehrlichia chaffeensis	+	+
Ehrlichia equi	+	+
Coxiella burnetii	+	
Spotted fever group rickettsiae	+	
Typhus group rickettsiae	+	

Table 2. *Continued*

Pathogen[a]	Test availability	
	IHC	ISH
Bacteria		
Bartonella henselae	+	
Bartonella quintana	+	
Brucella spp.	+	
Chlamydia spp.	+	+
Francisella tularensis	+	
Helicobacter pylori	+	
Legionella pneumophila (serogroups 1, 5, and 6)	+	
Leptospira spp.	+	
Listeria monocytogenes	+	
Mycoplasma pneumoniae	+	
Neisseria meningitidis (serogroup C)	+	
Streptococcus pneumoniae	+	
Treponema pallidum	+	
Yersinia pestis	+	
Parasites		
Acanthamoeba culbertsoni	+	
Balamuthia mandrillaris	+	
Naegleria fowleri	+	
Toxoplasma gondii	+	
Trypanosoma cruzi	+	
Fungi (*Aspergillus* spp.)	+	

[a]Abbreviations: HHV-1, human herpesvirus 1; HSV-1, herpes simplex virus type 1; VZV, varicella-zoster virus; EBV, Epstein-Barr virus; CMV, cytomegalovirus; HIV-1, human immunodeficiency virus type 1; HTLV-1, human T-cell lymphotropic virus type 1; SIV, simian immunodeficiency virus.

HANTAVIRUS PULMONARY SYNDROME

In May 1993, the deaths of several previously healthy individuals baffled health care workers in the southwestern United States and at CDC. These patients developed an influenza-like illness, followed by rapidly progressive pulmonary edema, respiratory insufficiency, and shock (8, 34, 40). Initial laboratory testing of patient specimens for bacterial, viral, and toxic causes failed to identify an etiologic agent. Patient specimens were subsequently forwarded to CDC for further studies.

CDC quickly performed batteries of immunoassays for numerous bacterial and viral pathogens in addition to toxicologic testing. The first clue came when antibodies reactive with hantaviruses were detected in the serum of the patients. However, the suggestion that a hantavirus was the etiologic agent of this outbreak was met with skepticism for several reasons. First, the pattern of serologic reactivity was atypical for known hantaviruses, and patients resided in a geographic area where hantavirus disease had not previously been documented. Second, all patients with hantavirus-associated illnesses known prior to this outbreak shared various degrees of fever and renal involvement, with or without hemorrhagic manifestations. Finally, and most importantly, the pronounced pulmonary involvement in patients involved in this outbreak had not been a prominent clinical feature for other patients with recognized hantavirus-associated disease.

An initial examination of coded specimens allowed correlation between the histopathologic features of patients with fatal disease and those patients with serologic evidence of hantavirus infection. Although this correlation led to increased confidence in the diagnosis during the initial days of the laboratory investigation, additional confirmation was needed to identify the nature of the hantavirus and to establish an etiologic relationship. Within days, demonstration of viral antigens in tissues from patients with HPS and amplification of genetic sequences from autopsy material established a previously unrecognized hantavirus as the causative agent (Color Plate 1A) (85). The newly identified agent, Sin Nombre virus (SNV), was subsequently isolated at CDC from a deer mouse, *Peromyscus maniculatus*, the natural reservoir and vector of this zoonotic virus (25). Although most cases of HPS in the United States are caused by SNV, other SNV-like hantaviruses have been implicated, including Bayou and Black Creek Canal viruses. Reports of HPS outside North America are increasing, primarily in South America (10, 68, 76, 78).

Correlation of clinicopathologic findings with the cellular tropism of SNV and its distribution within human tissues provided important insights into the pathogenesis of HPS (26, 28, 42). IHC analysis showed the widespread presence of hantaviral antigens in endothelial cells of the microvasculature, particularly in the lung. Hantaviral antigens were also observed within follicular dendritic cells, macrophages, and lymphocytes. The magnitude and extent of pulmonary microvascular involvement in HPS indicated that functional derangement of endothelial cells is central to the pathogenesis of the hemoconcentration, pulmonary edema, and shock seen in patients with HPS (82, 85).

Pathology was instrumental in answering questions early in the investigation related to the novelty of this infection. IHC analysis was used to identify retrospective cases in the United States that had occurred as early as 1978, predating the outbreak in the southwestern United States by 15 years (64, 83, 86). The occurrence of these earlier fatal cases of HPS caused by a virus or viruses antigenically related to SNV suggests that environmental and ecologic factors rather than genetic reassortment were responsible for the 1993 outbreak. These observations are in agreement with phylogenetic studies of the SNV genome.

LEPTOSPIROSIS

During the fall of 1995, more than 2,000 residents of northern Nicaragua contracted an acute febrile syndrome (16, 69, 91). Patients presented at local health centers with fevers, chills, headaches, and musculoskeletal pain. Among the most severely ill patients, additional clinical manifestations included severe abdominal pain, hypotension, respiratory insufficiency, and hemoptysis. At least 40 patients died with acute pulmonary hemorrhage and respiratory insufficiency. Because of hemorrhagic manifestations, the initial clinical speculation centered particularly on dengue hemorrhagic fever and other arthropod- and rodent-borne viral diseases. However, these conditions were excluded by using serologic, PCR, and IHC assays of serum and tissue specimens (91).

Tissue samples were referred to CDC for further evaluation. Because of the renal and hepatic histopathologic findings, tissues were tested for the presence of leptospires with IHC stains developed during the outbreak. These tests revealed intact leptospires and granular and filamentous leptospiral antigens in many organs, including lung, liver, and kidney (Color Plate 1B). The rapid identification of the etiologic agent allowed CDC and local health authorities to focus the investigation on leptospirosis-related risk factors, disease control, and therapeutic intervention measures. Subsequent culture and serologic studies supported the leptospiral etiology of this outbreak. However, results from these confirmatory assays were not available for several weeks after initial pathologic identification because of the slow growth of leptospires in culture and the time needed for seroconversion in patients.

Initially, leptospirosis was not considered in the differential diagnosis because the most impressive clinical findings in patients with severe disease were the marked pulmonary hemorrhage and respiratory difficulty, along with diffuse pulmonary infiltrates on the chest X rays. Furthermore, unlike the signs and symptoms of classic leptospirosis, there was no significant clinical evidence of renal involvement or jaundice. Similar reports of large outbreaks of leptospirosis associated with pulmonary hemorrhage have also been described in Korea and China.

A major outcome of this investigation was that it heightened awareness among members of the medical community of a disease with global endemicity, including the United States (14). In July 1997, an outbreak of leptospirosis was identified among triathletes in the midwestern United States. These patients presented with fever, myalgia, and headache. Unlike the clinical features seen in the Nicaraguan outbreak, prominent renal manifestations were observed among these patients. Leptospirosis, a waterborne disease, was initially suspected because of prolonged exposure to water during a swim in a lake. Laboratory confirmation was achieved through serologic and immunopathologic assays. Two of the participants whose serum had initially tested negative had cholecystectomies because of acute abdominal pain. IHC staining of gallbladder tissue revealed the presence of leptospires in these patients (14).

RICKETTSIAL AND EHRLICHIAL INFECTIONS

Rickettsial diseases are among the most ancient of described human illnesses; however, more than half of all known rickettsial diseases have been characterized in the last two decades. Historically, pathologists and the discipline of pathology have played pivotal roles in the discovery and characterization of the rickettsioses and, more recently, the ehrlichioses (71, 72). Because rickettsiae and ehrlichiae can be isolated only in cell culture and because the diseases that they cause mimic a variety of other infectious processes, direct visualization of these small gram-negative bacteria in patient tissues and body fluids has been fundamental in the initial recognition of rickettsial and ehrlichial infections. Newly available techniques in pathology provide more sensitive and specific methods for diagnosis and for reassessment of the magnitude of morbidity and mortality attributable to these agents.

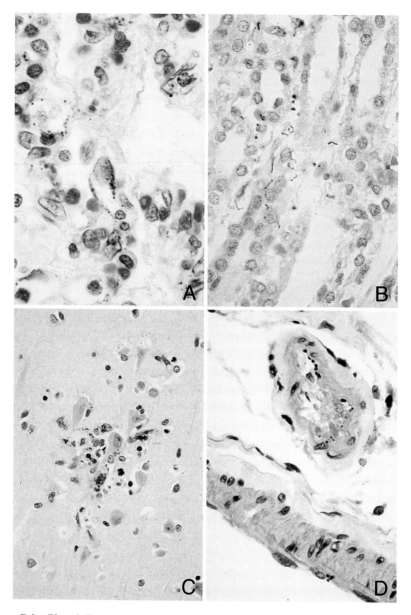

Color Plate 1. Emerging infectious diseases. Immunostaining of viral and rickettsial antigens in patient tissues by IHC is shown. (A) Hantavirus pulmonary syndrome, lung. Viral antigens are localized within the pulmonary microvasculature. (B) Leptospirosis, kidney. Intact and granular staining of leptospires within renal interstitium is shown. (C) Epidemic typhus, cerebral cortex. Staining of *Rickettsia prowazekii* within a characteristic glial nodule is shown. (D) Rocky Mountain spotted fever, leptomeninges. Spotted fever group rickettsiae are localized within the

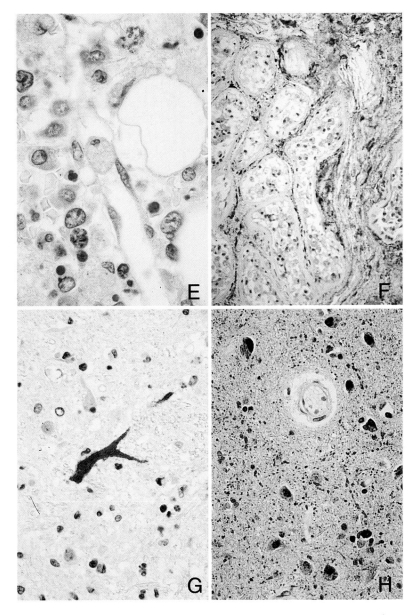

endothelia of medium-sized vessels. (E) Ehrlichiosis, bone marrow. Morulae of *E. chaffeensis* are stained within mononuclear cells. (F) Ebola hemorrhagic fever, skin. Abundant viral antigens in connective tissue surrounding a sweat gland in dermis are shown. (G) Enterovirus 71 encephalitis, central nervous system. Immunostaining of viral antigens within a neuron is shown. (H) Nipah virus encephalitis, cerebral cortex. Viral antigens are present within neurons and glial cells. Note the abundant extracellular antigen.

Epidemic Typhus

In January 1996, CDC alerted the international health community to an outbreak of epidemic typhus in Burundi by confirming a fatal infection with *Rickettsia prowazekii* in a European health care worker. The outbreak in Burundi ultimately involved over 43,000 persons (52). The sentinel patient was an International Red Cross nurse who provided care for inmates in the Ngozi Prison, situated in northern Burundi. During the last 2 months of her stay, an unexplained increase in mortality was observed among prisoners. Within days after returning to her home in Switzerland, she developed high fever, chills, and myalgias and was subsequently hospitalized. Because of her travel history and the rapid development of disseminated intravascular coagulopathy, the initial clinical differential diagnosis centered on exotic viral hemorrhagic fevers. The patient died 3 days after admission, and tissues obtained at autopsy were forwarded to CDC for evaluation. Histopathology revealed interstitial pneumonitis, myocarditis, portal triaditis, hepatic erythrophagocytosis, and glial nodules in the cerebral cortex, suggestive of a rickettsial infection. IHC staining for typhus group rickettsiae confirmed the diagnosis of typhus in this patient (Color Plate 1C), which was subsequently supported by detection of antibodies reactive with *R. prowazekii* in an acute-phase serum sample and by detection of *R. prowazekii* DNA in patient tissues by using PCR (92). This sentinel case and the subsequent epidemic in Burundi remind us that epidemic typhus remains endemic worldwide with the potential for periodic emergence.

Spotted Fever Rickettsioses

During 1996 and 1997, acute-phase serum samples and autopsy tissues from patients with suspected fatal Rocky Mountain spotted fever (RMSF) were submitted to CDC for confirmatory testing. RMSF was confirmed in 12 patients on the basis of IHC staining for spotted fever group rickettsiae alone or in combination with serologic testing and/or PCR. All 12 patients with laboratory-confirmed cases of disease had unequivocal evidence of rickettsiae and rickettsial antigens primarily in and around vascular endothelium (Color Plate 1D). Three of the 12 patients with fatal RMSF as confirmed by IHC additionally demonstrated a diagnostic titer of antibody reactive with *R. rickettsii* by using the indirect immunofluorescence assay (IFA). However, the remaining nine patients demonstrated positive IHC staining for rickettsiae in the absence of a confirmatory serologic result. This included seven patients from whom serum samples were obtained within 2 to 8 days after the onset of illness and two patients from whom serum samples were not available for confirmatory testing (45). IFA is the best recognized and most widely available serologic assay for RMSF, yet diagnostic antibody is lacking in more than 50% of patients in the first week of disease. Since at least half of all deaths as a result of RMSF occur in the first 8 days of the illness, serology alone will miss the majority of patients with fatal disease (45). In this context, immunopathology provides a powerful and much needed tool for better assessment of the magnitude of mortality attributable to *R. rickettsii*.

In recent years, the recognized emergence of several spotted fever group rickettsioses in new geographic areas has been facilitated by immunopathologic studies.

Between November 1993 and March 1994, a cluster of six pediatric patients with fever and rash was identified in Jujuy Province, Argentina. Although spotted fever had previously been documented in several countries in Central and South America, immunopathologic findings provided the first confirmatory evidence of the occurrence of spotted fever group rickettsial infections in Argentina (53).

The role of pathology in posttravel diagnosis of imported rickettsial disease is exemplified by the recognition of an emerging rickettsial infection that occurs in travelers from Africa. The disease, African tick bite fever, was described as a distinct entity in 1994 (33) and has recently been observed among U.S. travelers returning from southern Africa (12). In June 1997, a 66-year-old man returned to the United States after travel to Zimbabwe with fever, multiple skin lesions, and inguinal adenopathy. Skin biopsy specimens were forwarded to CDC for evaluation, by which IHC demonstrated abundant spotted fever group rickettsiae in areas of intense perivascular infiltrates and dermal necrosis. DNA of *Rickettsia africae*, the etiologic agent of African tick bite fever, was subsequently amplified from these tissues by PCR.

Infections Caused by *Ehrlichia* spp.

In June 1992, a 41-year-old human immunodeficiency virus-seropositive woman from Arkansas was hospitalized with an acute illness characterized by fever, diarrhea, and pancytopenia. Despite treatment with multiple broad-spectrum antibiotics, the patient died 2 weeks after the onset of her illness. Small, intracytoplasmic aggregates of bacteria were identified in the mononuclear cells in bone marrow, suggesting infection with an *Ehrlichia* sp. (46). IHC and PCR confirmed *Ehrlichia chaffeensis* as the etiologic agent (Color Plate 1E). Further confirmation of the etiologic agent was subsequently performed by using a novel ISH test for ehrlichiae (22). Ehrlichiae are small, obligately intracellular bacteria closely related to the rickettsia. Although well-recognized as pathogens of animals for over 60 years, these tick-borne agents have only recently been associated with disease in humans in the United States. These include ehrlichial infections caused by *E. chaffeensis* and the as-yet-unnamed agent of human granulocytic ehrlichiosis. As with the rickettsioses, these emerging infections can be difficult to diagnose by clinical criteria alone. Characteristically, the ehrlichioses require specialized serologic or molecular assays to confirm the disease. IHC and ISH have provided powerful adjuncts to the panel of confirmatory tests for ehrlichiae. In the past two decades, pathologists have played significant roles in the identification of these bacteria and in enhancing our knowledge of the expanding clinical spectrum of these diseases (72).

EBOLA HEMORRHAGIC FEVER

In April and May 1995, health authorities in Zaire identified an outbreak of a rapidly progressive hemorrhagic fever-like illness associated with a high rate of mortality. At least two clusters of patients in two different hospitals in Kikwit, a large city located several hundred kilometers east of the capital Kinshasa, were identified (11, 56). Patients experienced fever, asthenia, abdominal pain, nausea, vomiting, diarrhea, and headache (35). Initially, the disease was clinically diagnosed as epidemic dysentery; however, reports indicated that the disease had spread among health care workers involved in patient care and treatment, causing local medical providers to suspect a viral hemorrhagic fever (6, 35). Patient specimens were forwarded to CDC for laboratory testing. Immunoassay, PCR, and IHC testing identified Ebola virus as the etiologic agent of the outbreak (36, 87). The Kikwit epidemic of EHF was the first large outbreak of recognized filovirus disease among humans in nearly 20 years.

IHC and electron microscopic examination showed that endothelial cells, mononuclear phagocytes, and hepatocytes are the main targets for infection, and IHC showed an association of cellular damage with viral infection. However, while Ebola virus antigen can readily be detected by IHC in almost any part of the body, the amount and extent of immunostaining in the skin were remarkable in all patients with EHF examined (90) (Color Plate 1F). This finding provided an opportunity to develop and use an easy means of surveillance for EHF and, possibly, other hemorrhagic fevers.

Traditionally, laboratory diagnosis of EHF has been accomplished through virus isolation or serologic assays (36, 51, 84, 87, 89). Because of biosafety hazards associated with the handling and testing of Ebola virus, these assays can be performed only in a few specialized laboratories under biosafety level 4 containment conditions. Such testing requires transportation of potentially dangerous biological specimens to these laboratories from remote sites where the disease occurs by using a cold chain and rigorous international packaging and shipping procedures.

Small skin-snip biopsy specimens can be taken and placed in formalin, obviating the need for a cold chain and concerns about infectivity, and then moved to a central laboratory for IHC testing. In 1996, a surveillance program based on the test with skin-snip biopsy specimens was used to confirm an outbreak of EHF in Gabon and proved to be a more practical, cost-effective surveillance mechanism that could be managed easily in a large geographic area without on-site supervision and support (90).

Early detection of EHF is critical in stopping the spread of the disease. If EHF had been suspected or confirmed by the use of the test with skin-snip biopsy specimens for one of the patients with an early case of EHF in Kikwit, Zaire, from January to April 1995, the hospital might have taken steps earlier to improve infection control measures, such as the use of sterile needles, gloves, hand-washing, and isolation of suspected patients. These measures may not have prevented all cases of EHF transmission in the community, but they certainly may have helped protect the many health workers who contracted the disease (39).

ENTEROVIRUS 71 ENCEPHALOMYELITIS

CDC was involved in the investigation of two large outbreaks of hand, foot, and mouth disease in Malaysia and Taiwan in 1997 and 1998, respectively (13). Unique to these outbreaks was the rapid clinical deterioration and death (29 deaths in Malaysia, 55 deaths in Taiwan) among affected children. Initial clinical reports from Malaysia in 1997 suggested that myocarditis was the cause of death. However, no histopathologic evidence of myocarditis was observed in tissues forwarded to CDC for evaluation. Furthermore, histopathologic examination of central nervous system tissue revealed a fulminant brain stem encephalomyelitis. These findings suggested neurogenic pulmonary edema rather than a primary cardiac process as the cause of death in these children. Neurons in areas of inflammation and tissue necrosis were positive for enterovirus 71 (EV71) by IHC testing (Color Plate 1G). Isolation of EV71 from several patients further supported the diagnosis. These findings were helpful in guiding the epidemiologic and laboratory investigations of the subsequent outbreak in Taiwan in 1998.

The etiologies of the deaths in Malaysia and Taiwan are still under investigation, and further studies are needed to determine whether EV71 infection alone was responsible for all deaths reported from these outbreaks. Case-control studies are under way in Taiwan to further assess the associations between EV71 infections and rapid death and to identify other potential factors or cofactors (e.g., toxins, medicines, or environmental exposures) that might have contributed to the disease process.

NIPAH VIRUS ENCEPHALITIS

Between September 1998 and May 1999, over 250 residents of the states of Perak and Negri Sembilan in Malaysia contracted an acute febrile encephalitis. Over 100 deaths were associated with this outbreak (17, 18). A similar illness occurred among abattoir workers in Singapore during March 1999. In both Malaysia and Singapore, the disease occurred primarily among males who had been exposed to pigs. Concurrent with the human cases were illnesses and deaths among pigs from the same regions. Patients presented with 3 to 14 days of fever and headache, followed by drowsiness and disorientation. Patients with severe disease developed generalized seizures and coma within 24 to 48 h. In comparison, the disease in swine primarily involved the respiratory system, with manifestations including rapid and labored breathing and an explosive, nonproductive cough. Only a few pigs exhibited neurologic signs such as lethargy and aggressive behavior.

Initial clinical speculation focused on Japanese encephalitis (JE). However, several clinical and epidemiologic features of epidemic JE differed from the features of the outbreaks in Malaysia and Singapore, namely, (i) a predominance of cases in men, (ii) a strong association of disease with pig farming, (iii) the magnitude of disease in adult pigs, and (iv) a history of JE vaccination in many of the victims.

Virus isolates, serum samples, and autopsy tissues from several patients were forwarded to CDC for evaluation. Patient serum samples were negative for antibodies to JE virus. Electron microscopy studies of viral isolates revealed ultrastructural characteristics of a paramyxovirus. Immunofluorescent-antibody studies of infected cell cultures suggested infection with a Hendra virus ("equine morbillivirus") or a Hendra virus-like agent. Testing of patient serum samples by using a capture immunoglobulin M enzyme-linked immunosorbent assay demonstrated antibodies reactive with Hendra virus antigens. Histopathologic features of patients with fatal cases of disease, such as syncytial multinucleated endothelial cells and characteristic cytoplasmic viral inclusions, further supported the diagnosis of paramyxovirus infection. IHC studies showed systemic distribution of viral antigens within the vascular endothelium, as well as within several cell types in the central nervous system, including neurons and glial cells (Color Plate 1H) (17, 18, 48).

Molecular evaluation of viral isolates and human tissue by PCR and nucleotide sequencing revealed a virus related to, but distinct from, the recently described Hendra virus (30, 41, 44, 54, 62, 73). This new virus was tentatively named Nipah virus after the region where the first cases of disease were observed. Testing of swine specimens by molecular, serologic, and immunohistologic tests also demonstrated infection with the same virus. The molecular and immunologic reagents developed after the 1994 discovery of Hendra virus were instrumental in elucidating the etiology of this disease and illustrate the need for preparedness in confronting emerging infections.

CONCLUSIONS

A fundamental principle in the concept of emerging infections is recognition of disease. As illustrated in this chapter, disease recognition by infectious disease pathologists can play a key role in the study of emerging infectious diseases. It must be emphasized that pathologists from other disciplines, including medical examiners and academic, community, and veterinary pathologists, have also made important contributions to these studies. Improved collaboration among pathologists will undoubtedly advance this field.

This review provides several examples of the frontline role of pathology in guiding the early phases of epidemiologic investigations of infectious diseases. The sciences of pathology and epidemiology are complementary disciplines. Each is largely based on the recognition of shared patterns, albeit one from a microscopic perspective and the other from a macroscopic approach. The increasing role of pathology as an active partner in surveillance activities (90) highlights the logical and synergistic combination of these two disciplines in the study of emerging and reemerging infections.

It is important to consider that in an era of increased awareness of potentially new and emerging infections, contemporary pathologic methods can be used effectively in the identification and diagnosis of new emerging infectious diseases (88). The use of newly available molecular and immunologic assays also allows new insights into the pathogenesis and epidemiology of historically familiar diseases. These may include recognition of atypical presentations, such as pulmonary insufficiency caused by hantaviruses or pulmonary hemorrhage caused by *Leptospira*, or better definition of morbidity and mortality attributable to a disease, e.g., RMSF (45, 85, 91). However, with the realization that these new molecular and immunologic methods facilitate investigations that were never before possible, it is imperative that a continued role for standard pathology methods be maintained: the use of autopsies for unexplained deaths, the use of routine histopathology to help focus and guide the subsequent application of specific specialized tests, and the need for systematic archiving of frozen and paraffin-embedded biopsy and autopsy specimens from patients with diseases of unknown etiology to facilitate the study of new clinical entities and their associated etiologic agents (60).

Further challenges are difficult to predict, but it is certain that additional infectious diseases remain to be discovered. As in the past, successful identification and characterization of these diseases will rely on a multidisciplinary approach. The abilities of pathologists to diagnose infectious diseases have been expanded remarkably in the past decade. Continued advancements in this discipline will contribute to the field of emerging infectious diseases.

Acknowledgments. We are indebted to the many health care professionals both within and outside of CDC whose participation in the work related to different outbreak investigations helped make this chapter possible. We also thank John O'Connor and Lisa Coffield for editorial comments and Debbie Guess for secretarial support.

REFERENCES

1. **Anderson, B., K. Sims, R. Regnery, L. Robinson, M. J. Schmidt, S. Goral, C. Hager, and K. Edward.** 1994. Detection of *Rochalimaea henselae* DNA in specimens from cat scratch disease patients by PCR. *J. Clin. Microbiol.* **32:**942–948.
2. **Bakken, J. S., J. S. Dumler, S.-M. Chen, M. R. Eckman, L. L. Van Etta, and D. H. Walker.** 1994. Human granulocytic ehrlichiosis in the upper Midwest United States. A new species emerging? *JAMA* **272:**212–218.
3. **Blayney, D. W., E. S. Jaffe, W. A. Blattner, J. Crossman, M. Robert-Guroff, D. L. Longo, P. A. Bunn, and R. C. Gallo.** 1983. The human T-cell leukemia/lymphoma virus associated with American adult T-cell leukemia/lymphoma. *Blood* **62:**401–405.
4. **Boshoff, C., T. F. Schultz, and M. M. Kennedy.** 1995. Kaposi's sarcoma-associated herpesvirus infects endothelial and spindle cells. *Nature* **1:**1274–1278.
5. **Brynes, R. K., W. C. Chan, T. J. Spira, E. P. Ewing, and F. W. Chandler.** 1983. Value of lymph node biopsy in unexplained lymphadenopathy in homosexual men. *JAMA* **250:**1313–1317.
6. **Bwaka, M. A., M.-J. Bonnet, P. Calain, R. Colebunders, A. De Roo, Y. Guimard, K. R. Katwiki, K. Kibadi, M. A. Kipasa, K. J. Kuvula, B. B. Mapanda, M. Massamba, K. D. Mupapa, J.-J. Tamfun-Muyembe, E. Ndaberey, C. J. Peters, P. E. Rollin, and E. V. Enden.** 1999. Ebola hemorrhagic fever in Kikwit, Democratic Republic of Congo: clinical observations in 103 patients. *J. Infect. Dis.* **179:**S1–S7.
7. **Cali, A., D. P. Kotler, and J. M. Orenstein.** 1993. *Septata intestinalis*, ng, nsp, an intestinal microsporidian associated with chronic diarrhea and dissemination in AIDS patients. *J. Eukaryot. Microbiol.* **40:**101–112.
8. **Centers for Disease Control and Prevention.** 1993. Outbreak of acute illness—southwestern United States, 1993. *Morbid. Mortal. Weekly Rep.* **42:**421–424.
9. **Centers for Disease Control and Prevention.** 1994. *Addressing Emerging Infectious Disease Threats: a Prevention Strategy for the United States.* U.S. Department of Health and Human Services, Atlanta, Ga.
10. **Centers for Disease Control and Prevention.** 1995. Hantavirus pulmonary syndrome—Chile. *Morbid. Mortal. Weekly Rep.* **46:**949–951.
11. **Centers for Disease Control and Prevention.** 1995. Outbreak of Ebola viral hemorrhagic fever—Zaire, 1995. *Morbid. Mortal. Weekly Rep.* **44:**381–382.
12. **Centers for Disease Control and Prevention.** 1998. African tick-bite fever among international travelers—Oregon 1998. *Morbid. Mortal. Weekly Rep.* **47:**950–952.
13. **Centers for Disease Control and Prevention.** 1998. Death among children during an outbreak of hand, foot, and mouth disease—Taiwan, Republic of China. *Morbid. Mortal. Weekly Rep.* **47:**29–32.
14. **Centers for Disease Control and Prevention.** 1998. Outbreak of acute febrile illness among athletes participating in triathlons—Wisconsin and Illinois, 1998. *Morbid. Mortal. Weekly Rep.* **47:**585–588.
15. **Centers for Disease Control and Prevention.** 1998. *Preventing Emerging Infectious Diseases. A Strategy for the 21st Century.* U.S. Department of Health and Human Services, Atlanta, Ga.

16. **Centers for Disease Control and Prevention.** 1999. Outbreak of acute febrile illness and pulmonary hemorrhage—Nicaragua, 1995. *Morbid. Mortal. Weekly Rep.* **44:**841–843.
17. **Centers for Disease Control and Prevention.** 1999. Outbreak of Hendra-like virus—Malaysia and Singapore, 1998–1999. *Morbid. Mortal. Weekly Rep.* **48:**265–269.
18. **Centers for Disease Control and Prevention.** 1999. Update: outbreak of Nipah virus—Malaysia and Singapore, 1999. *Morbid. Mortal. Weekly Rep.* **48:**335–337.
19. **Chadburn, A., C. Metrka, and J. Mouradian.** 1989. Progressive lymph node histology and its prognostic value in patients with acquired immunodeficiency syndrome and AIDS-related complex. *Hum. Pathol.* **20:**579–587.
20. **Chang, Y., E. Cesarman, M. S. Pessin, F. Lee, J. Culpepper, D. M. Knowles, and P. S. Moore.** 1994. Identification of herpesvirus-like DNA sequences in AIDS-associated Kaposi's sarcoma. *Science* **266:**1865–1869.
21. **Connor, B. A., D. R. Shlim, J. V. Scholes, J. L. Rayburn, J. Reidy, and R. Rajah.** 1993. Pathologic changes in the small bowel in nine patients with diarrhea associated with a coccidia-like body. *Ann. Intern. Med.* **119:**377–382.
22. **Dawson, J. E., C. K. Warner, C. D. Paddock, U. G. Munderloh, J. H. Bartlett, P. W. Greer, and S. R. Zaki.** Unpublished data.
23. **Dumler, J. S., P. Brouqui, J. Aronson, J. P. Taylor, and D. H. Walker.** 1991. Identification of ehrlichia in human tissue. *N. Engl. J. Med.* **325:**1109–1110.
24. **Dumler, J. S., J. E. Dawson, and D. H. Walker.** 1993. Human ehrlichiosis: hematopathology and immunohistologic detection of *Ehrlichia chaffeensis*. *Hum. Pathol.* **24:**391–396.
25. **Elliott, L. H., T. G. Ksiazek, P. E. Rollin, C. F. Spiropoulou, S. Morzunov, M. Monroe, C. S. Goldsmith, C. D. Humphrey, S. R. Zaki, and J. W. Krebs.** 1994. Isolation of the causative agent of hantavirus pulmonary syndrome. *Am. J. Trop. Med. Hyg.* **51:**102–108.
26. **Foucar, K., K. B. Nolte, R. M. Feddersen, B. Hjelle, S. Jenison, J. McLaughlin, D. A. Madar, S. A. Young, S. R. Zaki, and L. Hughes.** 1994. Outbreak of hantavirus pulmonary syndrome in the southwestern United States. Response of pathologists and other laboratorians. *Am. J. Clin. Pathol.* **101:**S1–S5.
27. **Georges-Courbot, M. C., A. Sanchez, C. Y. Lu, S. Baize, E. Leroy, J. Lansout-Soukate, C. Tevi-Benissan, A. J. Georges, S. G. Trappier, S. R. Zaki, R. Swanepoel, P. A. Leman, P. E. Rollin, C. J. Peters, S. T. Nichol, and T. G. Ksiazek.** 1997. Isolation and phylogenetic characterization of Ebola viruses causing different outbreaks in Gabon. *Emerg. Infect. Dis.* **3:**59–62.
28. **Goldsmith, C. S., L. H. Elliott, C. J. Peters, and S. R. Zaki.** 1995. Ultrastructural characteristics of Sin Nombre virus, causative agent of hantavirus pulmonary syndrome. *Arch. Virol.* **140:**2107–2122.
29. **Guarda, L. A., S. A. Stein, K. A. Cleary, and N. G. Ordonez.** 1983. Human cryptosporidiosis in the acquired immune deficiency syndrome. *Arch. Pathol. Lab. Med.* **107:**562–566.
30. **Hooper, P. T., A. R. Gould, G. M. Russell, J. A. Kattenbelt, and G. Mitchell.** 1996. The retrospective diagnosis of a second outbreak of equine morbillivirus infection. *Aust. Vet. J.* **74:**244–245.
31. **Hughes, J. M.** 1999. Addressing the challenges of emerging infectious diseases: implementation of the strategy of the Centers for Disease Control and Prevention, p. 261–269. *In* W. M. Scheld, D. Armstrong, and J. M. Hughes (ed.), *Emerging Infections 1.* ASM Press, Washington, D.C.
32. **Institute of Medicine.** 1988. *The Future of Public Health.* National Academy Press, Washington, D.C.
33. **Kelly, P. J., L. Beati, L. A. Matthewman, P. R. Manson, G. A. Dasch, and D. Raoult.** 1994. A new pathogenic spotted fever group rickettsia from Africa. *Am. J. Trop. Med. Hyg.* **97:**129–137.
34. **Khan, A. S., R. F. Khabbaz, L. R. Armstrong, R. C. Holman, S. P. Bauer, J. Graber, T. Strine, G. Miller, S. Reef, J. Tappero, P. E. Rollin, S. T. Nichol, S. R. Zaki, R. T. Bryan, L. E. Chapman, C. J. Peters, and T. G. Ksiazek.** 1996. Hantavirus pulmonary syndrome: the first 100 US cases. *J. Infect. Dis.* **173:**1297–1303.
35. **Khan, A. S., T. F. Kwemingra, D. H. Heymann, B. LeGuenno, P. Nabeth, B. Kersteins, Y. Fleerackers, P. H. Kilmarx, G. R. Rodier, O. Nkuku, P. E. Rollin, A. Sanchez, S. R. Zaki, R. Swanepoel, O. Tomori, S. T. Nichol, C. J. Peters, T. Muyembe, and T. G. Ksiazek.** 1999. The reemergence of Ebola hemorrhagic fever, Zaire, 1995. *J. Infect. Dis.* **179:**S76–S86.

36. **Ksiazek, T. G., P. E. Rollin, A. J. Williams, D. S. Bressler, M. L. Martin, R. Swanepoel, F. J. Burt, P. A. Leman, A. S. Khan, A. K. Rowe, R. R. Mukunu, A. Sanchez, and C. J. Peters.** 1999. Clinical virology of Ebola hemorrhagic fever (EHF): virus, virus antigen, and IgG and IgM antibody findings among EHF patients in Kikwit, Democratic Republic of the Congo, 1995. *J. Infect. Dis.* **179:**S177–S187.

37. **LeBoit, P. E., B. M. Egbert, M. H. Stoler, J. A. Strauchen, T. G. Berger, T. S. B. Yen, T. A. Bonfiglio, C. K. English, and D. J. Wear.** 1988. Epithelioid haemangioma-like vascular proliferation in AIDS: manifestation of cat scratch disease bacillus infection? *Lancet* **i:**960–963.

38. **Lefkowitch, J. H., S. Krumholz, K. Fengehen, P. Grifin, D. Despommier, and T. A. Brasitus.** 1984. Cryptosporidiosis of the human small intestine: a light and electron microscope study. *Hum. Pathol.* **15:**746–752.

39. **Lloyd, E. S., S. R. Zaki, P. E. Rollin, T. G. Ksiazek, P. Calain, M. K. Konde, K. Tchioko, M. A. Bwaka, E. Verchueren, J. Kabwau, R. Ndambe, and C. J. Peters.** 1999. Long-term disease surveillance in Bandundu Region, Democratic Republic of the Congo: a model for early detection and prevention of Ebola hemorrhagic fever. *J. Infect. Dis.* **179:**S274–S280.

40. **Moolenaar, R. L., C. Dalton, H. B. Lipman, E. T. Umland, M. Gallaher, J. S. Duchin, L. Chapman, S. R. Zaki, T. G. Ksiazek, and P. E. Rollin.** 1995. Clinical features that differentiate hantavirus pulmonary syndrome from three other acute respiratory illnesses. *Clin. Infect. Dis.* **21:**643–649.

41. **Murray, P. K.** 1996. The evolving story of the equine morbillivirus. *Aust. Vet. J.* **74:**214.

42. **Nolte, K. B., R. M. Feddersen, K. Foucar, S. R. Zaki, F. T. Koster, D. Madar, T. L. Merlin, P. J. McFeeley, E. T. Umland, and R. E. Zumwalt.** 1995. Hantavirus pulmonary syndrome in the United States: a pathological description of a disease caused by a new agent. *Hum. Pathol.* **26:**110–120.

43. **Orenstein, J. M., J. Chiang, W. Steinberg, P. D. Smith, H. Rotterdam, and D. P. Kotler.** 1990. Intestinal microsporidiosis as a cause of diarrhea in human immunodeficiency virus-infected patients: a report of 20 cases. *Hum. Pathol.* **21:**475–481.

44. **O'Sullivan, J. D., A. M. Allworth, D. L. Paterson, T. M. Snow, R. Boots, L. J. Gleeson, A. R. Gould, A. D. Hyatt, and J. Bradfield.** 1997. Fatal encephalitis due to novel paramyxovirus transmitted from horses. *Lancet* **349:**93–95.

45. **Paddock, C. D., P. W. Greer, T. L. Ferebee, J. Singleton, D. B. McKechnie, T. A. Treadwell, J. W. Krebs, M. J. Clarke, R. C. Holman, J. G. Olson, J. E. Childs, and S. R. Zaki.** 1999. Hidden mortality attributable to Rocky Mountain spotted fever: immunohistochemical detection of fatal, serologically unconfirmed disease. *J. Infect. Dis.* **179:**1469–1476.

46. **Paddock, C. D., D. M. Suchard, K. L. Grumbach, W. K. Hadley, R. L. Kerschmann, N. W. Abbey, J. E. Dawson, K. Sims, J. Dumler, and B. Herndier.** 1993. Brief report: fatal seronegative ehrlichiosis in a patient with HIV infection. *N. Engl. J. Med.* **329:**1164–1167.

47. **Parsonnet, J., G. D. Friedman, and D. P. Vandersteen.** 1991. *Helicobacter pylori* infection and the risk of gastric carcinoma. *N. Engl. J. Med.* **325:**1127–1131.

48. **Paton, J. I., Y. S. Leo, S. R. Zaki, M. C. Wong, K. E. Lee, A. E. Ling, S. K. Chew, B. Ang, P. E. Rollin, T. G. Ksiazek, A. P. Auchus, T. Umapathi, I. Sng, C. C. Lee, E. Lim, A. Kurup, M. S. Lam, and S. Y. Wong.** Outbreak of Nipah virus infection among abbattoir workers in Singapore: description of a new infectious disease. *Lancet,* in press.

49. **Perkins, B. A., J. M. Flood, R. Danila, R. C. Holman, A. L. Reingold, L. A. Klug, M. Virata, P. R. Cieslak, S. R. Zaki, R. W. Pinner, and R. F. Khabbaz.** 1996. Unexplained deaths due to possibly infectious causes in the United States: defining the problem and designing surveillance and laboratory approaches. The Unexplained Deaths Working Group. *Emerg. Infect. Dis.* **2:**47–53.

50. **Perkocha, L. A., S. M. Geaghan, T. S. Yen, S. L. Nishimura, S. P. Chan, R. Garcia-Kennedy, G. Honda, A. C. Stoloff, H. Z. Klein, R. L. Goldman, S. V. Meter, L. D. Ferrell, and P. E. LeBoit.** 1990. Clinical and pathological features of bacillary peliosis hepatis in association with human immunodeficiency virus infection. *N. Engl. J. Med.* **323:**1581–1586.

51. **Peters, C. J., and S. R. Zaki.** Viral hemorrhagic fevers: overview. *In* R. L. Guerrant, D. J. Krogstad, J. A. Maguire, D. H. Walker, and P. F. Weller (ed.), *Tropical Infectious Diseases,* in press. Churchill Livingstone, Inc., New York, N.Y.

52. **Raoult, D., J. B. Ndihokubwayo, H. Tissot-Dupont, V. Roux, B. Faugere, R. Abegbinni, and R. J. Birtles.** 1998. Outbreak of epidemic typhus associated with trench fever in Burundi. *Lancet* **352:**353–358.

53. **Ripoll, C. M., C. E. Remondegui, G. Ordonez, R. Arazamendi, H. Fusaro, M. J. Hyman, C. D. Paddock, S. R. Zaki, J. G. Olson, and C. A. Santos-Buch.** 1999. Evidence of rickettsial spotted fever and ehrlichial infections in a subtropical territory of Jujuy, Argentina. *Am. J. Trop. Med. Hyg.* **61:**350–354.

54. **Rogers, R. J., I. C. Douglas, F. C. Baldock, R. J. Glanville, K. T. Seppanen, L. J. Gleeson, P. N. Selleck, and K. J. Dunn.** 1996. Investigation of a second focus of equine morbillivirus infection in coastal Queensland. *Aust. Vet. J.* **74:**243–244.

55. **Rosenblum, M. K.** 1990. Infection of the central nervous system by the human immunodeficiency virus type 1; morphology and relation to syndromes of progressive encephalopathy and myelopathy in patients with AIDS. *Pathol. Annu.* **1:**117–169.

56. **Sanchez, A., T. G. Ksiazek, P. E. Rollin, C. J. Peters, S. T. Nichol, A. S. Khan, and B. W. J. Mahy.** 1995. Reemergence of Ebola virus in Africa. *Emerg. Infect. Dis.* **1:**96–97.

57. **Schwartz, D. A.** 1997. Emerging and reemerging infections: progress and challenges in the subspecialty of infectious disease pathology. *Arch. Pathol. Lab. Med.* **121:**776–784.

58. **Schwartz, D. A., R. T. Bryan, and K. O. Hewan-Lowe.** 1992. Disseminated microsporidiosis (*Encephalitozoon hellem*) and acquired immunodeficiency syndrome. Autopsy evidence for respiratory acquisition. *Arch. Pathol. Lab. Med.* **116:**660–668.

59. **Schwartz, D. A., R. T. Bryan, and J. M. Hughes.** 1995. Pathology and emerging infections—quo vadimus? *Am. J. Pathol.* **147:**1525–1533.

60. **Schwartz, D. A., and C. J. Herman.** 1996. The importance of the autopsy in emerging and reemerging infectious diseases. *Clin. Infect. Dis.* **23:**248–254.

61. **Scott, M. A., T. L. McCurley, C. L. Vnencak-Jones, C. Hager, J. A. McCoy, B. Anderson, R. D. Collins, and K. M. Edwards.** 1996. Cat scratch disease: detection of *Bartonella henselae* DNA in archival biopsies from patients with clinically, serologically, and histologically defined disease. *Am. J. Pathol.* **149:**2161–2167.

62. **Selvey, L. A., R. M. Wells, J. G. McCormack, A. J. Ansford, K. Murray, R. J. Rogers, P. S. Lavercombe, P. Selleck, and J. W. Sheridan.** 1995. Infection of humans and horses by a newly described morbillivirus. *Med. J. Aust.* **162:**642–645.

63. **Sexton, D. J., P. E. Rollin, E. B. Breitschwerdt, G. R. Corey, S. A. Myers, M. R. Dumais, M. D. Bowen, C. S. Goldsmith, S. R. Zaki, S. T. Nichol, C. J. Peters, and T. G. Ksiazek.** 1997. Life-threatening Cache Valley virus infection. *N. Engl. J. Med.* **336:**547–549.

64. **Shefer, A. M., J. W. Tappero, J. S. Bresee, C. J. Peters, M. S. Ascher, S. R. Zaki, R. J. Jackson, S. B. Werner, P. E. Rollin, and T. G. Ksiazek.** 1994. Hantavirus pulmonary syndrome in California: report of two cases and investigation. *Clin. Infect. Dis.* **19:**1105–1109.

65. **Shieh, W. J., S.-M. Jung, C. Hsueh, T.-T. Kuo, and S. R. Zaki, for the Epidemic Working Group.** Pathologic studies on two fatal cases from an outbreak of hand-foot-and-mouth disease in Taiwan, 1998. Submitted for publication.

66. **Stoler, M. H., T. A. Bonfiglio, R. T. Steigbigel, and M. Pereira.** 1983. An atypical subcutaneous infection associated with acquired immune deficiency syndrome. *Am. J. Clin. Pathol.* **80:**714–718.

67. **Sun, T., C. F. Hardi, D. Asnis, A. R. Bresciani, B. Roberts, and S. Teichberg.** 1996. Light and electron microscopic identification of *Cyclospora* species in small intestine: evidence of the presence of asexual life cycle in the human host. *Am. J. Clin. Pathol.* **105:**216–220.

68. **Toro, J., J. D. Vega, A. L. Khan, K. J. Mills, P. Padula, W. Terry, Z. Yadon, R. Valderrama, B. A. Ellis, C. Pavletic, R. Cerda, S. R. Zaki, W. J. Shieh, R. Meyer, M. Tapia, C. Mansilla, M. Baro, J. A. Vergara, M. Concha, G. Calderon, D. Enria, C. J. Peters, and T. G. Ksiazek.** 1998. An outbreak of hantavirus pulmonary syndrome, Chile 1997. *Emerg. Infect. Dis.* **4:**687–694.

69. **Travejo, R. T., J. G. Rigau-Perez, D. A. Ashford, E. M. McClure, C. Jarquin-Gonzalez, J. J. Amadore, J. O. De Los Reyes, A. Gonzales, S. R. Zaki, W. J. Shieh, R. G. McLean, R. S. Nasci, R. S. Weyant, C. A. Bolin, S. L. Bragg, B. A. Perkin, and R. A. Spiegel.** 1998. Epidemic leptospirosis associated with pulmonary hemorrhage—Nicaragua, 1995. *J. Infect. Dis.* **178:**1457–1463.

70. **Visvesvara, G. S., F. L. Schuster, and A. J. Martinez.** 1993. *Balamuthia mandrillaris*, ng, nsp. agent of amebic meningoencephalitis in humans and other animals. *J. Eukaryot. Microbiol.* **40:** 504–514.

71. **Walker, D. H., and J. S. Dumler.** 1995. Will pathologists play as important a role in the future as they have in the past against the challenge of infectious diseases? *Infect. Agents Dis.* **4:**167–170.

72. **Walker, D. H., and J. S. Dumler.** 1997. Human monocytic and granulocytic ehrlichioses. Discovery and diagnosis of emerging tick-borne infections and the critical role of the pathologist. *Arch. Pathol. Lab. Med.* **121:**785–791.

73. **Wang, L. F., W. P. Michalski, M. Yu, L. I. Pritchard, G. Crameri, B. Shiell, and R. T. Eaton.** 1998. A novel P/V/C gene in a new member of the *Paramyxoviridae* family, which causes lethal infection in humans, horses, and other animals. *J. Virol.* **72:**1482–1490.

74. **Warren, J. R.** 1983. Unidentified curved bacilli on gastric epithelium in active chronic gastritis. *Lancet* **i:**1273–1275.

75. **Wear, D. J., A. M. Margileth, T. L. Hadfield, G. W. Fischer, C. J. Schlagel, and F. M. King.** 1983. Cat scratch disease: a bacterial infection. *Science* **221:**1403–1405.

76. **Wells, R. M., S. S. Estani, Z. E. Yadon, D. Enria, P. Padula, N. Pini, J. N. Mills, C. J. Peters, E. L. Segura, and The Hantavirus Pulmonary Syndrome Study Group for Patagonia.** 1997. An unusual hantavirus outbreak in southern Argentina: person-to-person transmission? *Emerg. Infect. Dis.* **3:**171–174.

77. **Will, R. G., J. W. Ironside, M. Zeidler, S. N. Cousens, K. Estibeiro, A. Alperovitch, S. Poser, M. Pocchiari, and A. Hofman.** 1996. A new variant of Creutzfeldt-Jakob disease in the UK. *Lancet* **347:**921–925.

78. **Williams, R. J., R. T. Bryan, J. N. Mills, R. E. Palma, I. Vera, V. F. De, E. Baez, W. E. Schmidt, R. E. Figueroa, C. J. Peters, S. R. Zaki, A. S. Khan, and T. G. Ksiazek.** 1997. An outbreak of hantavirus pulmonary syndrome in western Paraguay. *Am. J. Trop. Med. Hyg.* **57:**274–282.

79. **Winn, W. C., and R. L. Myerowitz.** 1981. The pathology of the *Legionella* pneumonias. *Hum. Pathol.* **12:**401–422.

80. **World Health Organization.** 1992. *Global Health Situations and Projections, Estimates 1992.* World Health Organization, Geneva, Switzerland.

81. **Wotherspoon, A., C. Ortiz-Hidalgo, T. Diss, M. R. Falzon, and P. G. Isaacson.** 1991. *Helicobacter pylori*-associated gastritis and primary B-cell gastric lymphoma. *Lancet* **338:**1175–1176.

82. **Zaki, S. R.** 1997. Hantavirus-associated diseases, p. 125–136. *In* D. H. Connor, F. W. Chandler, D. A. Schwartz, H. J. Manz, and E. E. Lack (ed.), *Pathology of Infectious Diseases.* Appleton & Lange, Stamford, Conn.

83. **Zaki, S. R., R. C. Albers, P. W. Greer, L. M. Coffield, L. R. Armstrong, A. S. Khan, R. Khabbaz, and C. J. Peters.** 1994. Retrospective diagnosis of a 1983 case of fatal hantavirus pulmonary syndrome. *Lancet* **343:**1037–1038. (Letter.)

84. **Zaki, S. R., and C. S. Goldsmith.** 1999. Pathologic features of filovirus infections in humans. *Curr. Top. Microbiol. Immunol.* **235:**97–116.

85. **Zaki, S. R., P. W. Greer, L. M. Coffield, C. S. Goldsmith, K. B. Nolte, K. Foucar, R. M. Feddersen, R. E. Zumwalt, G. L. Miller, and A. S. Khan.** 1995. Hantavirus pulmonary syndrome. Pathogenesis of an emerging infectious disease. *Am. J. Pathol.* **146:**552–579.

86. **Zaki, S. R., A. S. Khan, R. A. Goodman, L. R. Armstrong, P. W. Greer, L. M. Coffield, T. G. Ksiazek, P. E. Rollin, C. J. Peters, and R. F. Khabbaz.** 1996. Retrospective diagnosis of hantavirus pulmonary syndrome, 1978–1993: implications for emerging infectious diseases. *Arch. Pathol. Lab. Med.* **120:**134–139.

87. **Zaki, S. R., and P. H. Kilmarx.** 1997. Ebola virus hemorrhagic fever, p. 299–312. *In* C. Horsburgh, Jr., and A. M. Nelson (ed.), *Pathology of Emerging Infections.* ASM Press, Washington, D.C.

88. **Zaki, S. R., and A. M. Marty.** 1995. New technology for the diagnosis of infectious diseases, p. 127–154. *In* G. Seifert and W. Doerr (ed.), *Tropical Pathology.* Springer-Verlag, Berlin, Germany.

89. **Zaki, S. R., and C. J. Peters.** 1997. Viral hemorrhagic fevers, p. 347–364. *In* D. H. Connor, F. W. Chandler, D. A. Schwartz, H. J. Manz, and E. E. Lack (ed.), *Diagnostic Pathology of Infectious Diseases.* Appleton & Lange, Stamford, Conn.

90. **Zaki, S. R., W. J. Shieh, P. W. Greer, C. S. Goldsmith, T. Ferebee, J. Katshitski, K. Tchioko, M. A. Bwaka, R. Swanepoel, P. Calain, A. S. Khan, E. Lloyd, P. E. Rollin, T. G. Ksiazek,**

C. J. Peters, and the EHF Study Group. 1999. A novel immunohistochemical assay for detection of Ebola virus in skin: implications for diagnosis, spread and surveillance of Ebola hemorrhagic fever. *J. Infect. Dis.* **179:**S36–S47.

91. Zaki, S. R., W. J. Shieh, and The Epidemic Working Group at Ministry of Health in Nicaragua. 1996. Leptospirosis associated with outbreak of acute febrile illness and pulmonary haemorrhage, Nicaragua, 1995. *Lancet* **347:**535–536.

92. Zanetti, G., P. Francioli, D. Tagan, C. D. Paddock, and S. R. Zaki. 1998. Imported epidemic typhus. *Lancet* **352:**1709. (Letter.)

Emerging Infections 3
Edited by W. M. Scheld, W. A. Craig, and J. M. Hughes
© 1999 ASM Press, Washington, D.C.

Chapter 13

Medical Examiner and Coroner Surveillance for Emerging Infections

Kurt B. Nolte and Mitchell I. Wolfe

BACKGROUND

On 14 May 1993, Richard Malone, an investigator for the New Mexico Office of the Medical Investigator (OMI), was notified of the sudden death of a 19-year-old man from a rural northwestern New Mexico community. The man had collapsed while traveling to his fiancée's funeral in the nearby town of Gallup. Malone's investigation revealed that the man and his fiancée died after strikingly similar illnesses characterized by a flu-like prodrome including fever, chills, and body aches followed by the abrupt onset of cough and shortness of breath. Worried that both individuals may have died from plague, Malone arranged for immediate autopsies to be performed on both bodies that evening. The prosecting forensic pathologist, Patricia McFeeley, was struck by the similar autopsy findings for the two individuals and those of another young woman whom she had examined approximately 1 month earlier and who had died with the same symptoms in the same region of New Mexico. That evening, McFeeley notified the New Mexico Department of Health of an apparent cluster of fatal respiratory disease. Over the ensuing days and weeks, clinicians and pathologists recognized many more similar cases throughout the southwestern United States (5). Following a rapid investigation that involved the cooperation of several different state, tribal, and federal agencies, the hantavirus pulmonary syndrome was identified and described (16, 41). A vigilant and well-organized statewide medical examiner system was a crucial element in the recognition of this disease.

Kurt B. Nolte • Office of the Medical Investigator, University of New Mexico School of Medicine, Albuquerque, NM 87131-5091; Medical Examiner/Coroner Information Sharing Program, Division of Environmental Hazards and Health Effects, National Center for Environmental Health, Centers for Disease Control and Prevention, Atlanta, GA 30341; and Infectious Disease Pathology Activity, Division of Viral and Rickettsial Diseases, National Center for Infectious Diseases, Centers for Disease Control and Prevention, Atlanta, GA 30333. ***Mitchell I. Wolfe*** • Surveillance and Programs Branch, Division of Environmental Hazards and Health Effects, National Center for Environmental Health, Centers for Disease Control and Prevention, Atlanta, GA 30341.

Medicolegal death investigation systems, at first glance, may not seem relevant to emerging infectious disease surveillance. In most jurisdictions, laws authorize medical examiners or coroners to investigate deaths that are violent, sudden, suspicious, unexplained, or unnatural (14). These laws usually direct the medical examiner or coroner (ME/C) to determine the cause of death (disease or injury that initiates the fatal chain of events), manner of death (circumstances under which the death occurred, i.e., natural versus homicide, suicide, or accident), and the condition of the body. To do this most ME/Cs either are pathologists or forensic pathologists or contract with pathologists or forensic pathologists to conduct postmortem examinations of the victims of these deaths.

Not surprisingly, most medicolegal death investigation systems are biased toward the investigation of violent or unnatural deaths. However, sudden natural deaths, unexplained deaths, and deaths of public health importance also come under the scrutiny of forensic pathologists. These deaths are frequently due to infectious diseases (39) and represent the overlap between forensic pathology and emerging infectious diseases (Fig. 1). This overlap is not new. One of the earliest examples occurred in 1934, when Milton Halpern, a medical examiner for New York City, reported 17 fatal autopsy-recognized cases of malaria in intravenous heroin users (18).

CURRENT STATUS OF MEDICOLEGAL DEATH INVESTIGATION IN THE UNITED STATES

Currently, the United States has a patchwork of medicolegal death investigation systems (Fig. 2). As of 1997, 21 states and the District of Columbia had statewide or district- or county-based medical examiner-only systems. Eighteen states have

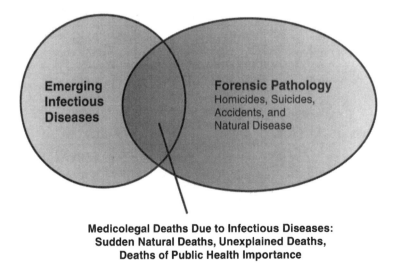

Figure 1. Overlap of forensic pathology and emerging infectious diseases.

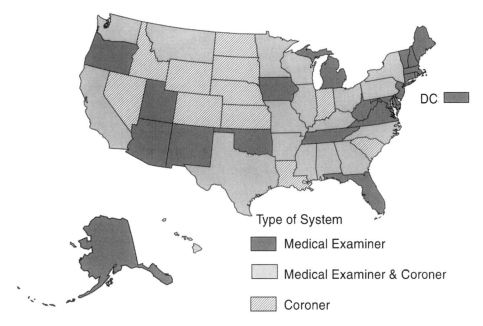

DC ▮

Type of System

▮ Medical Examiner

▯ Medical Examiner & Coroner

▨ Coroner

Figure 2. Death investigation system by state, United States, 1996.

mixed medical examiner and coroner systems. Eleven states have district or county coroner-only systems (21). Coroners are usually elected or appointed public officials who investigate deaths in their jurisdictions and who contract for autopsy services with pathologists. Medical examiners are usually appointed physicians who investigate deaths in their jurisdictions. The qualifications of coroners and medical examiners vary greatly. Most coroners are not required to have any medical training. Although most medical examiners are forensic pathologists (physicians who have completed training in pathology and subspeciality training in forensic pathology), some medical examiners are not required to have any forensic training (14). These organizational and personnel considerations alone do not mean that deaths will be inadequately investigated; however, there is no uniform national environment for medicolegal death investigation.

Presently, the vast majority of autopsies performed annually in the United States are forensic autopsies. The frequency of hospital-based autopsies, performed with the consent of the next of kin, has declined dramatically over the past several decades, from approximately 50% of all hospital deaths in 1950 to less than 10% in 1995 (25) (Fig. 3). Reasons for this decline include lack of reimbursement by hospitals and insurers, lack of incentive to perform autopsies due to the cost and time burden, decreased emphasis on the autopsy as an important learning tool in medical schools, and technological advances in diagnostic modalities. Furthermore, the lack of interest of pathologists in performing autopsies and the potential increased risk of occupational exposure of pathologists to dangerous pathogens have also contributed to the decline in the frequency of hospital-based autopsies (19).

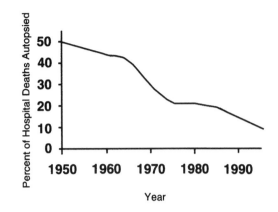

Figure 3. Hospital autopsy rates by year, United States, 1950 to 1995 (1, 25, 46).

As the hospital-based autopsy rates have decreased, the proportion of medico-legal autopsies has increased. In 1981, medicolegal autopsies comprised a large proportion and in some jurisdictions a majority of the total number of autopsies performed. Approximately 43% of these medicolegal autopsies were performed on victims of natural diseases (26). Since 1981, national hospital autopsy rates have continued to plunge, and medicolegal autopsies likely represent the majority of total autopsies in almost all areas of the United States. Consequently, to obtain autopsy-verified data on infectious disease deaths, ME/Cs are an excellent, if not the best, source of information. In the following sections of this chapter, we describe the use of ME/C data for public health surveillance, provide an overview of surveillance for fatal infectious conditions, and describe ongoing efforts aimed at identifying the most complete and accurate methods for incorporating ME/C-based autopsy data into state-based and national surveillance systems.

USE OF ME/C DATA FOR PUBLIC HEALTH SURVEILLANCE

ME/Cs investigate approximately 20% of all deaths in the United States (22). Data from these investigations are uniquely valuable in conducting mortality surveillance for many types of conditions. ME/Cs provide information from autopsies; toxicologic, microbiologic, and other laboratory tests; and investigations of the circumstances surrounding the death. Their jurisdictions are population based. They investigate and certify deaths that are not certified elsewhere (notably, deaths that occur outside of the hospital). Their data are timely: investigations begin immediately after they are notified of a death (22).

State law mandates which deaths are to be investigated. The circumstances of death that require investigation vary by state but generally include the following situations:

- deaths due to homicide, suicide, or accidental causes such as motor vehicle crashes, falls, burns, or the ingestion of drugs or other chemical agents;

- sudden or suspicious deaths, deaths from sudden infant death syndrome, and unattended deaths;
- deaths caused by an agent or disease constituting a threat to public health;
- deaths that occurred while the decedents were at work;
- deaths of people who were in custody or confinement; and
- deaths of people institutionalized for reasons other than organic disease (14).

Information regarding the usefulness of ME/C data for mortality surveillance is limited. Studies have looked at the usefulness of these data for analyzing natural-manner deaths, injury deaths, work-related injury deaths, maternal deaths, and poisoning deaths. In general, ME/Cs have been found to be a useful adjunctive source of data for the surveillance of specific causes of death (22). Surveillance systems that incorporate ME/C data include the Drug Abuse Warning Network for reporting of drug-related deaths, the Medical Examiners and Coroners Alert Project for reporting of deaths involving consumer products, the MedWatch Medical Products Reporting Program for reporting of adverse drug and medical product-related outcomes, the Fatal Accident Reporting System, the Medical Examiner and Coroner Information Sharing Program, the Occupational Safety and Health Administration surveillance for work-related deaths, and the Pediatric Toxicology Registry (22).

EXAMPLES OF EXISTING INFECTIOUS DISEASE MORTALITY SURVEILLANCE

Population-based surveillance for infectious disease mortality is a difficult endeavor. One retrospective descriptive study used the *International Classification of Diseases, Ninth Revision* (ICD-9), codes assigned to diagnoses on death certificates to classify deaths in the United States from 1980 through 1992 as infectious disease related. Using ICD-9 codes that they felt always represented infectious diseases, the investigators estimated that, in the United States, infectious diseases are the primary or contributing cause of death in 17% of all deaths and the underlying cause of death in 8% of all deaths (45). However, these rates may not accurately depict the true burden of infectious disease mortality because death certificates and ICD-9 codes have inherent flaws when they are used for surveillance. For example, ICD-9 codes are not assigned by persons who are directly associated with the deaths; they are usually assigned by specially trained persons (nosologists) at vital records departments in county or state offices. This situation may lead to misinterpretation of the physician's diagnoses or statements when assigning a code. ICD-9 codes are not designed to identify new infectious diseases; they either are assigned on the basis of known agents of syndromes or are assigned to "other" or "unspecified" categories. In addition, ICD-9 codes are not arranged in such a way as to facilitate aggregation of infectious disease mortality data. Only 67% (754 of 1,131) of the ICD-9 codes thought to represent infectious disease in all cases are in the code range 001 to 139 (codes for infectious and parasitic diseases) (45).

Death certificates themselves may not accurately represent the underlying or contributory cause of death for several reasons. Clinicians may lack proper training both in assigning a cause of death that can easily be translated into ICD-9 codes and in properly assigning a condition as underlying or contributory (37). In addition, the general autopsy rate is low, leading to a potentially large number of deaths with incorrectly classified causes. For example, in one study of paired death certificates and autopsy reports, 29% of the paired documents disagreed considerably with one another on the underlying cause of death. Another 26% agreed on the major disease category but disagreed on the specific disease (31). When autopsies are performed for nonmedicolegal deaths, the information is rarely used to correct the death certificates (31). Lack of autopsy-certified diagnoses certainly leads to inaccuracies in ICD-9 code assignment. Moreover, in 1995, the National Center for Health Statistics stopped collecting death certificate data that indicated whether or not an autopsy was performed. This information is now unavailable on a national basis, making it very difficult to perform death certificate analyses for autopsy-only cases or to measure the accuracy of the reported causes of death (20). By default, this information is now available only from ME/Cs or individual state vital records divisions.

In contrast to retrospective surveillance methods, the Centers for Disease Control and Prevention (CDC) in 1994 began active surveillance for infectious disease with the establishment of the Emerging Infections Program (EIP) at four sites in the United States. These sites are located in Oregon, Minnesota, Connecticut, and California and encompass a combined population of approximately 7.7 million persons. The selected sites conduct population-based surveillance, research, and outbreak response, addressing infectious disease issues important to public health (11).

In May 1995, CDC and the four EIP sites began conducting surveillance for unexplained deaths and severe illnesses possibly due to infectious causes in persons more than 1 and less than 50 years old. The objectives of this program are to identify new infectious agents that cause severe disease and death, to investigate clusters of unexplained illnesses or deaths, and to identify known pathogens that are causing illness not currently attributable to these organisms (11). The program is largely dependent on referrals from clinicians. Because the case definition includes only patients who die in a hospital, ME/Cs are usually not involved in the cases. While progress has been made in several program areas, no new infectious agents have been identified, and over 75% of deaths remain unexplained. One problem that the project has encountered with respect to finding a diagnosis has been the quality and quantity of pathologic specimens obtained from case patients (47). Integration of ME/C-based surveillance into the project would complement the current clinician-based referral system for case recognition and augment the tissues available for further diagnostic studies. In the following sections, we discuss issues related to the incorporation of ME/Cs into the overall surveillance for infectious diseases, including those from bioterrorist attacks, and describe the potential advantages and limitations of this data source.

ME/Cs AND EMERGING INFECTIOUS DISEASE SURVEILLANCE

CDC has four major goals in addressing emerging infectious disease threats: improving disease surveillance and outbreak investigation, improving applied research by integrating laboratory science and epidemiology techniques, improving communication of public health information to ensure prompt prevention and control efforts, and strengthening disease surveillance, prevention, and control infrastructure (6, 11). ME/Cs can and should be involved in achieving each of these goals (6). Specific areas of potential ME/C involvement include participation in sentinel networks to monitor syndromes and diseases, development of new approaches to improve the recognition of rare events, and integration of public health information and surveillance systems to link data collection with disease detection (11). Enthusiasm among medical examiners for participation in infectious disease mortality surveillance is high, as evidenced by their record attendance at the 1998 National Association of Medical Examiners annual meeting, which featured a special session, Emerging Infections and the Forensic Pathologist. One example of potential integration of ME/Cs into public health surveillance is the surveillance for infectious disease deaths and unexplained deaths.

ME/Cs use a definition of the term "unexplained death" that differs from that used in some surveillance projects. ME/Cs conclude that a death is of an "undetermined" cause or is "unexplained" after an exhaustive investigation of the circumstances surrounding the death and an autopsy and a laboratory evaluation yield no findings. When this is the case for intact (nondecomposed) bodies, the best explanation is usually an unrecognizable dynamic (physiologic) event that leaves no autopsy trace (e.g., seizure or cardiac arrhythmia), unrecognizable toxins, or unrecognizable environmental factors (e.g., heat or cold). Very few of these deaths are caused by infections. For the purposes of surveillance, CDC defines an "unexplained death" as having the "hallmarks of an infectious disease for which no cause is identified by preliminary testing" (43). After complete laboratory testing and in the absence of an identified pathogenic organism, most forensic pathologists would certify the cause of these deaths on the basis of the tissue reaction pattern (e.g., encephalitis).

It is important to recognize, however, that many tissue reaction patterns that commonly reflect an infection may also be the consequence of a toxin. For example, meningitis may be seen in ethylene glycol poisoning, fulminant hepatic necrosis in acetaminophen and *Amanita* mushroom poisoning, and diffuse pulmonary alveolar damage with a wide array of inhaled and ingested toxins (15, 24, 32, 34). In truly unexplained deaths, parallel laboratory testing should be directed toward potential unrecognized toxins as well as infectious agents. Understanding the pathologic effects of toxic agents is a strength of forensic pathologists.

Many of the deaths seen by ME/Cs, especially deaths from natural diseases, involve infectious diseases. In New Mexico, approximately 25% of autopsied natural deaths are infectious disease related (42). Because some of these deaths are caused by emerging infections, it is likely that ME/Cs could play an important role in surveillance for these conditions nationally. In recognition of this fact, CDC's 1994 emerging infections plan identifies medical examiners as an important sentinel surveillance network (6). There are several theoretical advantages to incorporating ME/Cs into the existing surveillance programs for infectious diseases and unexplained deaths: ME/Cs investigate deaths that occur outside of the hospital, death investigations by ME/Cs begin immediately after a death is reported, and ME/C jurisdictions are population based (22). In addition, ME/C surveillance is autopsy based. Many more infections are reported on autopsy reports than on death certificates because death certificates record only information on the cause of death and not information on incidental conditions. Some of these incidental conditions are emerging and reemerging infectious diseases such as hepatitis C and tuberculosis. Autopsy-based surveillance can also provide insights into the pathogenesis of infectious diseases that cannot be obtained from death certificates (41, 54). These insights could become critically important as new fatal infections emerge.

Although ME/Cs see a subset of all fatalities, their autopsy populations are enriched with groups that are associated with emerging or reemerging infectious diseases. For example, in 1994, the New Mexico OMI autopsy population encompassed several sentinel groups, including children under age 2 years (7%), alcoholics (>7%), intravenous drug abusers (>5%), and AIDS patients (1.3%). Intravenous drug abusers are clearly linked with AIDS and hepatitis C virus infections (10, 12). Alcoholics have an increased incidence of pulmonary infections such as tuberculosis (2). Infants and young children serve as sentinels for vaccine-preventable diseases (8). In addition, although the percentage of homeless people is unknown, the OMI autopsy population contains many homeless individuals who constitute a sentinel population for tuberculosis and other infectious diseases (9). Greater than 20% of New Mexico's ME/C autopsy population are members of groups known to be at risk for various infectious diseases.

It is important to note that the time needed by ME/Cs to detect specific organisms and disease processes varies depending on both the disease itself and the required diagnostic methods. Diseases that are suspected on the basis of clinical presentation or that have compelling gross autopsy findings, such as meningococcemia, may be immediately recognized and preliminarily reported to public health authorities while confirmatory tests are pending. Some diseases (e.g., rabies) may be histologically evident and results may be available in several hours. The time to receipt of results of culture, serology, and toxicology tests, immunohistochemistry tests, and tests with nucleic acid probes can take several days to weeks.

ME/C pathologists are often the first physicians to see an individual with a fatal disease. In this role, they can immediately report suspected and confirmed cases of infectious diseases. Because they have access to the broader array of tissue specimens available at autopsy, in addition to routine laboratory tests, they may be more likely than clinicians to detect some diseases and still do so within a reasonable time frame for disease control.

One potential system for the implementation of active surveillance for infectious disease mortality with ME/Cs is a death review team. This method has been implemented in New Mexico. A description of the methodology used and some of the results, strengths, and weaknesses of this system are described below.

New Mexico Infectious Disease Death Review Team

In late 1994, the New Mexico OMI created an infectious disease death review team (IDDRT) to systematically review autopsied deaths (42). The IDDRT's goals were to

- describe the burden of deaths due to infectious diseases and unexplained causes that are seen by the OMI and describe trends in infectious disease mortality;
- perform surveillance for clusters of events, outbreaks, emerging infections, and unexplained deaths, including monitoring of sentinel populations that have been associated with emerging or reemerging infectious disease; and
- improve detection and investigation of deaths from infectious diseases, mainly by increasing the proportion of infectious disease-related deaths that receive organism-specific diagnoses.

The OMI performs most (approximately 90%) of the autopsies in New Mexico and is the only forensic pathology agency in the state; therefore, OMI can be viewed as performing surveillance for autopsy-confirmed infectious disease-related mortality. The OMI is an important part of statewide infectious disease-related mortality surveillance. Of note, there are 22 medical examiner offices in the United States that have statewide jurisdiction, although some of these also contain local coroners or medical examiners (21). In these states, the medical examiner's office may also be able to perform statewide surveillance.

The IDDRT consisted of forensic and clinical pathologists, microbiologists, epidemiologists, infectious disease experts, and molecular diagnostic specialists. The team met quarterly and reviewed OMI-autopsied deaths. Of all 410 autopsied natural disease deaths during 1995, approximately 21% (85 of 410) were infectious disease related. IDDRT reviewed 106 total autopsied deaths with infectious diseases (including all manners of death: natural, homicide, suicide, and accidents) in 1995. Of the total infectious disease deaths, 73 (69%) were among persons between the ages of 1 and 54 years, for 37 (35%) no causative organism was identified, and for 25 (24%) both no causative organism was identified and the subjects were between the ages of 1 and 54 years (40). These data indicate that infectious diseases comprise a significant proportion of autopsied deaths investigated by ME/Cs. Many of these cases of infectious disease occur in younger persons, and for many a causative organism is never identified. Some of these cases may represent novel or emerging infections.

The IDDRT system proved to be useful in several respects. First, the quality and accuracy of death records improved through amendment of the cause-of-death portion of the death certificates. This improvement in accuracy is important because death certificates are used to compile mortality statistics, and these statistics serve as the basis for policy decisions regarding program and research funding (1, 31, 44). The IDDRT process maximizes the ability to detect specific causes of death, detect unusual causes of death, and obtain baseline data about infectious disease and unexplained deaths.

Second, the IDDRT process led to improved recognition and investigation of infectious diseases through various means, including the following:

- enhancing OMI pathologists' awareness of the importance of infectious disease deaths as a public health indicator and the importance of organism-specific diagnoses;

- generating baseline 10-year mortality data for several conditions including meningitis, encephalitis, myocarditis, and upper airway infections;
- designing a method for the prospective classification of OMI autopsies by role of infectious diseases in the death, including "infection suspected but not identified," to detect previously unrecognized emerging infections; and
- joining with other groups and agencies to initiate a study of the relationship between hepatitis C virus infection and cirrhosis in New Mexico.

Third, OMI improved its linkage with external agencies, mainly the New Mexico Department of Health, by reporting diseases of public health importance that were identified through IDDRT review of death records. Other anticipated uses of data from this system include detection of deaths from bioterrorism and comparison of IDDRT data to other data such as death certificates from vital statistics.

To facilitate the efforts of an infectious disease death review team, computer programmers may be able to develop sensitive computer-assisted search algorithms for infectious diseases that are inexpensive, that are easy to use, and that take only a few minutes to apply to a database. Computerized search tools could be used not only to identify trends and outbreaks retrospectively but could also be used for real-time detection of outbreaks. Ideally, an algorithm could be applied frequently to an ME/C system database or a collection of databases and generate lists of deaths for review by the death review team. This process could substantially reduce the number of deaths to be reviewed to a manageable number that an assigned reviewer could examine on a regular basis, perhaps weekly. Death review team members could then be notified when certain predetermined "flags" or unusual events (such as indicators of bioterrorist activity) occurred within the system. This technology might make an infectious disease death review team feasible for ME/C jurisdictions that otherwise would not have the resources to review all deaths for their relationship to infectious diseases. It could also create an opportunity to quickly and accurately review data from more than one ME/C office, allowing identification of trends and clusters that span an area larger than a single jurisdiction.

Other jurisdictions could form death review teams using IDDRT as a model to more effectively describe infectious disease-related mortality, detect trends, retrospectively identify clusters of disease, and identify important areas of study. The function of a death review team, however, is not necessarily limited to these important functions. Even though death review teams do exist in some locations, they usually review maternal or child deaths. The use of an ME/C-based death review team to perform surveillance for infectious diseases appears to be a unique endeavor. The New Mexico OMI's use of an IDDRT can be seen as a test of the usefulness of such a system. While the system had many accomplishments, its full usefulness has not yet been established because of its limited time of operation.

Bioterrorism

Any system that is implemented to conduct surveillance for acts of bioterrorism should involve medicolegal death investigators for several reasons. First, medical examiners and coroners may see cases of fatal unattended infections from acts of bioterrorism that other physicians, hospitals, or emergency rooms have not seen. It is not uncommon for individuals with infectious diseases to die at home or other locations away from medical facilities. Even individuals who do present for treatment may die precipitously and unexpectedly without a clear diagnosis and therefore may fall under the ME/C jurisdiction. Second, acts of bioterrorism may become mass-casualty events. The role of ME/Cs in mass-casualty events is often critical, as evidenced by their participation in the investigation of the Alfred P. Murrah Federal Building bombing in Oklahoma City in 1995 and many airline crashes (29, 52). Third, because deaths from acts of bioterrorism are homicides, state statutes dictate that they fall under the jurisdiction of ME/Cs. The potential role of pathologists in episodes of bioterrorism is best illustrated by the 1979 anthrax outbreak that occurred in Sverdlovsk, USSR (now Yekaterinburg, Russia), after release of a pathogen from a military bioweapons facility. Pathologists identified the cause of the outbreak by performing autopsies on 42 of the 66 persons who died in the outbreak, diagnosing anthrax, and providing the pathoanatomical confirmation that the form of anthrax was inhalatory (36, 51).

ME/C surveillance for acts of bioterrorism would best be accomplished by building such programs into a broader system of ME/C surveillance for emerging infections. ME/Cs would need to develop baseline infectious disease mortality data for specific potential organisms and syndromes so that case clusters could be more readily identified.

Current Barriers to ME/C Infectious Disease Surveillance

The use of ME/Cs in surveillance for infectious diseases has, like other sources of information, certain limitations. ME/Cs investigate and certify specific types of deaths. The laws and settings in which they operate determine the types of deaths that will come under their jurisdiction. Funding is a major factor in determining the proportion of deaths that receive an autopsy by an ME/C; therefore, in a particular jurisdiction the deaths that are autopsied by the ME/C office are highly selected and may not be representative of the deaths in the general population. This selection bias may increase or decrease the ability to detect emerging infectious disease mortality in a population.

Certain diseases or syndromes are more likely to be represented in the ME/C case population than in the general population. If an emerging infectious disease affects younger, healthier persons, it may be more likely to be seen by ME/Cs than if it affects older, sicker persons. For example, ME/Cs may investigate and certify the majority of deaths from infectious myocarditis, while they may certify a minority of deaths from pneumonia in the elderly. This variability in investigation of deaths by age group and likely cause of death limits the ability of ME/Cs to perform surveillance for all types of mortality but makes ME/Cs useful for analyzing mortality from specific syndromes.

The ability to perform a proper autopsy on an individual who has died from an infectious disease depends on the resources available to make organism-specific diagnoses and the capacity of autopsy facilities to ensure the safety of autopsy prosectors. These autopsy infrastructure issues are highly dependent on government funding and play critical roles in determining the level of infectious disease mortality surveillance that ME/Cs can provide.

Organism-Specific Diagnoses and Laboratory and Diagnostic Tests

Historically, forensic pathologists have been satisfied with general pathologic diagnoses rather than organism-specific diagnoses when certifying deaths from infectious diseases. For example, deaths are classified as "epiglottitis" rather than "*Haemophilus influenzae* epiglottitis." Frequently, the diagnostic tests necessary to achieve an organism-specific diagnosis, such as cultures and immunohistochemistry tests, are not performed. Unfortunately, this approach can limit the usefulness of medicolegal death investigation systems in recognizing emerging infectious diseases.

An autopsy is no guarantee that an infectious organism will be identified in an individual who has died from an infectious disease. To make organism-specific diagnoses, autopsy pathologists usually require additional tests beyond routine gross and histologic evaluations. The procedure most frequently used is culture of body fluids and tissue. However, the collection of samples for culture and the interpretation of postmortem cultures are fraught with difficulties, including artifactual postmortem proliferation of organisms in blood and tissues and contamination of specimens because of the use of nonsterile techniques (53). If autopsy pathologists change their sampling methods, then the level of contamination can be reduced (27). Serology and electron microscopy are also techniques used to identify infectious agents. However, detectable serologic immune responses to infectious agents may not yet have occurred at the time of death, and a search for organisms under an electron microscope is costly in terms of both time and resources and is dependent on proper preservation of tissue.

Use of a combination of autopsy and molecular pathology is a proven successful strategy for the identification of emerging infections (44). Recent advances in molecular biology have created an array of highly specific techniques for the identification of infectious agents in pathologic tissues. Immunohistochemistry tests of formalin-fixed, paraffin-embedded tissue can be used to identify specific antigens from pathogenic agents. The list of organisms detectable by this process is continually expanding and includes the herpes simplex virus, hepatitis B virus, measles virus, *Legionella*, group B streptococcus, influenza virus, and mycobacteria (48). Immunohistochemical methods were essential to the early understanding of hantavirus pulmonary syndrome (54). In addition, nucleic acid probes may be used on fresh, frozen, and formalin-fixed autopsy tissues, as well as clinical specimens, and can identify both known and unknown infectious agents, including viruses, fungi, bacteria, and parasites. In situ hybridization techniques can be used with archived tissue specimens in paraffin blocks (55). Unfortunately, many forensic pathologists remain unaware of these techniques or do not have access to the technology. Consequently, appropriate specimens are sometimes not retained at autopsy. Any effort to expand the involvement of forensic pathologists in the search for emerging infectious diseases will require the financial resources to increase their expertise in and access to these diagnostic techniques.

If an infection is suspected or if a death is unexplained, the prosecting pathologist should consider retaining serum, blood, and frozen tissues, in addition to obtaining standard specimens for culture. It is critical that representative samples of all major organs be embedded and saved as paraffin blocks for further histologic, immunologic, and molecular testing. To avoid antigenic or nucleic acid degradation, these tissues should not be kept in formalin for any more time than is necessary to ensure good histology (48). Those ME/C offices that maintain banks of archived tissue specimens coupled with computerized retrievable autopsy records are a valuable source of information when new infectious agents emerge.

Biosafety and Autopsy Infrastructure

Directing autopsy pathologists to search for emerging infections is not without some element of danger. The autopsy is a procedure that carries with it the risk of infectious disease transmission both for prosectors and for observers and other individuals in close proximity. Autopsy-transmitted infections have occurred by both direct cutaneous inoculation and aerosolization. For example, pathologists have died from streptococcal sepsis after sustaining minor cutaneous trauma during autopsies on individuals with the same disease (23). Several other infections can be transmitted by direct inoculation, including tuberculosis, blastomycosis, AIDS, hepatitis B, rabies, and some of the viral hemorrhagic fevers (3, 4, 13, 17, 33).

Mycobacterium tuberculosis is the prototypical organism transmitted by autopsy aerosols. Historically, large portions of medical school classes would become tuberculin positive after the autopsy training period of their curriculum (35). Recently, autopsy-transmitted outbreaks of tuberculosis occurred in the Syracuse Medical Examiner's Office, the Los Angeles Coroner's Office, the University of Arkansas School of Medicine, and the University of Health Sciences/Chicago Medical School (30, 38, 49, 50). Multidrug-resistant tuberculosis caused the outbreak in the Syracuse Medical Examiner's Office (50). Other infectious diseases that may be transmitted by autopsy aerosols include rabies, plague, meningococcemia, and anthrax (13).

Unfortunately, most ME/C and hospital autopsy facilities in the United States are not constructed to mitigate these risks. Many ME/C offices are located in aging facilities, often with shared ventilation between prosecting and administrative spaces. The majority of facilities barely meet biosafety level 2 standards. Very few autopsy facilities can function at biosafety level 3. Currently, the U.S. Army Medical Research Institute of Infectious Diseases in Fort Detrick, Md., houses the only autopsy facility in the United States that can function at biosafety level 4. This facility was designed for human autopsies but is currently used only for nonhuman primates (28). In addition, many forensic pathologists have been slow to come into compliance with precautions promulgated to prevent the transmission of both blood-borne and aerosolized pathogens (4, 7). Although some autopsy facilities can achieve biosafety level 3 standards by using power-assisted personal respirators, we need to have a better-prepared national infrastructure. To handle sporadic and generalized infectious disease outbreaks in the future, funding will be needed to bring autopsy facilities into compliance with accepted public health standards (4, 7, 13). All autopsy facilities should be able to function at biosafety level 3 and provide protection against aerosolized pathogens.

RECOMMENDATIONS FOR IMPLEMENTING AN EFFECTIVE ME/C INFECTIOUS DISEASE SURVEILLANCE SYSTEM

An ideal ME/C surveillance system would be able to increase the ease and accuracy of case identification and the ability to detect acute outbreaks of infectious disease mortality by

- developing a standard list of diagnoses and syndromes that represent infectious diseases;
- implementing an infectious disease coding form and computerized retrievable database for all cases to improve the collection of infectious disease variables;
- instituting methods including death review teams and computer search algorithms to review data and identify infectious disease deaths in an accurate, timely, and inexpensive way;
- increasing pathologists' awareness of the need for organism-specific diagnoses;
- implementing standardized, state-of-the-art methods for autopsy-based microbiologic diagnosis at either the local, regional, state, or federal level;
- banking serum, blood, and tissue specimens;
- improving the personal safety of pathologists when performing autopsies on individuals with potentially transmissible infectious diseases by providing biosafety level 3 autopsy facilities; and
- linking to health departments for the reporting of communicable diseases.

CONCLUSIONS

Because ME/C offices perform most of the autopsies in the United States, they are most likely the best sources of information regarding the causes of autopsy-verified deaths. A substantial proportion of these medicolegal autopsies is performed on individuals with infectious disease-related deaths. As a result, ME/C offices have been involved in the detection of emerging infectious diseases. ME/Cs are therefore an important source of data on fatal infectious diseases. Although efforts are under way to increase surveillance for infectious disease mortality, especially mortality due to emerging infectious diseases and bioterrorist events, ME/C offices remain a potentially rich but underused source of information. As hospital autopsy rates in the United States decline and the ability to study autopsy-confirmed diagnoses decreases due to changes in data collection procedures at the national level, ME/Cs will increasingly become vital primary sources of data that may not be available elsewhere.

The identification of causative agents in infectious disease deaths can be improved. The use of recent advances in laboratory techniques, combined with the use of established techniques on a more frequent and standardized basis, can help to increase the proportion of infectious disease deaths that receive organism-specific diagnoses. Increasing this proportion is a critical step toward improving surveillance for emerging infectious diseases in this country. The success of this strategy depends in large part upon ME/C pathologists becoming aware of and having access to improved laboratory techniques. In addition, the autopsy infrastructure of the United States can be improved to provide better safety for pathologists who encounter potentially transmissible infectious diseases.

REFERENCES

1. **American Medical Association Council on Scientific Affairs.** 1987. Autopsy: a comprehensive review of current issues. *JAMA* **258:**364–369.
2. **Carpenter, J. L., and D. Y. Huang.** 1991. Community-acquired pulmonary infections in a public municipal hospital in the 1980s. *South. Med. J.* **84:**299–306.
3. **Centers for Disease Control.** 1988. Management of patients with suspected viral hemorrhagic fever. *Morbid. Mortal. Weekly Rep.* **37:**1–15.
4. **Centers for Disease Control.** 1989. Guidelines for prevention of transmission of human immunodeficiency virus and hepatitis B virus to health-care and public-safety workers. *Morbid. Mortal. Weekly Rep.* **38:**1–37.
5. **Centers for Disease Control and Prevention.** 1993. Outbreak of acute illness: southwestern United States, 1993. *Morbid. Mortal. Weekly Rep.* **42:**421–424.
6. **Centers for Disease Control and Prevention.** 1994. *Addressing Emerging Infectious Disease Threats to Health: A Prevention Strategy for the United States.* U.S. Department of Health and Human Services, Atlanta, Ga.
7. **Centers for Disease Control and Prevention.** 1994. Guidelines for preventing the transmission of *Mycobacterium tuberculosis* in health-care facilities. *Morbid. Mortal. Weekly Rep.* **43:**1–132.
8. **Centers for Disease Control and Prevention.** 1995. Hemorrhage and shock associated with invasive pneumococcal infection in healthy infants and children: New Mexico, 1993–1994. *Morbid. Mortal. Weekly Rep.* **43:**949–952.
9. **Centers for Disease Control and Prevention.** 1995. Tuberculosis morbidity—United States, 1994. *Morbid. Mortal. Weekly Rep.* **44:**387–389.
10. **Centers for Disease Control and Prevention.** 1996. AIDS associated with injecting drug use—United States, 1995. *Morbid. Mortal. Weekly Rep.* **45:**392–396.
11. **Centers for Disease Control and Prevention.** 1998. *Preventing Emerging Infectious Diseases: a Strategy for the 21st Century.* U.S. Department of Health and Human Services, Atlanta, Ga.
12. **Centers for Disease Control and Prevention.** 1998. Recommendations for prevention and control of hepatitis C virus (HCV) infection and HCV-related chronic disease. *Morbid. Mortal. Weekly Rep.* **47:**1–39.
13. **Centers for Disease Control and Prevention and National Institutes of Health.** 1993. *Biosafety in Microbiological and Biomedical Laboratories,* 3rd ed. U.S. Department of Health and Human Services publication (CDC) 93-8395. U.S. Department of Health and Human Services, Atlanta, Ga.
14. **Combs, D. L., R. G. Parrish, and R. Ing.** 1995. *Death Investigation in the United States and Canada, 1995.* U.S. Department of Health and Human Services, Atlanta, Ga.
15. **Craig, J. R.** 1990. Liver, p. 1199–1320. *In* J. M. Kissane (ed.), *Anderson's Pathology.* The C. V. Mosby Co., St. Louis, Mo.
16. **Duchin, J. S., F. T. Koster, C. J. Peters, G. L. Simpson, B. Tempest, S. R. Zaki, T. G. Ksiazek, P. E. Rollin, S. Nichol, E. T. Umland, R. L. Moolenaar, S. E. Reef, K. B. Nolte, M. M. Gallaher,**

J. C. Butler, R. F. Breiman, and the Hantavirus Study Group. 1994. Hantavirus pulmonary syndrome: a clinical description of 17 patients with a newly recognized disease. *N. Engl. J. Med.* **330:**949–955.

17. Goette, D. K., K. W. Jacobson, and R. D. Doty. 1978. Primary inoculation tuberculosis of the skin (prosectors paronychia). *Arch. Dermatol.* **114:**567–569.

18. Halpern, M. 1934. Malaria among drug addicts in New York City. *Public Health Rep.* **49:**421–423.

19. Hanzlick, R. 1998. Case of the month: institutional autopsy rates. *Ann. Intern. Med.* **158:**1171–1172.

20. Hanzlick, R. 1998. National autopsy data dropped from the National Center for Health Statistics database. *JAMA* **280:**886.

21. Hanzlick, R., and D. L. Combs. 1998. Medical examiner and coroner systems: history and trends. *JAMA* **279:**870–874.

22. Hanzlick, R., and R. G. Parrish. 1996. The role of medical examiners and coroners in public health surveillance and epidemiologic research. *Annu. Rev. Public Health* **17:**383–409.

23. Hawkey, P. M., S. J. Pedler, and P. J. Southall. 1980. *Streptococcus pyogenes:* a forgotten occupational hazard in the mortuary. *Br. Med. J.* **281:**1058.

24. Hennigar, G. R. 1990. Drug and chemical injury—environmental pathology, p. 146–245. *In* J. M. Kissane (ed.), *Anderson's Pathology.* The C. V. Mosby Co., St. Louis, Mo.

25. Hill, R. B. 1996. College of American Pathologists Conference XXIX on restructuring autopsy practice for health care reform: summary. *Arch. Pathol. Lab. Med.* **120:**778–781.

26. Hirsch, C. S. 1984. Forensic pathology and the autopsy. *Arch. Pathol. Lab. Med.* **108:**484–489.

27. Hove, M., and S. D. Pencil. 1998. Effect of postmortem sampling technique on the clinical significance of autopsy blood cultures. *Hum. Pathol.* **29:**137–139.

28. Jaax, N. K. 1999. Personal communication.

29. Jordan, F. 1997. Investigating the Murrah Building explosion, p. 8. *In National Association of Medical Examiners Annual Meeting Abstract Book.* National Association of Medical Examiners, St. Louis, Mo.

30. Kantor, H. S., R. Poblete, and S. L. Pusateri. 1988. Nosocomial transmission of tuberculosis from unsuspected disease. *Am. J. Med.* **84:**833–837.

31. Kircher, T., J. Nelson, and H. Burdo. 1985. The autopsy as a measure of accuracy of the death certificate. *N. Engl. J. Med.* **313:**1263–1269.

32. Kuhn, C. I., and F. B. Askin. 1990. Lung and mediastinum, p. 920–1046. In J. M. Kissane (ed.), *Anderson's Pathology.* The C. V. Mosby Co., St. Louis, Mo.

33. Larson, D. M., M. R. Eckman, R. L. Alber, and B. G. Goldschmidt. 1983. Primary cutaneous (inoculation) blastomycosis: an occupational hazard to pathologists. *Am. J. Clin. Pathol.* **79:**253–255.

34. McClain, J. L., D. W. Hause, and M. A. Clark. 1989. Amanita phalloides mushroom poisoning: a cluster of four fatalities. *J. Forensic Sci.* **34:**83–87.

35. Meade, G. M. 1948. Prevention of primary tuberculosis infections in medical students: the autopsy as source of primary infection. *Am. Rev. Tuberc.* **58:**675–683.

36. Meselson, M., J. Guillemin, M. Hugh-Jones, A. Langmuir, I. Popova, A. Shelokov, and O. Yampolskaya. 1994. The Sverdlovsk anthrax outbreak of 1979. *Science* **266:**1202–1207.

37. Messite, J., and S. D. Stellman. 1996. Accuracy of death certificate completion. *JAMA* **275:**794–796.

38. Meyer, J. 5 April 1997. TB plagues office of L.A. coroner. *Los Angeles Times*, p. A1 and A27.

39. Neuspiel, D. R., and L. H. Kuller. 1985. Sudden and unexpected natural death in childhood and adolescence. *JAMA* **254:**1321–1325.

40. New Mexico Office of the Medical Investigator and Centers for Disease Control and Prevention. 1998. Unpublished data.

41. Nolte, K. B., R. M. Feddersen, K. Foucar, S. R. Zaki, F. T. Koster, D. Madar, T. L. Merlin, P. J. McFeeley, E. T. Umland, and R. E. Zumwalt. 1995. Hantavirus pulmonary syndrome in the United States: a pathological description of a disease caused by a new agent. *Hum. Pathol.* **26:**110–120.

42. Nolte, K. B., G. L. Simpson, and R. G. Parrish. 1996. Emerging infectious agents and the forensic pathologist: the New Mexico model. *Arch. Pathol. Lab. Med.* **120:**125–128.

43. **Perkins, B. A., J. M. Flood, R. Danila, R. C. Holman, A. L. Reingold, L. A. Klug, M. Virata, P. R. Cieslak, S. R. Zaki, R. W. Pinner, R. F. Khabbaz, and the Unexplained Deaths Working Group.** 1996. Unexplained deaths due to possibly infectious causes in the United States: defining the problem and designing surveillance and laboratory approaches. *Emerg. Infect. Dis.* **2:**47–53.

44. **Perkins, B. A., and D. Relman.** 1998. Explaining the unexplained in clinical infectious diseases: looking forward. *Emerg. Infect. Dis.* **4:**395–397.

45. **Pinner, R. W., S. M. Teutsch, L. Simonsen, L. A. Klug, J. M. Graber, M. J. Clarke, and R. L. Berkelman.** 1996. Trends in infectious disease mortality in the United States. *JAMA* **275:**189–193.

46. **Roberts, W. C.** 1978. The autopsy: its decline and a suggestion for its revival. *N. Engl. J. Med.* **299:**332–338.

47. **Tappero, J. W., and The Unexplained Illness Working Group.** 1998. Surveillance for unexplained deaths and critical illnesses due to possible infectious causes, p. 7–8. *In National Association of Medical Examiners Annual Meeting Abstract Book.* National Association of Medical Examiners, St. Louis, Mo.

48. **Taylor, C. R.** 1994. Principles of immunomicroscopy, p. 1–20. In C. R. Taylor and R. J. Cote (ed.), *Immunomicroscopy: A Diagnostic Tool for the Surgical Pathologist.* The W. B. Saunders Co., Philadelphia, Pa.

49. **Templeton, G. L., L. A. Illing, L. Young, D. Cave, W. W. Stead, and J. H. Bates.** 1995. The risk for transmission of *Mycobacterium tuberculosis* at the bedside and during autopsy. *Ann. Intern. Med.* **122:**922–925.

50. **Ussery, X. T., J. A. Bierman, S. E. Valway, T. A. Seitz, G. T. DiFernando, Jr., and S. M. Ostroff.** 1995. Transmission of multidrug-resistant *Mycobacterium tuberculosis* among persons exposed in a medical examiner's office, New York. *Infect. Control. Hosp. Epidemiol.* **16:**160–165.

51. **Walker, D. H., O. Yampolskaya, and L. M. Grinberg.** 1994. Death at Sverdlovsk: what have we learned? *Am. J. Pathol.* **144:**1135–1141.

52. **Wetli, C.** 1997. Investigating the TWA 800 crash, p. 8. *In National Association of Medical Examiners Annual Meeting Abstract Book.* National Association of Medical Examiners, St. Louis, Mo.

53. **Wilson, S. J., M. L. Wilson, and L. B. Reller.** 1993. Diagnostic utility of postmortem blood cultures. *Arch. Pathol. Lab. Med.* **117:**986–988.

54. **Zaki, S. R., P. W. Greer, L. M. Coffield, C. S. Goldsmith, K. B. Nolte, K. Foucar, R. M. Feddersen, R. E. Zumwalt, G. L. Miller, A. S. Khan, P. E. Rollin, T. G. Ksiazek, S. T. Nichol, B. W. J. Mahy, and C. J. Peters.** 1995. Hantavirus pulmonary syndrome: pathogenesis of an emerging infectious disease. *Am. J. Pathol.* **146:**552–579.

55. **Zaki, S. R., and A. M. Marty.** 1995. New technology for the diagnosis of infectious disease, p. 127–154. *In* W. Doerr and G. Seifert (ed.), *Tropical Pathology.* Springer-Verlag, Berlin, Germany.

Emerging Infections 3
Edited by W. M. Scheld, W. A. Craig, and J. M. Hughes
© 1999 ASM Press, Washington, D.C.

Chapter 14

The Role of the Public Health Community in Detecting and Responding to Domestic Terrorism Involving Infectious Agents

*James W. LeDuc, Stephen M. Ostroff, Joseph E. McDade,
Scott Lillibridge, and James M. Hughes*

The Tom Clancy novel *Executive Orders* includes a subplot that involves the release of Ebola virus as a biological warfare agent of mass destruction against the United States (11). The scenario begins with the acquisition of the virus by a rogue state from a patient infected during a small outbreak similar to those recently experienced in Gabon (19) and develops with propagation of the virus in a laboratory, experimental infection of prisoners, and finally, simultaneous release of the virus by aerosol spray by teams of terrorists at several different conventions where thousands of people have gathered. The resulting cases are quickly recognized by scientists at both the Centers for Disease Control and Prevention (CDC) and the U.S. Army Medical Research Institute of Infectious Diseases (USAMRIID), and the outbreak is eventually controlled through collaborations between these and other government agencies. While the scenario is clearly fictional, it illustrates the potential threat of bioterrorism and how such an emergency might be addressed. The following recent experiences indicate that these threats are real:

- World Trade Center bombing, New York, N.Y.
- Federal building bombing, Oklahoma City, Okla.
- Centennial Olympic Park bombing, Atlanta, Ga.
- Sarin release, Tokyo, Japan
- Anthrax hoaxes, Washington, D.C., Las Vegas, Nev., and other locations
- Embassy bombings, Kenya and Tanzania

James W. LeDuc, Stephen M. Ostroff, Joseph E. McDade, Scott Lillibridge, and James M. Hughes • National Center for Infectious Diseases, Centers for Disease Control and Prevention, 1600 Clifton Rd. NE, Mailstop C-12, Atlanta, GA 30333.

In reality, the recognition of and response to actual terrorist use of an infectious agent are likely to be far more complicated. In contrast to chemical agents or explosive devices, whose destructive impacts are immediately recognizable, covert delivery of biological agents in the absence of notification of intent would cause disease only after an incubation period during which exposed persons could be widely dispersed.

OUTBREAK DETECTION AND ASSESSMENT

Purposeful release of pathogenic microorganisms could result in an outbreak similar to a naturally occurring one. Alert health care providers will be critical for the timely recognition of such an event. Ill persons likely would first come to the attention of clinicians in outpatient settings or personnel working in emergency departments. Although it is not possible to predict which agents might be used by bioterrorists, clinicians should be familiar with the clinical manifestations of diseases caused by classic biological warfare agents (Table 1), available diagnostic techniques, patient isolation precautions, and recommended chemotherapy (17). Prompt diagnosis and treatment would minimize the impact of the event. Additionally, prompt reporting of cases to public health authorities would be essential to ensuring a follow-up investigation that would determine the scope and source of an outbreak (potential routes of exposure include aerosols, food, water, arthropod or rodent vectors, and medications), identify persons who are at risk, and facilitate consequence management.

Investigators may not immediately recognize that an outbreak is due to the intentional release of microorganisms. Epidemiologic investigations typically involve characterization of the clinical syndrome (Table 2), development of a provisional case definition, case finding activities, performance of appropriate diagnostic tests,

Table 1. Bioterrorism threats[a]

Core group
  Anthrax
  Botulism
  Brucellosis
  Plague[b]
  Q fever
  Smallpox[b]
  Staphylococcal enterotoxins
  Tularemia
  Viral encephalitides
  Viral hemorrhagic fevers[b]

Others
  Cholera
  Salmonellosis
  Shigellosis

[a]Adapted from reference 47.
[b]Person-to-person transmission occurs.

Table 2. Selected illnesses that may result from bioterrorism

Encephalitis
Hemorrhagic mediastinitis
Pneumonia with abnormal liver function tests
Papulopustular rash
Hemorrhagic fever
Descending paralysis
Nausea, vomiting, diarrhea

and identification of the source of infection and mode of transmission. The following list (adapted from Kadlec et al. [25]) summarizes some characteristics of outbreaks that should suggest the possibility of intentional use of an infectious agent, even though these features are clearly not specific.

- Outbreak of a rare disease
- Outbreak of a disease in an area of nonendemicity
- Occurrence of a seasonal disease (e.g., tick-borne disease) during the wrong time of the year
- Attribution of an outbreak caused by a known pathogen to a strain with an unusual antimicrobial pattern
- Unusual age distribution of persons involved in an outbreak
- Other unusual epidemiologic features of an outbreak due to a known pathogen (e.g., a typical food-borne pathogen found to be transmitted from person to person)
- Unusual clinical presentation associated with infection with a known pathogen (especially respiratory symptoms)

In contrast, Table 3 provides examples of naturally occurring outbreaks that could have been mistaken for terrorism involving biologic agents, emphasizing the need for rapid and thorough investigations.

Determination of whether an outbreak of unknown etiology is due to a previously unknown, indigenous pathogen or a known microorganism that has been modified for use as an agent of bioterrorism poses a special challenge. The experience with the initially unexplained illness now known as hantavirus pulmonary syndrome is relevant in this regard. Following recognition and reporting of severe unexplained illness by an alert clinician and medical examiner to public health authorities and negative results from initial diagnostic tests for likely etiologic agents, CDC assistance was requested. More than 20 candidate agents were considered, and diagnostic studies for each were begun at CDC once the specimens were received. Testing of patients' serum provided the first clue to a possible hantavirus etiology (28). PCR results obtained with primers and probes designed for known hantaviruses, and sequencing of the amplified product, documented that disease was attributable to infection with a newly recognized hantavirus (40). Experience with other hantaviruses in Europe and Asia indicated that a rodent res-

Table 3. Naturally occurring infectious disease outbreaks that could have been mistaken for bioterrorism

Event, location, yr	Comment	Reference(s)
Legionnaires' disease outbreak, Philadelphia, 1976	Severe pneumonia of unknown etiology occurred among a group of military veterans; discovery of the etiology took many months.	37
Rift Valley fever, Egypt, 1977	Outbreaks of Rift Valley fever were previously unknown in Egypt. Periodic political tensions in the Middle East could foster suspicions of biological warfare.	31
Urban Q fever, Nova Scotia, 1987	An outbreak of Q fever occurred in a factory in Nova Scotia. Domestic animal reservoirs were absent. Eventually, the outbreak was traced to contaminated clothing of a worker who owned an infected parturient cat.	36
Botulism, Egypt, 1991	A large outbreak of botulism occurred for the first time in Egypt during Ramadan among Copts at the time of the Gulf War. Despite initial suspicions of intentional release, fermented fish was found to be the source of infection.	48
Vibrio cholerae O139, Bangladesh and India, 1992	A new serotype was associated with epidemic cholera in Asia. The change in serotype resulted from a naturally occurring addition of DNA in an antigen gene of the virulent O1 strain and not the intentional addition of a virulence gene to an avirulent serotype. Both serotypes were subsequently detected in zooplankton in Bangladesh, suggesting that recombination could have occurred under natural circumstances.	1, 4, 12, 23
Hantavirus pulmonary syndrome, United States, 1993	The syndrome consisted of another outbreak of severe pneumonia of unknown etiology. Human illness with hantaviruses was unknown in the United States at that time, but hantaviruses were known to be endemic in Korea.	14, 28
Plague, India, 1994	An inability to trace the origins of pneumonic plague in Surat "fuelled speculation that the organism is being used as a biological warfare agent, most likely by the USA or Pakistan."	29
Food-borne cryptosporidiosis, Minnesota, 1995	A common-source food-borne outbreak was found to be associated with contaminated chicken salad; previous outbreaks were associated with drinking of contaminated recreational water, exposure to animals, and person-to-person contact.	7
Ebola virus infection, Zaire, 1995	A >99% sequence homology to Ebola virus which produced the 1976 outbreak raised the possibility of intentional reintroduction.	42
Antibiotic-resistant strain of the agent of plague, Madagascar, 1995	A naturally occurring strain was found, but it could have been attributed to genetic engineering for purposes of bioterrorism.	18

Table 3. *Continued*

Event, location, yr	Comment	Reference(s)
Monkeypox, Zaire, 1996	The monkeypox virus could have been mistaken for smallpox virus that was intentionally released.	8
Antibiotic-resistant strain of the agent of anthrax, India, 1997	A sporadic case of bacterial meningitis was caused by a *Bacillus anthracis* strain resistant to penicillin, cefuroxime, and cefotaxime.	30
Nipah virus encephalitis, Malaysia and Singapore, 1998–1999	An outbreak caused by a previously unrecognized virus that caused illness in pigs with transmission to humans raised questions of whether bioterrorism targeted pigs.	8b

ervoir was likely, the rodent was identified (9), and control strategies were developed and implemented (5).

Immunohistochemical staining of autopsy tissues (50) confirmed the existence of a previously unrecognized hantavirus approximately 1 month after the initial recognition of cases of the syndrome, but several months elapsed before the virus was finally isolated in cell culture (10, 43). This experience highlights the critical importance of highly trained field and laboratory personnel, appropriate biocontainment facilities, and the laboratory reagents and sophisticated molecular techniques, all of which must be available for the detection of candidate agents that terrorists might use. Fortunately, the hantavirus outbreak was relatively limited in scope, the centralized resources available at CDC and USAMRIID were able to meet the demands for laboratory testing, and the etiology was identified relatively quickly. Larger, more dispersed outbreaks might not be so effectively managed under current circumstances.

EFFECTIVE PUBLIC HEALTH RESPONSE

Ensuring an adequate response to bioterrorism will be extremely complex. In the event of such a scenario, there would be an immediate need for detailed advice on patient management from experts knowledgeable about the suspected disease. The availability of medical facilities that could provide appropriate supportive care might be limited locally. In addition, medical and emergency response personnel might also be exposed to and become ill from the agent that has been released. Collection of diagnostic specimens and the need to transport them to appropriate reference laboratories could overwhelm the system unless adequate laboratory surge capacities are available both locally and nationally. The availability and administration of appropriate antimicrobial drugs, antitoxins, and vaccines; advice on decontamination of potentially exposed persons and the environment; consultation on strategies for disease prophylaxis; communication with clinicians and public health personnel; and dissemination of current, accurate information to the public would present major logistical challenges (49). The public health response to a bioterrorist event would also be complicated by other factors, including the criminal investigation that would begin as soon as terrorism was suspected and the inevitable heightening of media interest, which is typically intense during investigations of large, naturally occurring infectious disease outbreaks. The complexity of such a response, even if the etiologic agent is promptly identified, in the predictable climate of uncertainty and potential hysteria should not be underestimated. Local and state public health authorities and emergency response personnel must be prepared to assess outbreak situations rapidly and to call for federal assistance if needed.

ROLE OF THE PUBLIC HEALTH SECTOR

The potential for bioterrorism emphasizes the urgency of strengthening the public health capacity to detect and respond to emerging infectious diseases, particularly the need to forge and strengthen partnerships between the public health and emergency response sectors (20, 21). The limitations of infectious diseases surveillance in the United States have been documented (2, 41), and the national security implications of a lack of preparedness have been emphasized (32, 33). The ability to detect and respond to a bioterrorism event then becomes an added value of this investment in public health (26). Examples on a relatively small scale are provided by recent reports of food-borne outbreaks in a hospital laboratory (27) and a community (45) caused by intentional microbial contamination of food. Twelve of 45 laboratory workers in a Dallas, Tex., medical center had severe diarrheal illness during the fall of 1996. Eight had positive stool cultures for *Shigella dysenteriae* type 2, and eating muffins or donuts in the staff break room was implicated as the likely source of infection. Pulsed-field gel electrophoresis patterns were indistinguishable for isolates from stools, isolates from the muffins, and the laboratory stock isolates. In The Dalles, Oreg., in the fall of 1984, 751 cases of *Salmonella* Typhimurium infection were detected among the residents of this small town. Consumption of food from salad bars in 10 separate restaurants was implicated as the likely source of infection. Subsequent criminal investigations implicated followers of Bhagwan Shree Rajneesh as the perpetrators, with their goal being to influence the outcome of a local election.

The role of CDC in responding to a suspected occurrence of bioterrorism is reasonably well defined (Table 4). For example, CDC's traditional public health roles, i.e., disease surveillance, epidemiologic and laboratory support, information

Table 4. CDC's collaborative role in combating bioterrorism

Provide information and training on clinical and epidemiologic features of candidate diseases
Ensure reliable and timely disease surveillance and reporting
Detect and investigate outbreaks
Develop protocols for rapid shipment of diagnostic specimens
Provide reference diagnostic services
Provide reliable clinical and public health information to health care professionals and the public
Ensure availability of certain antitoxins and other biological products (in collaboration with the U.S. Food and Drug Administration)
Address applied research priorities
Provide consultation on emergency response plans
Participate in scientific meetings on the issues

dissemination, consultation, and training, also apply in a bioterrorism scenario (8a). CDC maintains expertise in the detection of virtually all infectious agents pathogenic for humans and is able to use modern molecular techniques, traditional procedures for organism cultivation, and serologic methods in an attempt to rapidly identify known infectious diseases and accurately establish the specific etiology. Previously unknown bacteria, viruses, or other microbes would obviously be more difficult and take longer to identify, but as was seen during the first outbreak of hantavirus pulmonary syndrome, results can be obtained rapidly if additional resources can be quickly mobilized. However, even at the federal level, the laboratory surge capacity is extremely limited, especially when work at a biosafety level 3 or 4 biocontainment facility is required. The breadth of knowledge and experience that already exists within the laboratories of CDC could also play a role in the identification of engineered pathogens. However, relevant CDC laboratories are located in Atlanta, Ga., and Fort Collins, Colo. Depending on the location of the outbreak, shipment of specimens could present logistical problems, particularly if illnesses occurred over a large geographic area. The capacity for large-scale testing for likely threats needs to be developed locally at strategic sites. State public health laboratories are ideal locations where this capability can be developed.

Epidemiologic investigations are also a mainstay of CDC activities and would certainly be called into play in response to a suspected use of biologic agents. In fact, part of Alexander Langmuir's rationale for establishing the Epidemic Intelligence Service in 1951 was to improve the nation's capacity to detect and control a biologic warfare event (15). Establishing whether an outbreak was the result of an intentional act will be a critical early step in the national response and would draw heavily on the epidemiologic strengths of CDC. Subsequent studies would undoubtedly require predictions of possible mechanisms of transmission, the extent and rate of secondary spread, projected attack rates, identification of important risk factors, analysis of molecular epidemiologic data, and development of intervention strategies to interrupt secondary transmission. Historically, CDC epidemiologists have worked with their counterparts in local and state health departments on epidemiologic investigations. Similar collaborations with emergency response personnel, the Federal Bureau of Investigation, other law enforcement agencies, and U.S. Department of Defense units (46) will be essential in the event of a bioterrorist attack.

The CDC plan to address new and emerging infectious diseases has as one of its primary goals the strengthening of national and international surveillance and response to infectious diseases (6). This is being implemented in the United States through the establishment of Emerging Infections Programs, building of state health department epidemiology and laboratory capacities, and establishment of provider networks in settings such as infectious disease clinics, travelers' clinics, and emergency departments at teaching hospitals (3, 22). Internationally, the World Health Organization (WHO) has passed a resolution closely patterned after the CDC plan; that resolution likewise calls for improved global surveillance and response activities (34, 35). The WHO plan is being implemented under a recently reorganized division of communicable diseases. Among the many activities now under way at WHO are the routine electronic publication of outbreak summaries as they are recognized and the use of more detailed communications about disease incidents to international health officials via electronic mail. Most of the WHO regional offices have developed their own emerging infection plans, and each calls for greater surveillance activities and information sharing. Electronic dissemination of information on outbreaks has also improved under the ProMED system (38), whereby persons with Internet access can report outbreaks, observations related to epidemics, and general comments to a wide readership ranging from health professionals to interested lay parties. Collectively, these global efforts bring outbreaks of infectious diseases, both naturally occurring outbreaks and those caused by humans, to national and international attention sooner and facilitate timely investigation and intervention. As indicated in a recent commentary on the public health threats of biological weapons, "public health is the best form of civil defense" (13).

Prevention of biological warfare and terrorism is an area in which the role of CDC and other national agencies and organizations is less well defined. CDC was given the task of developing and implementing new regulations designed to minimize the risk of distribution of etiologic agents with the potential for use by terrorists (16, 44). These regulations resulted from the recognition that an individual with no apparent valid requirement had requested vials of *Yersinia pestis*, the cause of plague, from the American Type Culture Collection. This and other events which surfaced at about the time of the Persian Gulf War led the U.S. Congress to develop legislation that requires that full disclosure occur and that validated need and adequate research facilities exist before any etiologic agent on a list of those potentially useful to a terrorist is transported between laboratories.

In June 1996, Vice President Albert Gore announced Presidential Decision Directive NSTC-7, which called on federal agencies to work together to strengthen domestic preparedness to address emerging infections, implement the recommendations of the Working Group on Emerging and Re-emerging Infectious Diseases (39) in support of the WHO global strategy. Many governmental agencies are involved in various aspects of the national response to the challenges of emerging infections and bioterrorism. In May 1998, President Bill Clinton issued Presidential Decision Directives 62 (Table 5) and 63, which focus on terrorism issues.

CONCLUSIONS

Whether epidemics are the result of terrorism or natural factors, CDC and the public health community remain at the forefront of the global epidemic response. The specter of bioterrorism has intensified the need to provide such services within

Table 5. Goals of Presidential Decision Directive 62

Upgrade the public health system and medical surveillance systems
Train and equip emergency response personnel at the local, state, and national levels
Create a civilian stockpile of appropriate drugs, other therapeutics, vaccines, and equipment
Coordinate research and development efforts to capitalize on advances in genetic engineering and
    biotechnology

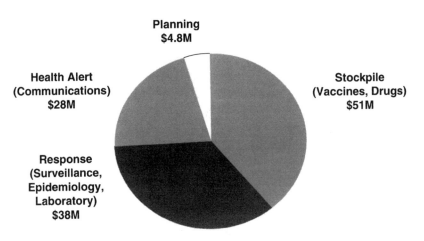

Figure 1. Fiscal year 1999 CDC bioterrorism funding. M, millions.

a rapid national response framework. Core elements in the public health response (namely, detection [surveillance], epidemiologic investigation and response, rapid laboratory diagnosis, stockpile development, and communications) have been identified, and CDC received a US$121.8 million appropriation in fiscal year 1999 to address these needs (Fig. 1). Many other federal agencies play critically important roles (24, 47). However, national preparedness for bioterrorism must work through selective improvements to the existing public health infrastructure if we are to fully protect the population. Specific measures to protect the public against epidemic diseases include the education of state and local public health officials about the public health issues associated with bioterrorism, improvements in disease detection and response capacity, enhancements to the nation's public health laboratory system, and strengthening of communication links between local, state, and federal public health agencies. Efforts are under way to address these needs and strengthen the national capacity to detect and control infectious diseases.

REFERENCES

1. **Albert, M. J., A. K. Siddique, M. S. Islam, A. S. Faruque, M. Ansaruzzaman, S. M. Faruque, and R. B. Sack.** 1993. A large outbreak of clinical cholera due to *Vibrio cholerae* non-O1 in Bangladesh. *Lancet* **341:**704.
2. **Berkelman, R. L., R. T. Bryan, M. T. Osterholm, J. W. LeDuc, and J. M. Hughes.** 1994. Infectious disease surveillance: a crumbling foundation. *Science* **264:**368–370.
3. **Berkelman, R. L., R. W. Pinner, and J. M. Hughes.** 1996. Addressing emerging microbial threats in the United States. *JAMA* **275:**315–317.
4. **Bik, E. M., A. E. Bunschoten, R. D. Gouw, and F. R. Mooi.** 1995. Genesis of the novel epidemic *Vibrio cholerae* O139 strain: evidence for horizontal transfer of genes involved in polysaccharide synthesis. *EMBO J.* **14:**209–216.
5. **Centers for Disease Control and Prevention.** 1993. Hantavirus infection—southwestern United States: interim recommendation for risk reduction. *Morbid. Mortal. Weekly Rep.* **42**(No. RR-11): 1–12.

6. **Centers for Disease Control and Prevention.** 1994. Addressing emerging infectious disease threats: a prevention strategy for the United States. Public Health Service, U.S. Department of Health and Human Services, Atlanta, Ga.

7. **Centers for Disease Control and Prevention.** 1996. Foodborne outbreak of diarrheal illness associated with *Cryptosporidium parvum. Morbid. Mortal Weekly Rep.* **45:**783–784.

8. **Centers for Disease Control and Prevention.** 1997. Human monkeypox—Kasai Oriental Zaire, 1996–1997. *Morbid. Mortal. Weekly Rep.* **46:**304–307.

8a. **Centers for Disease Control and Prevention.** 1999. Bioterrorism alleging use of anthrax and interim guidelines for management—United States, 1998. *Morbid. Mortal. Weekly Rep.* **48:**69–74.

8b. **Centers for Disease Control and Prevention.** 1999. Update: outbreak of Nipah virus—Malaysia and Singapore, 1999. *Morbid. Mortal. Weekly Rep.* **48:**335–337.

9. **Childs, J. E., T. G. Ksiazek, C. F. Spiropoulou, et al.** 1994. Serologic and genetic identification of *Peromyscus maniculatus* as the primary rodent reservoir for a new hantavirus in the southwestern United States. *J. Infect. Dis.* **169:**1271–1280.

10. **Chizhikov, V. E., C. F. Spiropoulou, S. P. Morzunov, M. C. Monroe, C. J. Peters, and S. T. Nichol.** 1995. Complete genetic characterization and analysis of isolation of Sin Nombre virus. *J. Virol.* **69:**8132–8136.

11. **Clancy, T.** 1996. *Executive Orders.* G. P. Putnam's Sons, New York, N.Y.

12. **Comstock, L. E., J. A. Johnson, J. M. Michalski, J. G. Morris, Jr., and J. B. Kaper.** 1996. Cloning and sequence of a region encoding a surface polysaccharide of *Vibrio cholerae* O139 and characterization of the insertion site in the chromosome of *Vibrio cholerae* O1. *Mol. Microbiol.* **19:**815–826.

13. **Danzig, R., and P. B. Berkowsky.** 1997. Why should we be concerned about biological warfare? *JAMA* **278:**431–432.

14. **Duchin, J. S., F. T. Koster, C. J. Peters, G. L. Simpson, B. Tempest, S. R. Zaki, T. G. Ksiazek, P. E. Rollin, S. Nichol, E. T. Umland, et al.** 1994. Hantavirus pulmonary syndrome: a clinical description of 17 patients with a newly recognized disease. *N. Engl. J. Med.* **330:**949–955.

15. **Eickhoff, T. C.** 1996. Airborne disease: including chemical and biological warfare. *Am. J. Epidemiol.* **144:**S39–S46.

16. **Ferguson, J. R.** 1997. Biological weapons and US law. *JAMA* **278:**357–360.

17. **Franz, D. R., P. B. Jahrling, A. M. Friedlander, D. J. McClain, D. L. Hoover, W. R. Bryne, J. A. Pavlin, G. W. Christopher, and E. M. Eitzen, Jr.** 1997. Clinical recognition and management of patient exposed to biological warfare agents. *JAMA* **278:**399–411.

18. **Galimand, M., A. Guiyoule, G. Gerbaud, B. Rasoamanana, S. Chanteau, E. Carniel, and P. Courvalin.** 1997. Multidrug resistance in *Yersinia pestis* mediated by a transferable plasmid. *N. Engl. J. Med.* **337:**677–680.

19. **Georges-Courbot, M. C., C. Y. Lu, J. Lansoud-Soukate, E. Leroy, and S. Baize.** 1997. Isolation and partial molecular characterization of a strain of Ebola virus during a recent epidemic of viral hemorrhagic fever in Gabon. *Lancet* **349:**181.

20. **Gore, A.** 1996. Emerging infections threaten national and global security. *ASM News* **62:**448–449.

21. **Henderson, D. A.** 1999. The looming threat of bioterrorism. *Science* **283:**1279–1282.

22. **Hughes, J. M.** 1998. Addressing the challenges of emerging infectious diseases: implementation of the strategy of the Centers for Disease Control and Prevention, p. 261–269. *In* W. M. Scheld, D. Armstrong, and J. M. Hughes (ed.), *Emerging Infections 1.* ASM Press, Washington, D.C.

23. **Huq, A., R. R. Colwell, M. A. R. Chowdhury, B. Xu, S. M. Moniruzzaman, M. S. Islam, M. Yunus, and M. J. Albert.** 1995. Coexistence of *Vibrio cholerae* O1 and O139 Bengal in plankton in Bangladesh. *Lancet* **345:**1249.

24. **Institute of Medicine, National Research Council.** 1999. *Chemical and Biological Terrorism.* National Academy Press, Washington, D.C.

25. **Kadlec, R. P., A. P. Zelicoff, and A. M. Vrtis.** 1997. Biological weapons control: prospects and implication for the future. *JAMA* **278:**351–356.

26. **Kaufmann, A. F., M. I. Meltzer, and G. P. Schmid.** 1997. The economic impact of a bioterrorist attack: are prevention and postattack intervention programs justifiable? *Emerg. Infect. Dis.* **3:**83–94.

27. **Kolavic, S. A., A. Kimura, S. L. Simons, L. Slutsker, S. Barth, and C. E. Haley.** 1997. An outbreak of Shigella dysenteriae type 2 among laboratory workers due to intentional food contamination. *JAMA* **278:**396–398.

28. **Ksiazek, T. G., C. J. Peters, P. E. Rollin, et al.** 1995. Identification of a new North American hantavirus that causes acute pulmonary insufficiency. *Am. J. Trop. Med. Hyg.* **52:**117–123.

29. **Kumar, S.** 1995. Surat plague caused by a novel strain. *Lancet* **345:**1626.

30. **Lalitha, M. K., and M. K. Thomas.** 1997. Penicillin resistance in *Bacillus anthracis*. *Lancet* **349:**1522.

31. **Laughlin, L. W., J. M. Meegan, L. J. Strausbaugh, D. M. Morens, and R. H. Watten.** 1979. Epidemic Rift Valley fever in Egypt: observation of the spectrum of human illness. *Trans. R. Soc. Trop. Med. Hyg.* **73:**630–633.

32. **Lederberg, J.** 1996. Infectious disease—a threat to global health and security. *JAMA* **276:**417–419.

33. **Lederberg J.** 1997. Infectious disease and biological weapons: prophylaxis and mitigation. *JAMA* **278:**435–436.

34. **LeDuc, J. W.** 1996. World Health Organization strategy for emerging infectious diseases. *JAMA* **275:**318–320.

35. **LeDuc, J. W.** 1996. WHO program on emerging virus diseases. *Arch. Virol.* **11**(Suppl.)**:**13–20.

36. **Marrie, T. J., D. Langille, V. Papukna, and L. Yates.** 1989. Truckin' pneumonia—an outbreak of Q fever in a truck repair plant probably due to aerosols from clothing contaminated by contact with newborn kittens. *Epidemiol. Infect.* **102:**119–127.

37. **McDade, J. E., C. C. Shepard, D. W. Fraser, T. R. Tsai, M. A. Redier, and W. R. Dowdle.** 1977. Laboratory investigation team. Legionnaires' disease. 2. Isolation of a bacterium and demonstration of its role in other respiratory diseases. *N. Engl. J. Med.* **297:**1197–1203.

38. **Mitchell, P.** 1997. ProMed-mail: outbreak intelligence or rash reporting? *Lancet* **350:**1610.

39. **National Science and Technology Council.** 1995. *Report of the NTSC Committee on International Science, Engineering, and Technology (CISET) Working Group on Emerging and Re-emerging Infectious Diseases.* Executive Office of the President of the United States, Washington, D.C.

40. **Nichol, S. T., C. F. Spiropoulou, S. Morzunov, P. E. Rollin, T. G. Ksiazek, H. Feldmann, A. Sanchez, J. Childs, S. Zaki, and C. J. Peters.** 1993. Genetic identification of a hantavirus associated with an outbreak of acute respiratory illness. *Science* **262:**914–917.

41. **Osterholm, M. T., G. S. Birkhead, and R. A. Meriwether.** 1996. Impediments to public health surveillance in the 1990s: the lack of resources and the need for priorities. *J. Public Health Manage. Pract.* **2**(4)**:**11–15.

42. **Sanchez, A., T. G. Ksiazek, P. E. Rollin, C. J. Peters, S. T. Nichol, A. S. Khan, and B. W. Mahy.** 1995. Reemergence of Ebola virus in Africa. *Emerg. Infect. Dis.* **1:**96–97.

43. **Schmaljohn, A. L., D. Li, D. L. Negley, D. S. Bressler, M. J. Turell, G. W. Korch, M. S. Archer, and C. S. Schmaljohn.** 1995. Isolation and initial characterization of a newfound hantavirus from California. *Virology* **206:**963–972.

44. **Tipple, M., R. C. Knudsen, S. Morse, J. Foster, and J. Y. Richmond.** 1997. New federal regulations for transfer of infectious agents and toxins. *ASM News* **63:**66–67.

45. **Torok, T. J., R. V. Tauxe, R. P. Wise, J. R. Livengood, R. Sokolow, S. Mauvais, K. A. Birkness, M. R. Skeels, J. M. Horan, and L. R. Foster.** 1997. A large community outbreak of salmonellosis caused by intentional contamination of restaurant salad bars. *JAMA* **278:**389–395.

46. **Tucker, J. B.** 1997. National health and medical services response to incidents of chemical and biological terrorism. *JAMA* **278:**362–368.

47. **United States Army Medical Research Institute of Infectious Diseases.** 1998. *Medical Management of Biological Casualties Handbook*, 3rd ed. United States Army Medical Research Institute of Infectious Diseases, Frederick, Md.

48. **Weber J. T., R. G. Hibbs, Jr., A. Darwish, B. Mishu, A. L. Corwin, M. Rakha, et al.** 1993. A massive outbreak of type E botulism associated with traditional salted fish in Cairo. *J. Infect. Dis.* **167:**451–454.

49. **Zajtchuk, R., and R. F. Bellamy (ed.).** 1997. *Textbook of Military Medicine. Medical Aspects of Chemical and Biological Warfare.* Part I. *Warfare, Weaponry, and the Casualty* (F. R. Sidell, E. T.

Takafuji, and D. R. Franz, specialty ed.). Office of the Surgeon General, United States Army, Washington, D.C.

50. **Zaki, S. R., P. W. Greer, L. M. Coffield, C. S. Goldsmith, K. B. Nolte, K. Foucar, R. M. Feddersen, R. E. Zumwalt, G. L. Miller, A. S. Khan, et al.** 1995. Hantavirus pulmonary syndrome: pathogenesis of an emerging infectious disease. *Am. J. Pathol.* **146:**552–579.

INDEX